Language in Mental Retardation

Language in Mental Retardation

Jean A. RONDAL
PhD (Psy.), D Ling

and

Susan EDWARDS
PhD, MSc, MRCSLT.

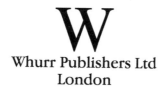

Whurr Publishers Ltd
London

© 1997 Whurr Publishers Ltd
First published 1997 by
Whurr Publishers Ltd
19b Compton Terrace, London N1 2UN, England

Reprinted 2000

British Library Cataloguing in Publication Data
A catalogue record for this book is available from the
British Library.

ISBN 1 86156 004 4

Printed and bound in the UK by Athenaeum Press Ltd,
Gateshead, Tyne & Wear.

Contents

opment of language in the mentally retarded • Language in mentally
retarded adults • Ageing and language in mental retardation

About the Authors

Jean Adolphe Rondal received his Ph.D. from the University of Minnesota (Minneapolis), specialising in Psycholinguistics, Child Development, and Educational Psychology. He did post-doctoral work at Harvard University, pursuing his specialization in developmental psycholinguistics. Later he obtained a doctorate in General and Applied Linguistics from the University of Paris-V (Sorbonne-René Descartes). Professor Rondal has taught and conducted research in a number of universities and research centers: the University of Minnesota at Minneapolis; l'Université Laval in Quebec City; the Schonell Centre of Queensland University, in Brisbane, Australia; l'Universidad Autonoma de Mexico, at Iztacala, Mexico; Hawaï University at Manoa (Honolulu); le Laboratoire de Psychologie du Langage of the Université de Poitiers; and l'Université Louis Pasteur of Strasbourg, in France.

Dr. Rondal is currently Professeur ordinaire de Psychologie and Psycholinguistique at the Université de Liège, Belgium, where he is in charge of the Laboratory for Psycholinguistics. He is Scientific Consultant and Adviser to a number of European organizations, including the Belgian Association on Down Syndrome (APEM). Dr. Rondal is also co-founder and past-President of the Scientific Council, and vice-President of the European Down Syndrome Association (EDSA). At the 1992 World Congress on Down Syndrome in Orlando, Florida, he received the distinguished Award of the National Down Syndrome Society of America for his work on language in Down's syndrome.

Dr. Rondal has published numerous journal and review articles written in English, French, Italian, Spanish, and Portuguese, invited chapters in edited books written in English and French; monographs in English and French, and more than twenty books written in French. A number of these books have been translated into Spanish and Italian. He is also the author of two noted books, written in English: *Adult-Child Interaction and the Process of Language Acquisition*. published by Praeger Press, New York, in 1985; and *Exceptional Language Development. Implications for the Cognition-Language*

Relationship, published by Cambridge University Press, New York, in 1995.

Susan Edwards received her Ph.D. (Linguistic Science) from the University of Reading. She is a Senior Lecturer in Clinical Linguistics and Language Pathology in the Department of Linguistic Science at the University of Reading. Her teaching and research activities are in the field of language disorders in both children and adults and, as a qualified speech and language therapist, she also has extensive clinical experience. Her clinical work has included working with children and adults with severe learning problems in both hospitals and schools and her doctorate thesis reported on a study of young children with severe learning problems. She has published book chapters and articles on a range of language disorders including language of children with severe learning disorders, dysfluency, motor speech disorders, and aphasia. She is currently involved in the redevelopment and restandardisation of a language test for young children and in the cross-linguistic study of aphasia in adults.

Preface

In writing this book, we have been influenced by many colleagues and people all over the world, through their writing, personal encounters and numerous exchanges over the years. The list is too long to be presented here. We will limit ourselves to acknowledging our debt to those people who were directly concerned with the realization of the manuscript. David Crystal insisted several times that the book be written, and without his enthusiasm it would probably never have started. Colin Whurr, our publisher and friend, was always a great pleasure to deal with. We are particularly grateful to him for his kindness and patience in waiting for the completion of the final manuscript.

A number of close colleagues and friends have been helpful at various stages of the preparation of the book. Lucien Koulischer, Professor of Genetics at the University of Liège supplied us with vital information on the genetic aspects of Down's syndrome, including his work on the prevalence of Down's syndrome in Belgium and the feasibility of large-scale maternal screening. Len Abbeduto, University of Wisconsin at Madison, kindly supplied us with a set of his fine publications on the pragmatic aspects of language and communication in mentally retarded people. Personal contacts and exchanges with Jon Miller and Robin Chapman, Waisman Center, University of Wisconsin, Mike Guralnick, University of Washington, Seattle, Lynn Nadel, Merrill Garrett and Cecile McKee, University of Arizona, Tucson, Bob Hodapp, University of California, Los Angeles, Mike Beveridge and Susan Gathercole, Bristol University, and Sue Buckley of Portsmouth University helped us to clarify a number of ideas on language, memory and other functions in mental retardation and Down's syndrome. In addition, we wish to acknowledge the lasting influence and permanent nurturing towards sophistication and excellence provided by old friends and mentors from the University of Minnesota at Minneapolis, Jim Turnure and John Rynders. Neil O'Connor, University of London, and former Head of the Developmental Psychology Unit of the Medical Research Council, kindly drew our attention to Neil Smith and Ianthi-Maria Tsimpli's excellent book *The*

Mind of a Savant, at an early stage. We are very appreciative of his long-time friendship.

Close to home, we acknowledge Annick Comblain, who allowed us to make use of data from her doctoral dissertation on language and working memory in Down's syndrome, reproduced here in Chapter 5. She was also very helpful in gathering relevant documents for the book. We are indebted to her in many ways. Brigitte Thewis, Bénédicte Morsomme and Mercedes George kindly helped with the preparation of the references and the indexes. Anastasia Piat-Di Nicolantonio was extremely helpful in word-processing the several copies, corrections, revisions of chapters, tables and figures, as well as in performing in her usual excellent way the numerous duties involved in preparing this type of large-scale manuscript for publication. We are very grateful to her.

Of course, any obscurities, infelicities, shortcomings and possible errors of interpretation in the present work are entirely our responsibility.

Note on Terminology

In this book, we use the terms 'individuals with mental retardation' and 'mental retardation' in line with the recommendations of the American Association on Mental Retardation, the American Psychological Association and the American Psychiatric Association. We are aware that these terms may have negative connotations in the United Kingdom, but we wish to emphasize that the choice of these terms reflects international usage and is in no way intended to denigrate this special population with whom we work and hold in high regard.

To Rick Cromer,
in memoriam.

Chapter 1
Outline and Rationale

This book proposes a synthesis of what we regard as the principal data in the area of language development and functioning in mentally retarded (MR) people, together with a discussion of questions relevant to theoretical issues in cognitive psychology, psycholinguistics and linguistics.

Language is a *developmentally organized process* and is modular. We therefore have structured our approach to this subject via a life-span perspective. Accordingly, we consider that remediation should conform to two major principles, namely it should follow developmental order and reflect the modularity of language.

1.1 Let us begin by specifying these principles in order to give the reader an idea of what is to come. Broadly, there are two divergent points of view about the way the mind works. One position (phrased here in a rather extreme form) holds that what exists in this respect is some kind of system of general intelligence, association, problem-solving, etc., which applies across all domains of the mind's activities. So, you apply that system to solving practical problems, to recognizing faces and voices, to constructing theories, to language, etc. A quite different idea is that the mind is modular. According to this view, the mind consists of discrete or, at least, semi-discrete subsystems, each with its own intrinsic structure, its way of functioning, developing, deteriorating, etc. The separate systems interact in complicated ways to create an intricate complex of highly specialized functions. The modular view applied to language is rapidly gaining empirical support. This view concerns both the relationship between language as a whole – assuming that this expression has a genuine denotation – and other major functions of the mind, and the relationships between the major components of the language system, i.e. phonetics and phonology, lexicon, semantics, morpho-syntax, pragmatics and discourse. The modular point of view applies to language pathologies as well. In fact, some of the clearest evidence favouring the modularity thesis comes from the study of pathological cases (aphasias, primary degenerative diseases, specific language impairments, mental retardation, autism, etc.). These indications carry

1

the hope of bringing about important clarifications as to the intrinsic organization of language and its relationships with other mental systems. At the same time, they have important implications for the pathological fields, including aspects of the remediation perspective.

1.2 The approach presented is *developmental-organizational* in the sense of Cicchetti and Beeghly (1990) and can be further defined as an instance of 'liberal' developmentalism in the sense of Hodapp, Burack and Zigler (1990), i.e. at variance with 'conservative' developmentalism (see Chapter 3). Many investigators in the recent past have conceptualized the developmental process of MR individuals as quantitatively and/or qualitatively different from non-retarded (NR) individuals. It is interesting to note that in the past (e.g. late nineteenth century), comparisons between MR and NR subjects were considered to be impracticable (e.g. Sollier, 1891, pp. 3–5). The practicability of systematic comparisons to determine what ages in normal development correspond to features associated with mental development observable in MR children and adolescents (and therefore based on the premise that retarded and normal developments have things in common) was only established following Binet and Simon's construction of the first psychometric scale (Binet and Simon, 1907, 1934; Binet, 1911). We shall discuss the quantitative–qualitative issue in this book, particularly in the discussion of the delay–difference question (Chapter 4).

However, beginning in the 1970s with the publication of a number of important studies on infants and children with Down's syndrome (DS), particularly in the perceptual–cognitive and the social–emotional areas (e.g. Fantz, Fagan and Miranda, 1975; Cicchetti and Sroufe, 1978), research increasingly showed that development and functioning in MR subjects are as organized, purposeful and adaptive as in NR subjects, albeit with limitations and difficulties. Henceforth, the quantitative and qualitative differences that are documented between MR and NR individuals tend to be viewed as *variations in basically similar processes or pathological distortions of otherwise normal phases of development*.[1] This is the core of the developmental–organizational perspective which expresses the hypothesis of a *continuity* (*similar sequencing*) and *structural similarity* between normal and pathological development.

This claim carries two major implications. The first is that it is theoretically and practically advantageous to characterize and assess development in MR individuals in comparison with NR subjects. The numerous data and theoretical interpretations available on normal development can be used with reference to MR subjects to establish to what extent the

---

[1] One of the first authors to have explicitly resorted to this conception in developmental psychopathology is Margaret Mahler (*circa* 1950, in the context of her studies of infantile psychosis) (see Puig-Vergès' 1993, interesting biographical analysis). The basic idea, however, goes back at least to Charcot (see Gasser, 1995), for whom pathological states were nothing but marked modifications of normal states obeying normal laws.

latter relate to normative indications. Comparisons between MR and NR subjects are not easy to make, however. They are beset with methodological difficulties (e.g. the procedures for matching MR and NR subjects) and conceptual caveats; for example, the temptation to characterize retarded development as a slow–motion picture of normal development.

The second major implication of the developmental–organizational perspective is that the study of retarded and abnormal development can markedly enhance our understanding of normal development and functioning. Theorizing about development without considering the deviations that may exist as a result of the action of pathological factors could certainly lead to an incomplete account of ontogenesis. But there is more to this question. Children and adults with mental retardation are an especially important population to consider. They constitute many 'experiments in nature' (in the sense of Bronfenbrenner, 1979; see Rondal, 1994b), experiments that would not be permitted on ethical grounds. Of course, there is a price to pay. In such cases, the 'experimenter' has no control over a number of independent variables.

Another important tenet of the developmental–organizational approach is that development may be conceived of as a series of reorganizations among and within the organismic systems. In this regard, normal development may be characterized by the harmonious integration of various competencies into adapted modes of functioning. In contrast, pathological development and functioning may be viewed as the lack of integration of various competencies, such as the social, cognitive, linguistic and emotional, thus making global adaptation more difficult to achieve. In addition, there may be insufficient integration of particular subskills and subcomponents within larger domains, such as language.

It could be asked whether pathology does not actually create artefactual or exotic dissociations which, although relevant to understanding pathological cases and processes, are of limited interest to theories of normal functioning. We believe that this is not the case and that the basic components and propensities out of which the mental organization (and, within it, the language organization) of MR individuals is constituted, are of the same kind as those of NR people. In other words, we are convinced, first, that the minds of MR individuals have the same cognitive features as all other humans; second, that the universal principles of ontogenetic development apply to MR persons; and third, that the differences which they exhibit, no matter how serious and debilitating, in no way call into question this basic *normality principle* (Cicchetti and Pogge–Hesse, 1982). The differences between NR and MR people remain relatively slight compared with their numerous and important similarities. In accordance with the outline above, we do not view the 'classical defect' approaches in the field of mental retardation, or their

modern successors, as necessarily in opposition to the developmental–organizational position. For a divergent point of view, see Zigler
(1967, 1969, 1973).[2] Some have suggested that MR subjects suffer from a
relative impermeability of the boundaries between regions in the cognitive areas, which is responsible for a high degree of mental rigidity
(Kounin, 1941a, 1941b); primary and secondary mental rigidity caused
by subcortical and cortical malformations (Goldstein, 1943); intrinsic
limitation in channel capacity – visual as well as auditory (Spitz, 1973);
impaired attention–directing mechanisms (Zeaman, 1959); relative
brevity in the persistence of stimulus trace (Siegel and Foshee, 1960);
and/or improper verbal regulation (directive function of speech) of the
thought system (Luria, 1956, 1961, 1963). These authors were often
reacting against the not uncommon tendency to tautology of their times
to attribute the abnormal behaviours of the retarded to a general cognitive inadequacy. They attempted to avoid this circularity by attributing
performance differences between MR and NR individuals not to the
global phenomenon of mental retardation itself, but to particular cognitive defects.

The general position that we advocate does not exclude the possible
existence of important quantitative and qualitative differences or
marked deficits in the mental organization of MR individuals. But we
insist that these problems are better situated with reference to normal
functioning.

Assuming, as we do, that pathological factors do not create artefactual
dissociations between and within psychological functions, but may
reveal the deep–seated architecture of these functions, there are additional advantages in studying MR subjects for clarifying theoretical
points in mental development. They are as follows. First, pathological
conditions bring about dissociations between functions and subsystems
that are normally intimately related to each other and hierarchically integrated. Henceforth, the particular contributions of the subsystems to the
integrated functioning should be easier to identify and to assess from a
'pathological vantage point'. It may be useful to specify that the organizational point of view presented above as one of the analytical principles
underlying the present approach, is not tied to the so–called orthogenetic principle (Werner, 1948) with which the organizational point of
view has often been associated (e.g. Cicchetti and Beeghly, 1990). The
orthogenetic principle states that the developing organism evolves from
a globally undifferentiated state to levels of greater complexity through
progressive differentiation. Although the modular point of view is not
tied to innatism out of logical necessity, most proponents of this view
share the premise that the initial mental equipment and functions are

---

[2] This position is analysed in Chapter 3, together with Zigler and Hodapp's new stand on the
problem.

fairly differentiated to begin with, which, of course, does not exclude further differentiation, regrouping and/or mutual interfacing. Second, the delayed pace of development and prolonged developmental transition in different domains make the study of mental retardation particularly useful for documenting important theoretical questions. A good case in point is the problem of the existence of sensitive or critical periods in ontogenesis. Third, the relatively large interindividual variability that characterizes the development and functioning of MR individuals (particularly in the extreme cases) may yield interesting information on the range of applicability, the plasticity and the dissociability of mental functions. In sum, the study of MR subjects, as well as other pathological cases, supplies a standpoint from which it is possible to understand better the functional architecture of the mind. When it comes to the relationships between non–language cognition and language development, the MR population is, of course, of irreplaceable benefit, as MR subjects by definition do not develop cognitively in normal ways.

1.3 The present approach is also *process–oriented*. Although research on language development in children with MR has long proliferated, it has been product–oriented for a long time. Modern linguistics and psycholinguistics place us in a better position to envisage the language of MR individuals in terms of the processes involved.

1.4 The present approach is structured according to *a life–span developmental perspective* (Rondal, 1988c). The general principles of this approach to human development have been defined (Goulet and Baltes, 1970; Baltes and Schaie, 1973; Mussen, et al., 1978). Huston–Stein and Baltes (1976) assigned to life–span developmental psychology the task of describing and explaining behavioural change from birth to death (p. 171). Some 30 years ago life–span preoccupations with moderately and severely MR individuals would have seemed futile, as so many MR subjects were assumed to die early. Indeed, a significant proportion did not live beyond the first years. According to Oliver and Holland (1986), the life expectancy of individuals with DS was 9 years in 1929, 12–15 years in 1947 and 18 years in 1961 (with two–thirds of the children dead by the age of 12 (Carter, 1958). Medical progress and enhanced social awareness and care have changed the picture markedly. (See, for example, Seltzer and Krauss, 1987). For Down's Syndrome approximately one eighth of infants die during the first 2 years of life from organic complications, including heart disease, severe gastroduodenal abnormalities or respiratory and liver problems, which are present at birth. However, as many as 60 per cent of individuals with Down's Syndrome can now expect to live beyond age 50; 44 per cent will survive to the age of 60 years; and 13.8 per cent to 68 years; compared with 86.4 per cent and 78.4 per cent, respectively, for the general population, irrespective of sex (Baird and Sadovnick, 1988;

Mann and Esiri, 1988; see Figure 1.1). This more optimistic life expectancy is partly spoiled, however, by the fact that beyond approximately 40 years, a number of DS individuals may develop primary degenerative diseases of the Alzheimer type – AZ (see Chapter 5).

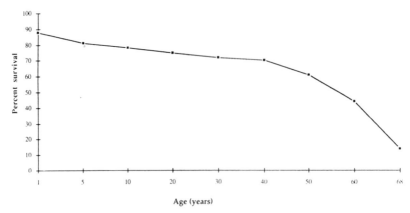

Figure 1.1 Life expectancy in Down's syndrome (based on Baird & Sadnovick, 1987)

The marked increase in life expectancy in MR people, coupled with the now well–established practice of deinstitutionalization or, better, non-institutionalization (legally enforced in some countries) makes it all the more necessary to understand better the various developmental aspects of the syndromes leading to mental retardation, and to design and implement efficient remediation practices. It is expected that between 1990 and 2010, the number of DS people over the age of 40 years will increase by 75 per cent and over 50 years by 200 per cent (Steffelaar and Evenhuis, 1989). Many specific data for establishing the empirical basis of a full life–span perspective in MR language and communicative functioning are still missing. A good deal of work is necessary, particularly with regard to late adolescence, adulthood and older ages. Specific studies of language in MR adults remain too rare despite the obvious fact that they are of great significance to professionals in occupational centres. These professionals need to know much more about the communicative abilities of MR adults. This would greatly help them to develop more efficient ways of stimulating and socializing MR individuals. Above all, it is imperative to develop in the professionals, as well as in the general public, a sense of life–continuation in the best possible conditions for MR people.

1.5 The book is also concerned with *language remediation in MR individuals*, but only in a secondary way. Chapter 6 will deal succinctly with this topic. It is clear that intervention programmes must rely more on the technical knowledge available regarding language development and functioning in MR subjects, incorporate the modular point of view and take into account individual and syndromic variations. MR children need efficient early and continued intervention programmes as their best hope to develop better linguistically.

1.6 No one chapter will be devoted to the topic of language assessment. There is no good reason to believe that this assessment should be basically different from that in NR individuals or in other developmental disorders. A number of useful books or annotated catalogues on language assessment have been published in recent years, to which one can direct the interested reader. See, for example: D. Crystal, *Profiling Linguistic Disability* (Arnold, 1982); D. Crystal, P. Fletcher, and M. Garman, *Grammatical Analysis of Language Disability* (Whurr, 1989); M. Kersner, *Tests of Voice, Speech and Language* (Whurr, 1992); J. Beech and L. Harding, *Assessment in Speech and Language Therapy* (Routledge, 1992); and C. Weir, *Communicative Language Testing* (Prentice Hall, 1990).

Chapter 2
Historical Sketch

According to Rondal (1975) and the bibliographies compiled by Rondal and Rondal (1975, 1976) on speech and language studies in mental retardation, approximately 750 studies[1] were published in English between 1900 and 1975. Most of these works were published between approximately 1950 and 1975 (see Figure 2.1). Peins (1962) signalled that 51 reports of research (in the USA) on speech and language associated with mental retardation appeared in the period between 1934 and 1957. It is known that research concerning MR children began to proliferate in the United States particularly in the early 1960s, when President Kennedy established the National Commission for Mental Retardation. The Commission declared that any child with mental retardation had the right to be educated to his or her best potential (proposal legalized in 1975 by Public Law), which led to an intensification of research and intervention studies in order to meet these objectives.

No complete count of studies on speech and language in mental retardation is available for the period between 1975 and the present time. A search through the 1994 Thesaurus of Psychological Index Terms of the American Psychological Association (covering the years from 1967 until the last updating on 26 November 1993) yields 817 entries for language or language development and mental retardation – 117 for language or language development and Down's syndrome – out of a total of 17,564 for language or language development, 20,065 for mental retardation and 1,480 for Down's syndrome. These data are reported in Figure 2.1. The APA indications are conservative estimates as they do not take into account books and chapters in books, as well as the journal articles and monographs published in sources not reviewed by the APA. There may be

---

[1] Conservatively counted. No work was included that dealt primarily with the role of speech and language in conceptual development, discrimination learning, problem-solving, verbal learning (e.g. serial and paired–associate learning) and verbal mediation theory. Similarly, no work was included that referred primarily to written language development or reading in the retarded. Also no unpublished doctoral dissertation or master's thesis, and no unpublished paper presented at conventions or symposia, or otherwise unpublished manuscripts were included.

some overlap (which is impossible to quantity without further analysis) between Rondal and Rondal's (1976) bibliography and that part of the APA Thesaurus, for the years 1967 to 1976. A reasonable estimate of the number of publications in English on language in mental retardation is about 1000, and 175 – 200 on language in Down's syndrome.

What follows is a personal sketch of the major trends of research in speech and language of MR individuals from the early 1950s to the early 1970s (later studies are presented and discussed in the non-historical chapters). Its aim is to give an idea of the major conceptual changes which have taken place in the field within this period.

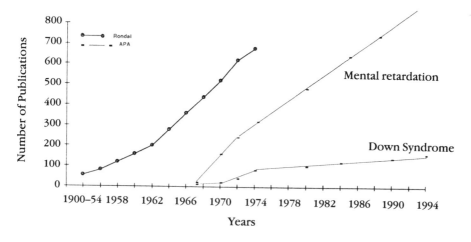

Figure 2.1 Cumulative record of the number of publications in English on speech and language in mental retardation between 1900 and 1974 (after Rondal, 1975); updated with quantitative indications from the *Thesaurus of Psychological Index Terms* (American Psychological Association, 1994) covering the period between 1967 and 1993

2.1 Early speech studies

Early studies appear to have been primarily concerned with speech (articulation, voice, hearing problems, stuttering) and with words and lexical matters. For the researchers in those decades, communication and language in MR individuals were viewed mainly as a question of hearing and articulating sounds, making words and associating words sequentially. Morphosyntactic, semantic and pragmatic aspects were little considered unless in association with other variables representing global categories, such as verbal expression and/or verbal comprehension.

2.1.1 A large number of works conducted in the 1950s and 1960s concerned quantitative aspects of *the production of speech sounds* by MR subjects. Reviews of this literature have been published at different times (e.g. Goertzen, 1957; Spradlin, 1963; Webb and Kinde, 1967; Zisk and Bialer, 1967; Keane, 1972). For example, Spradlin (1963) signalled that 70 per cent of moderately and 90 per cent of severely MR subjects presented articulatory difficulties vs 8 per cent for the mildly retarded, and 5 per cent in the NR population. It was also suggested that articulatory problems are more prevalent among DS individuals than in MR subjects of other diagnostic groups (e.g. Levinson, Friedman, and Stamps, 1955; Schlanger and Gottsleben, 1957; Blanchard, 1964).

2.1.2 *Hearing problems* were suspected a long time ago to be a contributing factor in articulatory difficulties of MR individuals. Depending on the particular study and the criterion used, from 10 to 60 per cent of (bilateral) hearing loss pertaining to the major speech frequencies (i.e. 500, 1000 and 2000 Hz) have been reported (Birch and Matthews, 1951; Foale and Patterson, 1954; Johnson and Farrel, 1954; Kodman, 1958; Rigrodsky, Prunty and Glovsky, 1961; Lloyd and Reid, 1965). These studies were conducted using standard tonal audiometry techniques. It is difficult to parcel out how much attention, motivation and task comprehension contributed to these results. Glovsky (1966) noted that the auditory behaviours of some MR subjects appear to be highly variable. However, better adapted investigation techniques such as play audiometry for the younger subjects, as well as a range of electrophysiological techniques, have confirmed a higher prevalence of hearing loss in MR individuals, and particularly in DS subjects. West (1947) suggested that many DS individuals present an VIIIth cranial nerve abnormality and the inflectionless voice characteristic of this type of deafness. In Rigrodsky et al.'s report (1961), hearing impairment was shown to affect approximately 60 per cent of the institutionalized DS sample. The losses were mainly in the mildly to moderately impaired range (mean decibel range 25–55) with about half perceptive or mixed, and half conductive impairment in the speech frequencies. Other reports (e.g. Clausen, 1968) signal somewhat lower figures of hearing loss in DS subjects and prevalent rates of conductive losses over perceptive or mixed ones. More recent work with brain stem auditory evoked potentials (BAEP) (e.g. Gigli et al., 1984; Ferri et al., 1986) confirms the existence of conductive problems in a large proportion of the DS subjects studied. Moreover, many DS children exhibit BAEP abnormalities suggestive of a brainstem conduction dysfunction.

2.1.3 *Stuttering problems* in MR subjects were also of great concern to the researchers of this time. Schlanger (1953) reported 20 per cent of stutterers in a group of 74 institutionalized MR subjects. In another study of 516 cases undertaken together with Gottsleben, Schlanger found 17 per cent stutterers (Schlanger and Gottsleben, 1957). Schaeffer and Shearer's (1968) sample of more than 4300 MR subjects in state institutions had an incidence of 7.6 per cent of stutterers. Gens (1951) and Gottsleben (1955) suggested that there is a higher incidence of stuttering among DS than non–DS MR subjects. Schlanger and Gottsleben (1957) reported 45 per cent of stuttering for individuals with Down's syndrome. It may be that the varying rates of stuttering in some of these studies conducted with mixed samples of MR subjects are partly related to the representation of DS individuals in the samples. Some researchers have expressed doubt about whether it is a question of genuine stuttering or just stuttering–like behaviours in DS subjects (e.g. Evans and Hampson, 1968). In particular, it was asked whether these behaviours should not be better classified as instances of *cluttering* (Cabanas, 1954). According to Weiss (1964), cluttering is the rhythmic manifestation of a central language imbalance which affects all channels of communication. It is specifically characterized by a short attention span, impaired articulation and excessive speed of delivery. Weiss's definition of cluttering, which claims a disturbance of the central processes preliminary to speech, is questionable and not necessarily shared by other authors concerned with cluttering (e.g. Cabanas, 1954). Cluttering could be a more peripheral problem, involving the distribution of the speech units over intervals of time, therefore concerning final processes more than antecedent thought processes. The question of the exact nature of stuttering–cluttering symptoms was not clarified until Preus's study (1972). In day institutions in Oslo, Preus identified 67 individuals above the age of 7 years (CA) with DS. Those below the age of 7 were found to be unsuitable for the study as they presented with insufficient speech proficiency to participate in the screening test for stuttering and cluttering. The results of the study indicated that approximately one third of the DS subjects sampled stuttered on 5 per cent of the words in a spontaneous speech sample of 200 words. About one third of the subjects had a clear tendency to clutter. Approximately 20 per cent of those subjects who cluttered were also stutterers. However, statistical analyses showed the occurrence of stuttering and cluttering in individual subjects to be mostly uncorrelated. It appears, therefore, that significant proportions of DS subjects have a marked tendency either to stutter or to clutter, and some do both but not in temporal proximity.

2.1.4 The prevalence of *voice (phonation)* defects in MR subjects, and particularly in DS individuals, and the possible reasons for these problems were also debated in those decades. As we have indicated, West (1947) stated that many children with Down's Syndrome have voice problems, primarily manifested by hoarseness. Schlanger and Gottsleben (1957), as well as Blanchard (1964), found that approximately 50 per cent of their institutionalized DS subjects presented with abnormal voice qualities (e.g. low–pitched, harsh, monotone). Benda (1949) had noted that DS subjects often have a characteristic voice. According to him, a blind diagnosis of Down's syndrome[2] should be possible on that basis alone. Strazzulla (1953) confirmed that DS children often exhibit abnormally low–pitched

---

[2] The genetic basis of Down's syndrome and its aetiological relationship with chromosome 21 was only ascertained in the late 1950s (Jacobs et al., 1959; Lejeune, Gautier & Turpin, 1959; Lejeune, Turpin & Gautier, 1959).

voices. Jones (1963; summarized in Zisk and Bialer, 1967) attempted to validate Benda's claim regarding the identification of Down's syndrome by voice quality alone. One–minute tape–recorded samples of the voices of a group of DS and non–DS MR subjects were presented to three speech pathologists who were asked to judge whether each voice belonged to a DS or to a non–DS individual. On the whole, the judges were able to differentiate the DS voices from the non–DS ones reliably. However, the voices of the youngest DS girls and those of the oldest DS boys were particularly difficult to differentiate from NR subjects. Similar experiments conducted by Michel and Carney (1964) and Hollien and Copeland (1965) did not confirm Jones' data nor Benda's suggestion. These researchers found that the pitch levels of their male and female DS subjects (aged 8-10 years CA) approximated the norms for NR 10–year-olds. They concluded that characteristics other than pitch contribute to the auditory impression DS voices may give.

2.2 Early language studies

Many early language studies with MR individuals reflected theoretical trends in psycholinguistics at the time, e.g. Skinner's (1957) treatment of the referential aspects of language, as well as Osgood's (1953, 1957a), Jenkins and Palermo's (1964) and Jenkins' (1965) associative and mediational.

   2.2.1 However, attempts at explaining language in associative terms were abandoned after Chomsky's demonstration (Chomsky, 1957a) that probabilistic models give no particular insight into the problem of linguistic structures. Similarly, explanations of language and language behaviour in terms of conditioning processes virtually came to an end (with the notable exception of Staat's work, e.g. 1971) after Chomsky's devastating criticism of Skinner's *Verbal Behaviour* (Chomsky, 1957b) which he showed came nowhere near to meeting the sufficiency condition and was largely irrelevant to any serious study of grammar. Notwithstanding conditioning, particularly operant conditioning, approaches to language remediation were attempted on a relatively large scale in the United States and in certain other countries for a number of years (see below). It is correct to note that the proponents of these procedures did not always claim that the theory behind their practice was explanatorily adequate. They often justified their procedures in terms of the results obtained, even if it involved building behavioural entities possibly removed from natural language mechanisms.

   2.2.2 Karlin and Strazzulla (1952) and Strazzulla (1953) reported on the ages of appearance of conventional words in MR children. They signalled comparable data for DS and non–DS MR children, i.e. around 33 months chronological age (CA). They cautioned, however, that there were important individual differences. These data seem more favourable than those reported by Engler (1949), which indicated that by the age of 3 years, roughly 50 per cent of the institutionalized DS children had begun to produce conventional words, 62 per cent of the children by the age of 4 years, and about 81 per cent by the age of 5 years.

Begining in the early 1950s, several studies attempted to answer more specific questions regarding lexical development in MR children. For example, Papania (1954) undertook qualitative analyses of the responses on the Vocabulary subtest of the Stanford–Binet Intelligence Test with a group of institutionalized mildly MR children aged 6 – 10 years–CA. He reported that MR children can define as many words as NR children of comparable mental ages (MA), but at a markedly lower level of abstraction. Waters (1956) administered the same test to three groups of MR children: organic, familial and of unknown aetiologies. They were matched for MA (7 years). The subjects' responses were analysed according to the following scheme: mere repetition, physical demonstration, descriptive definition based on use, synonym and verbal explanation. No significant difference was observed in total vocabulary scores between the groups. Significant differences held in the descriptive definition category only. The familial MR subjects produced fewer such responses than the other two groups.

2.2.3 Another question asked was whether DS individuals develop language in the same way as other MR individuals. Using the Gesell Developmental Examination (Gesell and Amatruda, 1941), Share and his colleagues (Share et al., 1963; Fishler, Share, and Koch, 1964; Share, 1975) reported that language in DS children was the area of slowest progress, compared to motor ability, adaptive and personal–social behaviour. Since then it has often been asserted that DS individuals as a group are characterized by a specific deficit in language development. The question is still with us, as we shall see in Chapter 3.

2.2.4 In the early 1960s, O'Connor and associates supplied additional analyses of the lexical functioning of moderately and severely MR subjects. Mein and O'Connor (1960) compared the productive vocabularies of a group of institutionalized moderately and severely MR children aged 3–7 years–CA, using pictorial material as a starting point for small conversations. MR children produced an average number of words comparable to that of NR children (i.e. 359 words). However, they had larger 'core' vocabularies (defined as the words produced most often by at least half the subjects in the sample) and, consequently, smaller 'fringe' vocabularies (i.e. lexical items less frequently produced). In another study using the same methodology, Wolfensberger, Mein and O'Connor (1963) showed that, together with increases in CA and/or MA, the absolute size of the core vocabularies is greater in MR subjects whereas the percentage of core words in the entire vocabulary decreases. MR individuals produce a more diversified set of words in their descriptions as CAs and MAs increase. Mein (1961), using conversa-

tional interviews and picture description tasks, classified his MR subjects
into four MA groups (MA 3.6, 4.8, 5.6 and 6.5 years, respectively). He
observed that as MA increased, the proportions of nouns produced in
free speech decreased relative to other formal classes. This means that
with increased MA, there is a beginning of diversification of word classes
in the language of MR subjects, although less marked than in NR children. When compared to NR children and to MR children of similar MAs
but different aetiologies, DS children are observed to produce more
nouns but fewer articles in obligatory contexts, which indicates that
their nominal phrases could be slightly less developed at corresponding
MAs. A confounding possibility, however, is that as DS subjects have
poorer articulatory skills, their production of less audible article forms
could have been missed by the judges more often than was the case for
non–DS MR subjects.

2.2.5 Lyle (1959, 1960a, 1960b, 1961a, 1961b) showed in a series of
studies that the social and physical environment of some institutions
and hospitals has a negative effect on language development in moderately and severely MR children. Research by Papania (1954), Badt
(1958), Rheingold and Bayley (1959) and Haggerty (1959) confirmed a
lower level of language development (particularly lexical development)
in institutionalized compared to non–institutionalized MR individuals.
Other studies by Centerwall and Centerwall (1960) and by Shotwell and
Shipe (1964) indicated that the finding applies equally to DS children.
Even when carefully matched with non–institutionalized peers for IQ,
MA and/or CA, institutionalized MR children tend to use shorter
sentences and produce fewer words per minute. They obtain lower
scores on the Illinois Test of Psycholinguistic Abilities (ITPA). It could be
the practical organization within the institutions that is responsible for
discouraging rather than enhancing language development (Haviland,
1972). Daily routines and the tranquillizing use of radio and television
may contribute to rendering speech signals less salient (Spradlin, 1968).
In addition, there were often poor adult–child ratios and infrequent
adult–child contacts, which reduced the child's opportunities for verbal
interaction. Curiously, however, at this time, the demonstration that
institutionalized children were at a significant disadvantage with respect
to their opportunities for developing language did not motivate research
into the language environment of the MR child cared for at home.

2.3 More theoretically oriented studies

2.3.1 Some of the studies undertaken in the 1950s and the 1960s were
more 'theory oriented'. One theoretical impetus came from the *Russian
studies on semantic conditioning and generalization*, which were
inspired by Pavlov's late writings on what he called the second signalling
system (i.e. speech stimuli) (Pavlov, 1954, 1962; see also Ivanov-

Smolensky, 1951). An example of this orientation is Shvarts' experiment. Shvarts (1954) established a Pavlovian conditioned association between a vasoconstrictive reflex and words such as *dom* (*house*, in Russian) and *doctor* (*doctor*), using as an unconditional stimulus a temperature of 10° celsius applied on the forearm. Transfer of the conditioned reaction was undertaken to homonyms such as *dym* (*to smoke*) and *diktor* (*speaker*), and to synonyms such as *house* (the subjects had a good command of English) and *vrach* (*physician*). Generalization tests took place at the beginning and at the end of the conditioning procedure, and following the administration of a dose of chloric hydrate. Shvarts (1954) observed that semantic generalization dominates phonetic generalization, but that the latter is always latent and may appear or reappear in states of reduced functional efficiency (for example, within the first half–hour following drug administration). Riess (1946) had already demonstrated that semantic generalization tended to dominate phonetic generalization with age increasing in the child. He claimed that 10 years of age is the decisive developmental stage in this respect. Luria and Vinogradova (1959) confirmed Riess's findings in a series of experiments showing the predominance of semantic generalization in NR children aged 11 and 12 years. Luria and Vinogradova (1959) applied the same paradigm to subjects with severe learning problems. They reported that mildly MR children (aged CA 10–15 years) display generalization to words similar in meaning and words similar in sounds to the test words, whereas moderately and severely MR children (with corresponding CAs) are limited to phonetic generalization. The Russian investigators concluded that pathological cortical states such as those found in severe forms of mental retardation, result in qualitative changes in the system of word association.

O'Connor and Hermelin (1959a, b) discovered, however, that moderately and severely MR subjects (CA range 9–16 years) were not completely devoid of the capacity to generalize along a semantic lexical basis. Their subjects were able to associate and connect by meaning words they knew well. Verbal generalization in MR subjects appeared to follow basically the same course as in NR subjects at similar MAs. O'Connor and Hermelin found that Luria and Vinogradova's conclusion was too pessimistic, although there were methodological variations between the two series of studies that could account at least in part for the difference in the data obtained.

A large-scale experimental study of speech and thought in moderately and severely MR subjects by O'Connor and Hermelin (1963) embodied two of the major tenets of the developmental–organizational perspective central in the present approach to mental retardation. These were, first, that the study of pathological development may significantly enhance our understanding of non-pathological development, and, second, that pathological development is best characterized with direct reference to

non-retarded development. O'Connor and Hermelin (1963) demonstrated that moderately and severely MR children are able to use
concepts as organizing principles for their classifications, although they
may be unable to verbalize these concepts, which leaves the organization of perceptual and motor responses in a state of instability. Reinforcing verbalizations usually leads to a more stable response 'set',
which once consolidated may be difficult to modify. MR subjects exhibit
limited but real transfer and generalization capacities attesting to some
preserved 'dynamism' in their symbolizing and semantic organization.
For instance, naming can be transferred from a picture to the written
word designating it. Symbols can be taught to evoke the same verbal
response as the things that they symbolize.

2.3.2 Let us consider further the relationships between thought and
language as proposed by the Russian School (Luria, 1959, 1961, 1966a,
1966b; Luria and Yudovich, 1959; Vygotsky, 1962; O'Connor, 1966) and
the influence of these writings on developmental studies with MR individuals. According to Vygotsky, man's psychological nature originates in
social relations which are internalized to form the structures of personality. Speech and language, which are social functions *par excellence*,
play a most important role in this formative evolution. Vygotsky distinguishes a first developmental stage that is non-verbal. Any speech
existing during this period is considered to be 'non-intellectual'. Gradually, language develops, and as soon as it is developed to a 'sufficient'
extent, language and thought converge and fuse into each other in such
a manner as to become practically impossible to disentangle. From that
moment on, language becomes 'intellectual' and thought verbal, which,
according to Vygotsky, constitutes the double key characteristic of the
human species. Initially, the above convergence can only manifest itself
at the level of external (social) speech. Later, it will also take place at the
level of inner speech which develops from private external speech
(so–called egocentric speech).

In a series of elegant experiments, Luria (1961) applied Vygotsky's
model to the progressive control of motor behaviour by the second
signalling system (the *directive function of speech*). He stated (e.g.
Luria, 1966a) that true (i.e. genuinely human) voluntary activity is
evoked by a spoken self–instruction or at least by an intention requiring
the 'closest participation' of speech. Luria identified several stages in the
above development and presented empirical data validating his conception. According to Luria, an elementary form (externally guided) of
verbally regulated behaviour is achieved by about 1½ years when the
infant becomes able to respond to simple commands. At this stage,
however, the child is still unable to respond properly to more complicated instructions such as 'When you see the light, press the rubber
bulb', which requires that he, first, refrains from pressing before the
light appears, then, presses the bulb when the light does appear, and

finally, stops pressing until the next light appears. In handling such a situation, the child may take advantage of self–vocalizations accompanying performance on the motor task. For children younger than 3 years, any combination of motor and verbal responses is difficult and of little regulatory value. With children in a second stage, i.e. between 3 and 4 years, a clear regulation of motor reactions is obtained when a verbal accompaniment corresponds rhythmically to the motor task regardless of the meaning of the words employed (for example, when the child is required to say 'go' while pressing the bulb once, or 'go, go' while pressing it twice). Luria labelled this type of verbal regulation 'impulsive' or 'rhythmic'. When the rhythmic correspondence between verbal and motor responses is removed, the child is no longer able to perform the motor task correctly. For children in the third stage, i.e. by 5 years of age, the meaning of the verbal accompaniment comes to predominate over its rhythmic aspect so that if the two aspects, meaningful and rhythmic, are in conflict, the meaningful aspect dominates inducing correct motor performance (meaningful verbal regulation of behaviour).

Luria's thesis and developmental sketch was widely accepted (somewhat uncritically) in the early 1960s and his experiments were quickly integrated into the literature concerning the notion of mediational deficiency (Flavell, 1977). However, when the first replications were attempted in the West, in the early 1970s, they led to varying results and conclusions compared to those of Luria (see Wozniak, 1972, for a review of these studies).

Luria (1961) also suggested that the bond between verbal system and non-verbal behaviour is insufficiently developed in MR individuals, causing a number of cognitive and behavioural problems. A series of studies conducted by Tikhomirova, Nepomnyashchaya, Lubovsky, and Marcinovskaya (summarized in Luria, 1956, 1961) reveal major difficulties in the reflection of objects and events in the second signalling system of MR subjects, and, consequently, in their verbal control of thought and behaviour. Regarding the latter point, more particularly, moderately and severely MR children (labelled 'oligophrenic' by the Russian researchers), and even MR adolescents (until CA 16 years, in the studies performed), are not able properly to coordinate motor responses and spoken verbal responses corresponding to the motor responses. As a rule, when they produce the motor response, they fail to utter the verbal one, and vice versa. When, eventually, following specific training, they become capable of coordinating the two types of response, it is the impulsive aspect of the verbal regulation that predominates over the meaningful one. For instance, when the target is to say 'don't push' while refraining from pressing the rubber bulb given a specific stimulus, MR subjects usually are led into pressing the bulb by the meaningfully negative but rhythmically 'positive' verbal response. It is only when the verbal response is in direct 'impulsive correspondence' with the motor response that a verbal regulation can be obtained. For example, a verbal response: 'push, push' and a motor response consisting in pressing the rubber bulb twice for each presentation of a light, would be successful. Experimental data obtained by Hermelin and O'Connor (1960) (discussed in O'Connor and Hermelin, 1963) and by Cornil (1970) confirmed the findings of Luria and associates. It would seem, therefore, that moderately and severely MR individuals are indeed restricted to impulsive types of verbal regulation of their behaviour.

However, the Western replications of Luria's experimental work with NR subjects have generally failed to confirm the Russian findings related to the meaningful type of verbal regulation, which seriously puts in question the conceptualization proposed by Luria (Miller, Shelton and Flavell, 1970; Bronckart, 1973). One of us (Rondal, 1976) has shown, however, that meaningful short–term planning and regulation of motor behaviour can be demonstrated in NR adults, using a combination of retroactive introspective reporting and electromyographic recording, for example, at the level of the orbicularis oris muscle. Most importantly, when spontaneously used at the level of inner speech, meaningful verbal self–accompaniments do not persist. They tend to appear at the beginning of the task and then disappear to an extent and with a speed depending on the subject's relative ease with the task. Errors in task performance are likely to be followed by verbalizations which help the subjects signal to themselves defects in their performance and concentrate their attention on correcting them in the subsequent course of the task. Such reactions are often followed by a momentary returning to verbal self–accompaniment. If the role of meaningful verbal regulation is of that sort, it is likely that requesting the subjects to accompany themselves verbally during the whole motor task may not be the optimal strategy for revealing the efficiency of such a regulation, and may even be enough to nullify the regulating effect on motor behaviour. The process of meaningful verbal regulation of behaviour in adults is probably mostly through inner speech. The same may be true of children over 6 or 7 years of age, i.e. as soon as they have matured enough to use efficient ways of covertly regulating their own activities. This may be the major reason why this type of regulation, as advocated by Luria, could not be confirmed in subsequent experiments. To the best of our knowledge, there has been no experimental study conducted with children using the Lurian paradigm but where inner speech has been controlled for. However, convincing data on the role of inner speech in the regulation of mental activities obtained by the use of electromyographic techniques with adult subjects have been reported (McGuigan, 1966; Sokolov, 1972).

The same reasoning can also be applied to MR individuals. Studies of their covert language processes could reveal that they have access to meaningful types of verbal regulation of their behaviours, just like NR subjects, at a given level of mental development. No electromyographic study of inner speech in moderately and severely MR subjects is known to us. Some observations (see Rondal, 1995a) suggest that moderately and severely MR individuals make little or no spontaneous use of inner speech or private external speech. When they do, or are pressed to do so by the examiner, such speech usually seriously disrupts ongoing behavioural activities rather than helping them. It is likely, therefore, that meaningful verbal regulation of thinking and behavioural activities is largely out of reach of most moderately and severely MR individuals.

2.3.3 Other studies conducted with MR subjects in the 1950s and 1960s were influenced by another important developmental theory, *i.e.* *Piaget's*. Contrary to the Russian theorists, Piaget sees mental development, which he often terms logico–mathematical development, as largely independent of language development at least up to the level of so–called propositional or formal operations, which are reached at adolescence. According to Piaget (1970; see also Flavell, 1963; Furth, 1969), language cannot be a sufficient or even a necessary condition for the formation of intellectual operations. Conversely, this is language that depends on intellectual evolution for its development. The capacity to represent, Piaget claims, depends on the same knowledge structure that permits the construction of reality. The representative capacity gradually emerges in the second half of the sensorimotor period (i.e. between 12 and 18 months). It manifests itself, first, in the symbolic play and mental imagery of the child (Piaget, 1968). Language is also the product of this general representational function. Thus, lexical, semantic, as well as grammatical development is considered to depend largely on cognitive development. Piaget's thesis is, at least partly, false as can be judged from a number of recent empirical data which will be considered in Chapter 4 (see also Rondal, 1995a, for a full discussion).

For the time being, let us simply signal the existence of studies aimed at specifying Piagetian developmental patterns for moderately and severely MR children, particularly in their speech and language aspects. Woodward (1959, 1963) and Woodward and Stern (1963) obtained observational data compatible with Inhelder's hypothesis (1944). This hypothesis can be summarized in the following way. Mildly MR subjects, as a rule, reach the stage of concrete operations, but not the stage of formal operations, upon completion of their mental development. Moderately and severely MR subjects eventually reach only the intuitive and preoperational stages. And profoundly MR individuals do not advance beyond the sensorimotor stage (so–called sensorimotor intelligence).

Woodward (1959) showed that the sequence of substages in sensorimotor development, which Piaget observed in NR infants, takes place also in low–grade MR subjects. Woodward and Stern (1963) documented the early development of 83 moderately and severely MR children aged from 11 months to 8 years 7 months, comparing their evolution in different areas and examining the relation of various aspects of development to Piaget's sensorimotor stages. Locomotor development was found to be significantly in advance of speech development. Some acquisition in language, drawing, performance ability and social skills was associated with the attainment of the latest sensorimotor substages, suggesting that the achievement of the end of this period constitutes an important step in the development of MR children.

2.3.4 *The Illinois Test of Psycholinguistic Abilities* (ITPA; McCarthy and Kirk, 1961; revised version: Pareskevopoulos and Kirk, 1969) was developed on the basis of the *Differential Language Facility Test* devised by Sievers (Sievers and Essa, 1961). Both tests were inspired by Osgood's model of human communication. Osgood (1957a, b) distinguished two major channels of communication: auditory–vocal and visual–motor; three basic processes: decoding, association and encoding; and two levels of organization of the communication process: representational level and level of automatic processing. The representational level is semantic whereas the automatic level regulates more sequential aspects of language. The ITPA was one of the first attempts to assess systematically various language functions and to provide individual profiles of underlying abilities. In its experimental version, the test consisted of nine subtests: auditory decoding, visual decoding, auditory–vocal association, visual–motor association, vocal encoding, motor encoding, auditory–vocal automatic, auditory–vocal sequential and visual–motor sequential. Three subtests were added in the revised version: visual closure, auditory closure and sound blending. Some modifications were also brought to the subtest auditory–vocal automatic relabelled grammatical closure, and to the subtest visual–motor sequencing relabelled visual-sequential memory. The differences between the experimental and the revised version of the ITPA have been analysed by Marinosson (1974) and Waugh (1973), the latter author with comparative empirical data. Conclusions were that the two versions of the test could be used interchangeably for most practical purposes.

The ITPA has been employed with mildly, moderately and severely MR subjects, aged between 6 and 16 years–CA, living in institutions or in families (Carr, 1964; Mueller and Weaver, 1964; Bateman and Wetherell, 1965; Bilovsky and Share, 1965; McCarthy, 1965; Brown and Rice, 1967; Roberts, 1967; Glovsky, 1970; Caccamo and Yater, 1972; Ogland, 1972; Marinosson, 1974). A consistent picture emerged from these studies. Briefly stated (see Rondal, 1977, for a detailed analysis), MR children exhibit a deficit at the entire automatic–sequential level of functioning. They have marked difficulties in correctly reproducing sequences of digits presented auditorily and series of symbols presented visually, although there is relative strength at the semantic level. MR subjects also have fewer difficulties in dealing with visual–motor than with auditory–vocal tasks. This holds true for the decoding, encoding, and associative processes. Performance on the ITPA usually reveals relatively good performance in motor encoding, such as explanations for the use of objects (both real or represented in pictures) and weaknesses in grammatical functioning. One ITPA study (McCarthy, 1965) compared DS and non–DS MR children matched for CA (mean CA 9 years 4 months), MA and IQ. DS children received slightly higher scores in motor encoding and slightly lower scores in grammatical closure.

The ITPA has been criticized on several grounds. These criticisms probably led to the test being gradually abandoned. Weener, Barritt and Semmel (1967) charged that the model underlying the test failed to integrate adequately the various dimensions of language and, consequently, could not supply a relevant explanation for relationships between subtests as well as between subtests and other language variables. Mittler (1970a) remarked that the test failed to take into account advances in linguistics and developmental psycholinguistics. Spradlin (1968) criticized the test for its lack of interest in functional or social–behavioural aspects of language.

2.4 Lenneberg's studies

Eric Lenneberg's influence on developmental psycholinguistics has been most important. He contributed to the affirmation of a new paradigm in which language is seen primarily as a system characterized by the existence of *a priori* information, species–specific structures, and particular maturational constraints. These constraints include a critical period for development and predictable lines along which disintegrating pathological forces operate. According to Lenneberg (1967), natural language is essentially a phenomenon with biologically determined principles. The indices revealing a maturationally controlled emergence of language are the following: (1) regularity in the sequence of appearance of the developmental milestones, all well correlated with concomitant development facts, such as physical growth and motor development; (2) evidence that the opportunity for environmental stimulation remains constant throughout development, but that the child makes different use of such opportunities as he or she grows up; and (3) emergence of the behaviour, either in part or entirely, before it is of functional use to the individual.

2.4.1 One of Lenneberg's most interesting contributions is his suggestion of the existence of *a critical period* for language development. According to Lenneberg (1966, 1967), there is a critical period for language acquisition extending from approximately 2 years until puberty. It corresponds to the gradual establishment of the dominance of the left cerebral hemisphere for language functions. Lenneberg claimed that at birth the two cerebral hemispheres are functionally equivalent for the language to come. This is the equipotentiality hypothesis. At puberty, cerebral language laterality is definitively established. As a consequence, the plasticity of the neural organization underlying language substantially decreases and further basic language development becomes increasingly difficult. In fact, two versions of Lenneberg's critical period hypothesis can be extracted from his writings: (1) *a strong version*: humans cannot acquire a first language naturally, i.e. by mere exposure, after puberty; and (2) *a weak version*: normal (i.e. complete) language development cannot occur naturally beyond the critical period.

The critical period hypothesis was based on three series of data: first, language development in NR children and the developmental regularities and relative independence of those regularities from direct environmental influence; second, recovery in cortical pathologies of language, particularly in aphasic cases; and third, the study of brain development from birth until puberty. Lenneberg (1967) defined the effect of age in the following way: a cerebral lesion occurring before 14 or 15 months may determine a delay in early lexical development no matter whether it is located in the right or the left hemisphere; whereas after 15 months or so, the functional dominance of the left cerebral hemisphere for language is progressively established. Accordingly, the incidence of aphasias following lesions to the right hemisphere is more frequent in children than in adults and in adolescents. After puberty, the incidence of aphasias following lesions to the right hemisphere is equivalent to the very low incidence in adults. Basing his observations on language recovery following hemispheric lesions or hemispherectomy in childhood (Basser, 1962), Lenneberg concluded that the hemispheric lateralization of language function is completed by puberty. He observed that postlesional recuperation varies with the age at which the lesion occurs (and, of course, with the site and the importance of the lesion). Before 8 or 9 years, he claimed, recuperation is usually complete. After puberty, permanent losses are observed. Studying brain development, Lenneberg (1967) observed that the set of neurobiological parameters of cerebral growth (e.g. cerebral weight, histological development, myelogenesis, biochemical components of the brain metabolism) present a temporal profile that roughly parallels language development. There is rapid initial growth followed by a gradual slowing down of the development pace. As puberty occurs, the brain behaves as if it were set in definitive ways. Maturation is attested in the structural, biochemical and electrophysiological changes culminating in the brain at that time. The definitive brain setting goes along with a marked decrease in the functional plasticity of the central nervous system for the demands of language acquisition, with the important consequence that 'basic language skills not acquired by that time remain deficient for life' (Lenneberg, 1967, p. 158).

Lenneberg's hypothesis regarding the existence of a critical period for language acquisition, must of course, be assessed in the light of more recent data in neurolinguistics and developmental psycholinguistics (see Chapter 5).

2.4.2 Lenneberg is also to be credited with a major impulse towards placing the language study of MR individuals in line with the work in theoretical linguistics and psycholinguistics. He was convinced that language development in MR children follows general laws of evolution that are no different from the unfolding of language in healthy children (1967, p. 309). The study of language development in MR subjects therefore affords the opportunity to study language development in slow motion. Capitalizing on this insight, Lenneberg, Nichols and Rosenberger (1964) undertook the study of a group of 61 DS children raised by their own parents. An interesting question concerned the *role of intelligence* in language acquisition. Lenneberg et al. (1964) claimed that there is a certain intelligence threshold value that must be attained for language to develop. Individuals below this threshold (e.g. profoundly retarded subjects) have little language in the strict sense. Above this threshold, however, Lenneberg et al. found that standard intelligence figures correlate poorly with language development. The relation between physical growth and language maturation appears to be roughly similar to that of NR children. For example, there is a much greater likelihood for language acquisition after gait is established than before. Also right–handedness emerges at the same time as early language unfolds. This, of course, is much later in MR children than in NR children. Among MR children, CA is a better predictor of early language development than IQ. This relationship was later confirmed and quantified by Rondal et al. (1988) with samples of American–English DS subjects aged 3–10 years. They found statistically significant product–moment correlations between CA and mean length of utterance (MLU) with MLUs between 1 and 2.5 words plus grammatical morphemes. Miller and Chapman (1981) reported corresponding findings with a sample of 123 NR children aged 1 year 5 months to 4 years 11 months (MLU range 1–5). De Villiers and de Villiers (1973) with a sample of 21 NR children aged 16–40 months (MLU range 1–4), and Rondal et al. (1987) with samples of American–English NR children ranging in CA from 1 year 8 months to 2 years 5 months (MLU range 1–2.5) also found significant correlations between CA and MLU.

The data analysed by Lenneberg et al. (1964) confirm that for all the DS subjects studied, *the sequences of emergence for various language aspects* (e.g. understanding, quantitative aspects of vocabulary development, language imitation and comprehension, productive language development: few phrases only, few primitive sentences only – not clearly defined on formal grounds, many primitive sentences, and simple sentences mostly correct – none of the DS subjects was producing complex sentences) remain undisturbed by the pathological condition.

Lenneberg's contribution has opened the modern approach to language acquisition and language development pathologies, particularly in the case of mental retardation and Down's syndrome. He anticipated the contemporary interest in carefully documenting pathological conditions interfering with normal processes. Further, in pointing out that stages of language development are more significantly related to general maturation than to intellectual development per se, Lenneberg initiated the move that has led to the present day insistence on the relative autonomy of language as a system and its modularity properties.

Lenneberg, Nichols and Rosenberger (1964) also suggested that language teaching could not be efficient unless certain maturational stages had been reached. Language training should follow and be properly integrated in the developmental sequences. Such recommendations were largely ignored in the conditioning wave that 'submerged' language intervention in the 1950s and 1960s.

2.5 Psycholinguistically oriented work

Contemporary with or following Lenneberg's classic work and influenced by the new developing *Zeitgeist* in psycholinguistics are a number of studies on the language development of MR individuals, which appeared in the late 1960s and the early 1970s. By this time, the particular research questions and objectives had changed thereby reflecting changes in psycholinguistics. Many researchers were no longer concerned with speech and elementary lexical abilities. Instead, they tended to focus more on grammar and morphosyntax. It is easy to recognize in these efforts the influence of transformational grammar (Chomsky, 1957a) and the works in experimental psycholinguistics that were devoted, albeit somewhat naïvely and counterproductively (see Chomsky, 1994), to testing predictions derived from early transformational models (e.g. Mehler, 1963; Miller and McKean, 1964).

2.5.1 Lovell and Dixon (1967) used the test of imitation, comprehension, and production of sentences (ICP) designed by Fraser, Bellugi and Brown (1963) with a group of 20 NR children (CA range: 2 years and 6 months to 6 years and 6 months) and to a group of 40 mildly MR children (CAs between 6 and 7 years; IQs around 60 points). Fraser et al.'s claims regarding the relative order of development of comprehension and production of language were found to hold also for mildly MR children. In addition, it was found that MR subjects exhibited the same rank difficulty of the morphosyntactic contrasts across tasks and age levels. Corresponding results were published by Graham and Gulliford (1968). The latter authors added that the ability of a child (retarded as well as normally developing) to repeat any particular sentence depends on the syntactic type of sentence as well as the child's short–term memory (STM) capacity. Graham (1968) confirmed the differential effect of sentence types at different levels of STM in mildly MR children (aged 6 to 11 years–CA). He suggested that STM limitations might account for some language deficiencies in MR subjects. Along similar lines, Semmel and Bennet (1970) demonstrated weak recoding abilities in mildly MR children (CA range: 9–14 years; mean MA 8 years; mean IQ 70) and a reduced and inconsistent use of word–associative probabilities and syntactic patterning in processing linguistic material.

Lovell, Hersee and Preston (1969) administered a test of syntactic similarity (designed after Brown and Berko, 1960) to 20 mildly MR children (CAs 8–15 years; IQs between 60 and 70). The performance of mildly MR children in recognizing syntactic similarity appeared comparable to that of younger NR. Mittler (1970b) used a comprehension task, consisting of identifying grammatical constructions by pointing to their correct visual referents. This was presented to 50 severely MR children (mean CA 8 years 10 months) and 50 NR children matched for MA (mean MA 3 years and 7 months) with the MR children. No significant difference appeared between the two groups of subjects concerning the rank order of sentence difficulty. The error analysis indicated that the difficulty in comprehension resided more in sentence structural complexity than in sentence length per se. Another work on sentence comprehension, also using pictures, was conducted by Semmel and Dooley (1971). These researchers tested 40 DS children aged CA 6–14 years. The children correctly comprehended simple active declarative affirmative sentences but negative sentences were correctly interpreted less often than would be expected by chance. Comprehension of passive declarative affirmative and negative sentences was at chance level.

More directly in line with Lenneberg's general position on language development is Lackner's work (1968). This author studied five MR children (MA range: 2 years and 3 months to 8 years and 10 months) diagnosed as suffering from congenital or early acquired encephalopathy. He compared their performance with that of five NR children (CA range: 2 years 8 months to 5 years 9 months). A random selection of 1000 sentences produced in free–play conversation was obtained from each child. Lackner (1968) observed that the development of syntax progressed through the gradual use of declarative sentences, interrogatives, passives and negative passive interrogatives tended to follow with increased CA in NR children and with increased MA in MR children. The MA level required for the production of the last type of sentence seemed to be within the range of 8 to 10 years. Simple declarative sentences were produced by NR and MR children with MAs of 2 or 3 years. Simple negative and interrogative sentences were also observed to occur at this level but less often. MR children as well as NR children could understand

and correctly imitate sentences constructed from their own vocabulary and corresponding to the sentence types appearing in their spontaneous speech, but they were usually not able to understand or imitate sentences of more advanced syntactic types.

Lovell and Bradbury (1967) initiated the experimental study of grammatical morphology with MR children using Berko's technique (Berko, 1958). This technique consists in presenting pictures illustrating meaningful or nonsensical words and asking the child to apply some morphological rules to the words, such as plural marking, e.g. 'Here is a wug. Here are two of them. They are ... (wugs)'. Lovell and Bradbury administered this task to 160 mildly mentally retarded children (CA range: 8 to 15 years, mean IQ 70). Comparing their results with Berko's original data obtained from NR children, they concluded that their older MR subjects (aged 14 and 15 years CA) performed more poorly on morphological marking with nonsensical words than NR children age 6. Newfield and Schlanger (1968) administered Berko's test to a group of 30 moderately and mildly MR children (CA range: 8–12 years, IQ range: 44–76 points) and to a group of NR children (CA range: 4–8 years) matched for MA with the MR children. For meaningful words, the order of acquisition of the allomorphs in the morphological constructions presented was virtually identical for the NR and MR children. However, MR children scored significantly lower than their MA–matched non-retarded peers with nonsensical items, demonstrating an inferior ability to generalize from familiar words to new items. Bartel (1970) administered pre– and post–tests of morphological usage and generalization following Berko's technique to 18 moderately and mildly MR children (CA range: 9 years 1 month to 11 years 8 months; MA range: 3 years 8 months to 8 years 5 months; IQ range: 33–77 points). Between pre– and post–test, a 6–week training period took place on half the test items. Results indicated that mildly as well as moderately MR children made equivalent gains on the non–trained part of Berko's test, suggesting that both types of MR children are able to generalize from language training (in this case, grammatical morphological training) and apply these morphemes to novel linguistic forms. Bartel's data are consistent with those of Bradbury and Lunzer (1972), who reported virtually no difference between mildly MR children (CA range: 9–10 years; mean MA 6 years) and NR children matched for MA on a task consisting in learning grammatical inflections on a modified version of Berko's test of morphological development. However, the MR children had a reduced capacity in a transfer task when items were presented only once. Lastly, Dever (1972) cautioned against generalizing from the MR children's performance on Berko's test to free speech. He tested a group of 30 mildly MR children (CA range: 8 years 9 months to 12 years 9 months; MA range: 6–9 years; IQ range: 60–74) on Berko's test and then analysed a sample of free speech obtained from each child. The correlation between the scores for bound grammatical morphemes with nonsense items and for corresponding forms in free speech did not differ significantly from zero. Real–word stimuli, though affording a somewhat better prediction of performance in free speech than nonsensical stimuli, still did not predict it very well.

2.5.2 Cloze–task procedures were used to study the lexico–syntactic abilities of mildly MR children and adolescents. Semmel, Barritt, and Bennet (1970) proposed a productive cloze–task to four groups of 20 subjects. Institutionalized MR subjects were matched with MR subjects from state-run schools on CA, IQ and sex (CA range: 10–14 years; IQ range: 60–80 points). A first group of NR subjects was matched on CA with the MR subjects, and a second group of NR children was matched on MA with the MR subjects. Institutionalized and state-run schools MR subjects demonstrated significantly lower performance as compared to the CA– and MA–matched groups of NR subjects. As noted by the authors, this observation suggests more than a simple lag in language development due to mental retardation.

Additional data were provided by Goodstein (1970) who administered two cloze–task procedures (production and recognition) to a group of 56 mildly MR subjects (mean CA 14 years 2 months; mean MA 9 years 5 months; mean IQ 67 points), matched on MA with a group of NR children. His findings confirmed those of Semmel et al. (1970) regarding the difficulty of verb deletion in productive cloze-tasks. This may reflect the restricted cohort of semantico–syntactically appropriate verbs from which the retarded child can draw in such tasks. However, selecting the appropriate verb fillers in recognition cloze tasks proved much easier for the mildly MR subjects, suggesting that they are not devoid of relevant semantical and syntactic knowledge.

In conclusion, the studies in the late 1960s and early 1970s opened the way to theory–dependent empirical work on the language of MR subjects. They were particularly concerned with morphosyntactic aspects of language behaviour.

New topics were addressed in the psycholinguisitics of the 1970s. They relate to the semantic basis of language (and its cognitive counterpart) and to pragmatics or the study of the interpersonal aspects of language use. In addition, theoretical considerations appeared regarding the learnability of language, together with attempts to map the language input and feedback received by the language–learning child, and a renewed interest in the innate basis of grammar development. These questions have also had an important impact on the study of language and language development in the retarded. We consider that the contemporary period in this domain, which will be fully analysed in the next chapters, begins in the 1970s with those studies influenced by the new orientations just listed.

2.6 Intervention studies

2.6.1 Fifty years ago, speech training with moderately and severely MR children was generally regarded as a waste of time (Backus, 1943). This point of view was accepted by many speech specialists until the late 1950s. Copeland and Schiefelbusch (1961) report that fewer than 5 per cent of MR children were receiving speech and language training in the United States. In a survey of the US state departments of education, at that time, ten states reported no speech and language therapy for MR subjects. When language rehabilitation really started, in the early 1960s or slightly earlier (Kolstoe, 1958), it was most often equated with articulatory training and lexical learning. The research emphasis ranged from the particular methodology used in articulatory improvement to the amount of time a programme should be administered (e.g. Schlanger, 1958; Harrison, 1959). There were attempts to extend speech training to classroom situations with the cooperation of school teachers (e.g. Freeman and Lukens, 1962) and to train mothers to aid in speech correction (e.g. Sommers and Shilling, 1959; Tufts and Holliday, 1959; Sommers, 1962; Carrier, 1970). Results indicated that MR children whose mothers were trained to assist in the correction of misarticulations made significantly greater progress than children whose mothers were not trained. This line of research was meant to meet the problem of generalization of the articulatory gains obtained in the speech clinics to family setting and other loci of activities. Brookshire (1967) defined generalization of therapeutic improvement from clinic to ordinary environment as a problem of stimulus control and claimed that correct responses should be trained in the environment in which they are expected to be used. Other researchers attempted to apply speech improvement programmes with the institutionalized mentally retarded and reported some success (Rittmanic, 1958; Shubert, Vanden Heuvel and Fulton, 1966).

No particular theorizing seems to have been involved at the time, except that articulatory training was based on available knowledge in articulatory and physiological phonetics as well as on general indications regarding phonological development; for example, the universal sequence of phoneme acquisition proposed by Jakobson (1941, 1968). Snyder–McLean and McLean (1987), referring to this period, speak of a traditional approach to articulatory remediation followed (if not completely superseded) by a distinctive feature approach. The traditional approach sought to identify errors in a child's phonemic repertoire by having the child produce a collection of words containing the various phonemes of the target language. Errors were classified by type (i.e. omission, substitution or distortion) and their extent was further specified (i.e. the words and phonemic contexts in which they typically occur). Therapeutic procedures included direct modelling, verbal instruction, tactile cues and manipulations by the therapist of movable elements of the articulatory apparatus (e.g. lips, tongue). The distinctive feature approach, derived from the distinctive feature theory of phonology proposed by Jakobson, Fant and Halle (1963), analyses sound production in terms of a set of distinctive features shared by the phonemes, which are correctly or incorrectly produced by the child (e.g. nasal, voiced). The implication of this model resided in the expectation that features learned in one sound should generalize and, therefore, not have to be retrained, to other sounds sharing the same features; an expectation that did not always materialize. Regarding lexical training, common sense and general indications as to word frequency in the target language and psychosemantic development, served as a basis for intervention work (Schiefelbusch, 1965). One exception was Smith's (1962) experimental language development programme for mildly MR children based on McCarthy and Kirk's experimental version of the ITPA (1961).

2.6.2 Things began to change towards the end of the 1950s and the early 1960s, with the affirmation of the paradigm of behaviour modification based on operant conditioning and its application to language intervention with MR individuals. Robinson and Robinson (1965) note that the number of studies of learning in which MR children were used as subjects increased dramatically. In view of this development, it is surprising that no coherent picture of the learning capacities and deficits of MR children emerged. The advances made towards understanding the learning behaviour of MR remained fragmented.

With operant conditioning, spontaneous behaviour is subjected to functional control through the manipulation of reinforcing conditions or contingencies of reinforcement (Skinner, 1938). The evidence from studies of this type suggests that the behaviour of MR subjects follows the same laws as other human subjects (see Ellis, Barnett and Pryer, 1960; Orlando and Bijou, 1960). Some differences linked to mental retardation exist, however. These are a longer time needed for conditioning and for extinction; more variability from one learning session to the next; and a greater difficulty in establishing secondary reinforcers (Girardeau, 1962).[3] Bijou and Baer (1961, 1965) have supplied a behaviouristic account of child development. Following Skinner (1957), they define 'verbal behaviour' as the class of vocal behaviour which is reinforced through the action of another person. They insist that the development of language has much in common with the development of other skills.

On this basis, it was possible to envisage language delay as inadequate development due to improper learning and establish remediation as a general procedure aimed at fostering specific language learning through the use of appropriate stimulus presentation and reinforcement

---

[3] Corresponding results have been reported with classical (i.e. Pavlovian) conditioning (see Lipman, 1963, for a review).

procedures. During the 1960s and the early 1970s, a number of experimental studies carried out with MR children and adolescents attempted to do just that. (For reviews of this literature, see Peterson, 1968; Sherman, 1971; Garcia and DeHaven, 1974.) Researchers in this line of work agreed that the development of functional speech in non-verbal or severely language delayed children was to be furthered in two phases of training. The first phase was directed towards the establishment of imitative verbal behaviours. The child was taught to reproduce a verbal stimulus presented by the therapist. In the second phase, the child was trained to produce functional speech (e.g. labelling objects appropriately, putting words together in sentence form, asking and answering questions) and encouraged to use it across a variety of settings. Operant procedures were used systematically to achieve these objectives. Language training programmes were consistent in stating how to do the training, the use of reinforcement, social or concrete, and modelling, shaping and fading techniques. For example, Hollis and Sherman (1967) demonstrated that the free vocalizations of institutionalized non-verbal profoundly MR children could be placed under the control of specific reinforcement schedules. The techniques consisted in shaping imitative vocal repertoires. Patients were given physical help to imitate responses demonstrated by models. The responses were reinforced. Physical prompts were faded and more accurate responses required until the sole demonstration was sufficient to produce the matching response. Some researchers begun with motor imitations before training vocal imitations, claiming that motor imitative skill facilitates vocal imitation. For instance, Baer, Peterson and Sherman (1967) first trained three non-verbal non-imitative severely MR children (CA range 9–12 years) to imitate hand movements before succeeding to train vocal imitations. Sloane, Johnston and Harris (1968) included mouth and tongue imitations among the motor responses trained before establishing vocal imitations in MR children who were initially non-verbal and non-imitative. However, other researchers who also reported success in remedial speech training, did not include the motor imitative component in their programmes. For example, Risley and Wolf (1967) established functional speech in echolalic autistic and MR children by directly training imitative vocalizations.

Vocal imitation training was usually followed by vocal labelling and by question–answer training procedures designed according to the same principles as the vocal training studies described above. An interesting concept was that of 'generative response class'. Such a class was defined as a group of responses that could be controlled by applying specific control procedures to some responses of that group only (Skinner, 1938; Risley, 1966). According to this concept, if a training procedure is successful in modifying given members of such a class, all members of the same response class should be affected without further training. The problem is to identify correctly the assumed generative response classes. Grammatical morphological and syntactic subclasses of elements seemed, without further theoretical elaboration from those researchers, to supply the appropriate candidate categories for the status of generative response classes.

Guess et al., (1968) claimed to have established generative use of the plural morpheme in the vocal repertoire of a severely MR girl (CA 10 years) who, prior to training, showed no signs of plural usage. They reinforced the girl for imitating the therapist verbally labelling single objects or pairs of objects. The subject ended up correctly labelling new objects in plural form. Guess (1969) trained two moderately MR adolescents (CAs 13 years 10 months and 13 years 8 months, respectively; IQs 40 and 47, respectively; both, MAs 4 years 5 months) in order to understand the use of plurals. This was done by pointing to the single or paired objects. The subjects were then encouraged to use plurals in expressive speech. Neither subject spontaneously generalized from receptive training to expressive plurals. Sailor (1971) reported successful training of plural allomorphs in two moderately and severely MR children (CAs 8 years and 15 years, respectively; IQs 51 and 36 points, respectively). Guess and Baer (1973a) also reported successful teaching of four severely MR children to use appropriate pluralization rules on nouns, by concurrently training expressive and receptive language. Other experimental studies reported the successful generative training of other grammatical aspects of language with MR subjects. These included converting action verbs into nouns (Guess and Baer, 1973b), adjectival inflections (Baer and Guess, 1971), verb inflections (Schumaker and Sherman, 1970), sentence 'form' (Wheeler and Sulzer, 1970), production of strings of words corresponding to basic grammatical relations (Stremel, 1972), syntactic usage (i.e. responding to a question asked by the therapist when a picture was presented) (Garcia, Guess, and Byrnes, 1973), sentence answers to three forms of WH–questions involving changes in verbs inflections (Clark and Sherman, 1975), sentence usage (i.e. producing sentences with correct subject–verb agreement to describe pictures) (Lutzker and Sherman, 1974), and so–called conversational speech (i.e. sequences of three chained verbal responses associated with the display of a picture and prompted by questions asked by the experimenter related to that picture) (Garcia, 1974). Guess and Baer (1973a) have supplied a review of some the above experimental studies.

2.6.3 It could have seemed at the time that an efficient remediative technology had been implemented with regard to speech and language training in MR subjects. In fact, this conditioning technology raised many theoretical and practical questions which were never properly answered. This situation led to its being progressively abandoned. A discussion of some of the problems associated with operant conditioning technology as applied to language remediation now follows. These problems concern the claim by language conditioners that generative language had been established, the issue of generalization, the non-developmental way in which language remediation was conceived of and the fundamental concepts of language adhered to by the proponents of the operant approach.

Assuming 'something like true language' had been established through the use of the experimental procedures described in the preceding pages, one of the major problems concerns the generalization of the improvement brought about by training outside the training setting. Spontaneous generalization of linguistic structures from experimental setting to non-training environments has never been clearly demonstrated, although diverse attempts to improve this aspect of the conditioning approach were made (Stokes and Baer, 1977). Attempts at extending speech and language training effects into the individual's daily environments have been reported. For example, Guess et al. (1970) and Guess, Smith and Ensminger (1971) analysed the role of non-professionals (e.g. two psychiatric aides in an institution for severely MR children); Wheeler (1972) trained institution attendants to build a verbal repertoire in a profoundly MR adolescent; Garcia and Batista–Wallace (1977) taught parents to assist in teaching speech to normal toddlers using the operant technology. The feasibility of conducting speech conditioning within a preschool classroom was assessed by Appelman, Allen and Turner (1975). These authors also examined the process of transfer of learned verbalizations from training sessions to classroom free–time. It is not known that these generalization procedures met with marked success. Certainly, they have not been adequately generalized to the contexts of home, school, ward or the wider society.

There are several reasons for this unsatisfactory situation. Individual differences in generalization have been acknowledged but not explained (Guess and Baer, 1973b). Most importantly, the correct application of operant technology may be particularly difficult to set up properly in social, professional and/or familial contexts. Additionally, the extreme rigidity, at times the harshness, characteristic of operant methodology, coupled with the sort of 'conceptual imperialism' (Hogg, 1975) exhibited by many operant researchers, did not facilitate the diffusion and the application of these practices beyond a limited number of experimental 'sanctuaries'.

Also seriously in question is the claim of operant researchers to have established in their subjects generative use of a series of grammatical devices through the application of modelling–imitation–feedback procedures. The use of the word generative with reference to this work may be misleading. The term does not correspond to the meaning of 'generate' or 'generative' in linguistics (where the objective is to explain the realization of a linguistic form from underlying linguistic representations: Chomsky, 1984). It probably corresponds to the more general sense of 'bringing into existence, producing' (*Concise Oxford Dictionary of Current English*, 1964). What the operant researchers meant by their concept of 'generative response class' (Risley, 1966) was something akin to the notion of productivity in developmental psycholinguistics. This is seen as the systematic application of a rule, or rule–like mechanism, to a class of linguistic structures in obligatory contexts. Nowhere in the learning literature reviewed does one find a clear demonstration that the operant responses taught to MR children spontaneously applied across entire response classes defined in linguistic terms, and, therefore, that they reflected genuine productive mechanisms.

What is observed repeatedly across the training procedures is the gradual conditioning of specific response items, for example, adding the –*er* morpheme to a limited number of action verb stems presented by the experimenter together with a picture illustrating the action referred to (in Baer and Guess's training study, 1971), or adding the plural morpheme to a limited series of nouns in response to the question 'What do you see?' when presented with pairs of familiar objects (in Guess et al.'s experiment, 1968). Other examples include marking past and third–person singular forms on action verbs in response to verbal requests of the type 'Now the man is painting. Yesterday he ...?' presented with corresponding pictures (in Schumaker and Sherman's training study, 1970); gradually adding sentence components, i.e. subject, auxiliary and present participle of action verbs, to form sentences describing pictures presented to the subjects (in Lutzker and Sherman's study, 1974). A related question (Yule and Berger, 1972) is, does operant training concern better speech, language, or both? Critics (Weiss and Born, 1967) maintain that only speech was taught. Specific verbal forms were taught, but there was no demonstration of any true generative or productive capacity.

2.6.4 The discussion above brings us to perhaps the major problem with the conditioning/learning approach to language remediation. This is the very notion of language advocated by the proponents of this orientation. Behaviourists viewed language acquisition as

> an essentially linear process starting from a primitive form of behavioral control involving tangible reinforcement through a succession of approximations involving major shifts in the topography (i.e. the external form) of the responses, the antecedent controlling stimuli, and the subsequent reinforcing stimuli, until the behavior has the form and emission pattern that typifies adult verbal behavior in a particular language community.
>
> *(Lynch and Bricker, 1972, p. 14)*

The modern study of language dismisses every one of these notions as false, or void of non-trivial content. Contemporary linguistics has clearly established that language production and understanding is only linear in appearance. Language organization actually is hierarchical. This is particularly obvious at the syntactic level (Bickerton, 1984). Further, language has been demonstrated to involve specific processes, making it a particular system of mind evolved through natural selection (Pinker and Bloom, 1990) and unique to humans (Pinker, 1993). This establishes language as qualitatively distinct from animal communication, pre– or para–speech symbolic expression in humans (including gestural expression; see Petitto, 1987, for a discussion), and, therefore, unrelated to anything starting from a primitive form of behavioural control involving major shifts in the topography of responses, as specified in the behaviouristic definition.

The notion of language 'response', language 'antecedent controlling stimulus' and 'subsequent reinforcing stimulus', as implied in Lynch and Bricker's definition, and basic to every behaviouristic account of language and language acquisition (from Skinner, 1957, to Staats, 1971, 1975) is not without problems, and these have never been openly examined in the learning tradition. Chomsky (1957b) stressed that when labels such as 'response, stimulus, or reinforcement' are used with reference to language, they lose any precise operational meaning which they may have in the context of describing simple conditioning events. Furthermore, Chomsky repeatedly claimed that there is no demonstration, and actually no good reason to expect, that language is controlled, shaped or elicited, in any strict sense, by particular environmental events. Within the behaviouristic tradition, it has actually been demonstrated that no reinforcement was necessary for the acquisition of linguistic forms (see Ribes, 1977, 1979, for data and discussions). It can be noted also that in the tradition of observational learning (Bandura, 1976), the problem of the explanatory status of reinforcing stimuli is largely eschewed in appealing to the notion of self–reinforcement, a notion in clear danger of circularity. It is our belief that some of the practical limitations of the conditioning methodology as applied to language remediation have much to do with a misplaced confidence in pseudo–explanatory concepts, such as controlling stimulus, response and reinforcing stimulus, when applied to language acquisition and disorders.

A recurrent problem in the learning tradition is the forceful refusal to take into account language structures (see Skinner, 1957, for the boldest claims in this respect), or their assimilation to simple linear associative devices dealt with by appealing to conditioned dependencies (e.g. Staats, 1971, 1976). Chomsky (1957b) has demonstrated that Markovian processes or other simple linear devices cannot, in principle, account for the structural characteristics of human languages. Lynch and Bricker (1972) suggested that linguistic theory and operant procedures might be used in a complementary manner to improve language training programmes for the mentally retarded. They proposed that linguistic theory could specify the content of instruction while the behaviouristic approach would take care of the instructional procedures to teach that content efficiently. However, besides attracting the operant conditioners' attention to the formal properties of language, Lynch and Bricker's position paper achieved little that was concrete. There are two reasons for this. First, the paper contained no suggestion on how the two orientations could be integrated. Second, you can only integrate things that can be integrated. It is not clear how conceptions of language as divergent as the operant and the generative could be meaningfully integrated. The problems with the operant approach to language acquisition, use and remediation were more serious than Lynch and Bricker (1972) anticipated. These caveats eventually proved fatal to the operant approach.

A last criticism of the learning approach to language remediation with MR subjects to be considered regards its *non-developmental character*. Nowhere within this orientation are the normal sequences of development taken into consideration when designing remediative interventions. Prerequisites for the acquisition of specific linguistic forms or structures were not systematically verified or taught before training took place. Nor was this viewed as necessary, the assumption being that linguistic forms were not organized in the mind in any systemic way, according to complex mental networks, but, on the contrary, depended entirely on external events, those claimed to be controlled through the conditioning procedure. Of course, nothing requires that language remediation should completely recapitulate normal language development. Prosthetic devices may be useful while differing from natural functioning. However, one may think that a non-developmental conception of language intervention is less than optimal. More recent approaches to language remediation with MR children insist on the developmental perspective.

Contemporary language intervention programmes are not only developmental in their conception, they also have a number of other definitional characteristics. These include early start, linguistic base, interactive and true communicative character, and being carried over for younger children with reference to the familial setting. At times, they involve multicommunication channels. They are closely related to the emergence of semantic functions and to the child's cognitive level and evolution. They are not divorced from the pragmatic dimension of language. Particular programmes, of course, may or may not exploit all these possibilities. The evolution towards this state of affairs is traced in Schiefelbusch (1974) and Schiefelbusch and Lloyd (1974).

Chapter 3
IQ, Sex, Social Class, Syndrome Considerations and the Question of Specificity

3.1 IQ, levels of mental retardation and language

3.1.1 The Classification Manual of the American Association on Mental Retardation (Grossman, 1983) suggests four psychometric levels of mental retardation following the major scales of intellectual development (Table 3.1).[1]

Table 3.1 IQ ranges and levels of mental retardation (after the Classification Manual of the AAMR, Grossman, 1983)

MR level	IQ range
Mild	50–55 to approximately 70
Moderate	35–40 to 50–55
Severe	20–25 to 35–40
Profound	Below 20 or 25

According to the Classification Manual, mental retardation refers to 'significantly subaverage intellectual functioning *resulting in or associated with concurrent impairments in adaptive behavior* (and manifested during the developmental period' (p. 11). By 'significantly subaverage intellectual functioning', an IQ of 70 or below on standardized measures of intelligence is implied. It is customary to consider that

[1] In the latest AAMR manual to date (Luckasson et al., 1992), the classification by IQ ranges and levels of mental retardation (i.e. mild, moderate, severe, profound), reproduced in Table 3.1 here, has disappeared. Also, in Luckasson et al.'s manual, *significantly subaverage intellectual functioning* is defined as an IQ score of approximately 70–75 or below vs 70 or below in Grossman's (see text). Luckasson et al.'s increased IQ cut-off, as well as their forsaking of the MR levels of intellectual functioning, have been sharply criticized (e.g. MacMillan, Gresham & Siperstein, 1993; Jacobson & Mulick, 1993; see also Reiss's (1994) reply to some of these criticisms). In the present work, we will keep with the widely accepted definition of mental retardation proposed by Grossman (1983) and with the usual levels of MR, because these levels have demonstrated descriptive, concurrent and predictive validity, and correspond to genuine *quantitative* differences in characteristics between forms of mental retardation.

the standard error of measurement is approximately 3 points on the WISC (Wechsler Intelligence Scale for Children) and 4 points on the Stanford-Binet. Hence, an IQ of 70 may be considered to represent a zone of about 66–74 (i.e., a confidence interval with a 0.66 probability of containing the correct IQ) or 62–78 (0.95 probability) (Grossman, 1983). Impairments in adaptive behaviour are defined as 'significant limitations in an individual's effectiveness in meeting the standards of maturation, learning, personal independence and/or social responsibility that are expected for his or her age level and cultural group, (p. 11).

The validity of the adaptive behaviour component of the AAMR definition has been criticized. For example, Zigler and Hodapp (1986) remarked that there are non-retarded individuals with adaptive behaviour problems and mentally retarded individuals who can satisfactorily adapt to the various demands of everyday living. This is certainly correct. In the second of the above two situations (i.e. individuals with retarded intellectual functioning but non-retarded adaptive behaviour), the AAMR suggests not retaining the label mental retardation (Grossman, 1983, p. 12), which is questionable – at least, cognitively. Why not simply talk of cognitively retarded individuals with no adaptation problem? It can certainly be argued that social adaptation is no more intrinsic to mental retardation than to intellectual normality.

Developmental period is defined as the period of time between conception and the 18th birthday. It is generally estimated that MR subjects defined in this way constitute between 1 and 2 per cent of the general population (Rosenberg and Abbeduto, 1993). The per-centage figure varies slightly depending on the surveys, the criteria used and the particular age spans on which the prevalence statistics are computed. Although the preceding characterization of mental retardation is not without its detractors, it enjoys considerable acceptance, and this is the scheme that we are using in this book for classificatory purpose. This use should not be taken to mean that we share the view that standardized intelligence tests (even associated or combined with Piagetian measures) 'tell the whole story' regarding the intellectual capacities and achievement potential of people with MR. This is not the case. Traditional intelligence tests have been criticized on the ground that they assess too narrow a range of mental abilities (Sternberg, 1988a). Piagetian assessments are also questionable as indices of intellectual functioning because they are based on the premise that intelligence, at its core, is a logicomathematical trait cutting across performance on a variety of tasks (Piaget, 1968). We will not enter into a discussion of human intelligence theories for lack of space and because this is not the topic of this book. It will be enough to recall that some theorists have adopted the view of a hierarchical representation of intelligence combining general abilities and more specific ones (see Vernon, 1971). See Zigler and Hodapp (1986) for a discussion of these theories in relation to mental retardation. Sternberg (1988b) has proposed a theory of human intelligence stressing the importance of three kinds of component: (1) metacomponents or *higher order* processes controlling the planning, monitoring and evaluation of performance in a task; (2) performance components or *lower order* processes used to execute various strategies in a task performance; and (3) knowledge acquisition components involved in learning new information and storing it in the memory. We know of no application of Sternberg's triarchic scheme to mental retardation. Traditional psychometric (hierarchical or not), Piagetian or Sternbergian accounts of the structure of intelligence are still examples of 'horizontal faculties' in the sense of Fodor (1983), that is general purpose mechanisms. This is less so in the factorial tradition which followed Spearman (1904, 1927); see, for example, Thurstone (1938) and the eight primary mental abilities that he identified. Should full modular theories of mind come to prevail, i.e. views of the mind as composed of sets of cohesive, special-purpose algorithms devoted to particular tasks (Pinker, 1993), the above-mentioned accounts of intelligence would have to be revised. Modular accounts of intelligence may be more in agreement with proponents of conceptions of mental retardation as being fundamentally a disorder of specific cognitive processes (e.g. Ellis and Cavalier, 1982) as opposed to holistic conceptions such as those of Piaget or Zigler.

3.1.2 As discussed, estimates of the prevalence of mental retardation fall at about 1.5 per cent of the general population. This is a relatively high prevalence for a chronic condition. In the United States it represents over 3 million people (Jacobson and Mulick, 1993). Mildly MR people constitute approximately 85 per cent of the MR population (DSM-III-R, 1989); moderate mental retardation represents about 10 per cent; approximately 3 per cent of the MR population fall in the severe range, and profoundly MR individuals constitute about 2 per cent of the MR population.

Down's syndrome is estimated to be the aetiology of about 30 per cent of the moderately and severely MR subjects (Clarke, Clarke and Berg, 1985). The incidence of this condition is estimated by Dolk et al. (1990) to be 1/750 lifebirths in both sexes, with an apparent reduction in some countries, for instance, down from 1/616 to 1/917 lifebirths in the Liverpool and Bootle areas of England, between 1961 and 1979. This reduction was explained by the fall in mean maternal age (Owens, et al., 1983). A similar trend was reported in Spain (Martinez-Frias, 1992). These prevalence figures may have to be modified further in the future as induced abortions following early prenatal diagnosis of chromosomal anomaly increase, particularly for DS cases with maternal age 35 and over (Cuckle, Wald and Lindenbaum, 1984; Dolk et al., 1990).

This issue is a complex one, however. According to other analyses in a number of countries (e.g. Nicholson and Alberman, 1982; Goodwin and

Huether, 1987; Malone, 1988; Bell, Pearn and Firman, 1989), the combination of age structure, current age-specific fertility rates, joint use of maternal serum alpha feto-protein, free oestriol and chorionic gonadotrophin (i.e. the most efficient maternal screening procedure with dried blood samples and non-radioactive methods; see Verloes et al., 1995), would lead to DS livebirth prevalence still close to 1/1000 for the year 2000 and beyond. This projection assumes a 60 per cent utilization of the screening policy, which is not a particularly conservative estimate, and people's desire for such screening and termination of pregnancy, which is not without controversy, as is known. The prevalence figure for DS given above, coupled with the markedly increased survival rates and life expectancy for people with DS, led Nicholson and Alberman (1982) to predict that in the twenty-first century the prevalence of DS will actually be higher. Likewise, Steele and Stratford (1995), using two projection methods (the prevalence-based projection which involves applying age-specific prevalence rates to population projections in 5-year age bands, and the incidence- and mortality-based projection method), report no indication of a marked reduction in the future DS population in the United Kingdom from a current level which they estimate to be 6.7 cases per 10 000 live births (i.e. 1/1493), representing approximately 30 000 affected individuals.

Conventional opinion may still have it that DS occurs more often in males than in females. This opinion may be based on the outcome of previous studies reporting higher institutional admission rates for DS males (e.g. Malzberg, 1953), which corresponded to a tendency to institutionalize more MR males and to institutionalize them earlier than females. Although the DS sex ratio at birth is roughly equivalent for both sexes and corresponds to the sex ratio in the general population (i.e. 51.57 per cent males), regional and temporal fluctuations may be observed. For example, Koulischer and Gillerot (1984; see also Koulischer and Gillerot, 1980) observed an 'excess' of DS males (56.41 per cent) in Wallonia (the French-speaking south Belgium region) between 1971 and 1974, whereas the opposite trend was noted between 1975 and 1978 (45.80 per cent DS males). From 1979 to 1981, the DS sex ratio in Wallonia (51.13 per cent males) approximated the ratio in the general population. The next largest aetiological group in mental retardation is the 'Fragile-X' group. Fragile-X is the aetiology of approximately 10 per cent of MR individuals. There are various estimates for this syndrome: 1/1350 in males and 1/2033 in females (Webb et al., 1986), 1/1250 in males and 1/1500 in females (Einfeld, 1993), or 1/750 to 1/1000 males and 1/500 to 1/750 females (Gustavson, Blomquist and Holgren, 1986; Sherman, 1992).

3.1.3 As analysed by Kanner (1964) and Foucault (1961) (see also Perron, 1969; Netchine 1969; and, more recently, Michelet and Woodill, 1993), most people in the seventeenth and eighteenth centuries, as well as in the Middle Ages and before, did not care to make social distinctions or deal specifically with delinquents, fools, hysterics, epileptics,[2] idiots, prostitutes, etc. These creatures were rejected with the same oppro- brium and confined in asylums and general hospitals. This confusion reflected not only a serious lack of knowledge but also the dominant ethical ideas of the times. Most people appeared to believe that such individuals were morally at fault and constituted a real danger to society. It was thought in some circles that such social calamities favoured each other in a certain way. Morel (1859) suggested a degeneration theory according to which, from generation to generation, laziness and minor delinquency unavoidably led to perversity, hysteria, epilepsy, and from there to dementia and deeper intellectual deterioration (feeble-minded- ness, imbecility and idiocy). An acute fear of large-scale degeneration (in the etymological sense) seems to have infected Western societies, partic- ularly in the second half of the nineteenth century and the first decades of the twentieth century. Lombroso, following Morel, insisted that a genetic basis to criminality exists. Langdon Down's (1887) belief that the clinical entity known today as trisomy 21 (Down's syndrome) actually involved a regression towards morphological characteristics of primitive races, such as that of the Mongols (hence the term Mongolism used for a long time to refer to trisomy 21), also belonged to the same preoccupa- tion with degeneration, mixed in this case with ethnical prejudice (also quite common in those times).

It took a good deal of the nineteenth century before there was an acceptance of a more specific definition of severe and profound mental retardation as distinct from dementia. The French physician Esquirol (1838) was among the first to suggest that mental retardation actually corresponded to a state of arrested development of the intellectual faculty, and that it was incurable. The first part of Esquirol's definition is still with us in some sense, but the contemporary position has rejected the idea that mental retardation is incurable. This sort of therapeutic nihilism (Zellweger, 1990) was shared by many physicians at the time (e.g. Down, 1866, 1887; Fraser and Mitchell, 1976) but not by Seguin (1846). Incidentally, it is interesting to note that Esquirol's pronounce- ment on incurability was already being contradicted at the very time it was expressed by the results of Itard's most remarkable educative work with Victor, 'the wild child from Aveyron' (see Itard, 1801, 1807; Kanner, 1960; Malson, 1964). In contrast to mental retardation, Esquirol (1838) claimed that dementia consisted in a regression from a prior normal intellectual state. He coined the term *idiocy* (from the Greek *idios* meaning private or particular) and proposed degrees of intellectual retardation. He suggested two categories along a continuum of mental underdevelopment: the imbeciles (from latin *imbecillus*, i.e. feeble,

---

[2] See Lebrun's interesting essay on 'The language of epilepsy' (1992).

lacking potency) and the idiots in the strict sense. In the following decades, particular clinical entities leading to mental retardation began to be identified. Esquirol (1838) himself seems to have been the first physician actually to describe what is now called Down's syndrome (also Seguin, 1846). But Langdon Down's (1866, 1887) subsequent clinical description of cases and regression hypothesis are better known. This clinical movement eventually led to the definition of the 60 or so general aetiological categories of mental retardation (Grossman, 1983).

Mildly MR individuals (sometimes labelled feeble-minded or morons; in French 'débiles': Zazzo, 1969) were not explicitly distinguished from non-retarded individuals until the beginning of the twentieth century. They were not dealt with separately from the latter during school age before the establishment of special schools for the mentally retarded in the course of the twentieth century (after World War II in many countries). In France, for instance, a law promulgating obligatory primary schooling for all children was passed in 1882. One of its side-effects was to bring in to school many mildly MR children who would not have attended previously or would have dropped out of school after a few years. This state of affairs led to the nationwide creation of classes and schools of 'perfectionnement' (improvement) for MR children, in 1909. This is the context in which Binet and Simon developed their first 'Echelle Métrique de l'Intelligence' (Metric Scale of Intelligence) (Binet and Simon, 1907, 1934; Binet, 1911). (See Vial (1990) for a well-documented analysis of the origins of special education in France and the particular role played by Binet in this development.)

3.1.4 Some more recent accounts have supported *the dichotomy between mild and other forms of mental retardation*. One of these theories is Zigler's two-group approach. In a number of publications, Zigler (1967, 1969 and 1973 for comprehensive summaries), distinguishes between so-called cultural-familial mentally retarded, with IQs between 50 and 70 points, and biomedical or organic MR subjects, with IQs below 50 points. The subnormality of the cultural-familial retarded is considered to be a reflection either of limited inherited capacities and the product of a large number of genes operating in a normal manner, or of adverse social and educational experiences characterizing the life of many children growing up in culturally disadvantaged homes, or a combination of both of the foregoing conditions. Familial retarded come predominantly from low socioeconomic families in which the incidence of retardation may be relatively high. In contrast, the subnormality of the organic retarded reflects genetic anomalies, infection, trauma, biochemical imbalances, etc.; in short, 'a genuine' pathological condition. If general intelligence, as measure by IQ tests, is normally distributed across the population, MR subjects in the first group may be viewed as psychometrically normal, in the sense of constituting an integral part of the distribution of IQs that is expected from the normal manifestation of the genetic pool. They are as integral a part of the normal distribution of IQs as the 2.2 per cent of the population considered as superior with reference to the WAIS, for example. MR individuals, in the second group, those with known neurophysiological defects, represent a distribution of intelligence with a mean that is considerably lower than that of the familial retarded.

A cornerstone in Zigler's formulation is the belief that mildly MR subjects are exempt from the neurological defects that characterize moderate, severe and profound mental retardation. We seriously question this axiom. There is no question that the neurological problems of moderately and severely (and profoundly) MR persons are more pervasive than those of mildly MR persons; but neurological problems the latter must have too. They suffer from brain underdevelopment and dysfunction (see Jellinger, 1972; Huttenlocher, 1975). The milder and more diffuse character of the brain problems in mildly MR subjects probably explains why neurological research still has to document these problems in detail. Current standard neurological examination cannot characterize many subtle forms of neurological dysfunction which are detectable by other methods (e.g. neuropsychological examination; see Lashley, 1930, on this question).

A sharp distinction between mild and other (organic) forms of mental retardation is basic to Zigler's cognitive-motivational theory, which he applied to the cultural-familial retarded (see below). According to this formulation, familial MR and NR individuals with similar MAs should perform similarly on cognitive tasks. This contention was a direct consequence of both Zigler's adhesion to a stage-conception (horizontal organization) of mental development and his faith in the validity of psychometric measures such as MA, as a correct reflection of the level of cognitive development.

On most, if not all cognitive tasks, however, MR subjects tend to score consistently lower than MA-matched normals. Zigler claims that it is of no explanatory value to say that the retarded do less well than MA-matched normals because they are less intelligent. This circularity can be avoided by attributing the performance differences between MR and NR individuals not to the global phenomenon of mental retardation per se, but to particular defects in MR subjects. In the past, as indicated in Chapter 2, theoretical proposals by Luria, O'Connor and Hermelin, Spitz, Ellis, and others, insisted that MR subjects suffer from particular defects (see Routh's (1973) edited book for a detailed presentation of these stands) 'over and above their slower general rate of cognitive development' (Zigler, 1967, p. 294).

Zigler offered his developmental position in opposition to these defect accounts of MR. According to Zigler, the remaining differences in cognitive performance between MA-matched NR and mildly MR subjects have to be attributed to motivational variables resulting from the retardeds' particular personal histories. The global formulation is to be understood as a cognitive-motivational theory. Zigler never contended that the distinctive aspect of mental retardation is motivational. Motivational variables are called upon to explain why mildly MR persons perform cognitively below the level that could be expected on a MA basis.

Zigler and associates now seem willing to abandon the restriction of the cognitive-motivational theory to mildly MR subjects and to extend their developmental perspective to moderately and severely MR subjects (see Hodapp, Burack and Zigler, 1990; Hodapp and Zigler, 1990; Hodapp and Zigler, 1995). This on the ground that studies demonstrate that the latter subjects progress in many domains in the same sequences as those of NR children (e.g. sensorimotor, cognitive functioning, conservation, space, time, moral judgement concepts, play, social abilities, communicative development) (for reviews, see Weisz and Zigler, 1979; Hill and McCune-Nicholich, 1981; Abbeduto and Rosenberg, 1987; Cicchetti and Mans-Wagener, 1987; and Cicchetti and Beeghly, 1990). Hodapp and Zigler (1990) insist, however, that 'The bulk of the evidence seems to suggest that Down's syndrome children, like other organically retarded groups, *do not possess a similar structure to their intelligence* as that found in nonretarded children of the same cognitive level (i.e. MA)' (p. 11, emphasis added).

This new position, amounting to something like conservative developmentalism in mental retardation, appears self-contradictory. It suggests applying the developmental perspective to moderately and severely MR subjects while at the same time refusing them a similar mental structure status. We wonder, on logical grounds, how MR subjects could pass through the same sequence of developmental steps as mildly MR and NR subjects, and yet construct fully idiosyncratic mental structures. Hodapp and Zigler (1990, 1995) propose the notions of 'local homologies of shared origin' and 'cross-domain relations' in attempts to explain the above contradiction. Borrowed from Bates et al. (1979) and Mundy, Seibert and Hogan (1984), the notion of local homology means that subsets of skills may be sustained by common underlying capacities and go together in development. Such a notion may have the advantage of justifying the existence of some sort of 'structures de groupement' (Piaget, 1968), while not resorting to the hypothesis of complete horizontal organizations in development. For example, the ability to use one object as a means to retrieve something else (e.g. using a stick as a rake) is structurally similar to using one person as a means to attain social effects. A single underlying scheme could be manifested by different behaviours. According to Hodapp and Zigler (1990, 1995; see also Hodapp, Burack and Zigler, 1990), local homologies of shared origin also apply to MR subjects including the organic ones. This could explain how these subjects demonstrate some degree of coherence in their development while not constructing structures similar to those of NR subjects and familial retarded.

The notion of local homologies, or further the idea that mental domains may be modular, that is, have individual structures and behaviours holding together within given systems, but various systems functionally separated one from another (an idea pervading much recent thinking in psychology), is appealing. However, such a notion does nothing to justify the paradoxical interpretation 'similar sequence–different structure' in the development of moderately and severely MR subjects. On the contrary, it would seem to us that the existence of local homologies, and possibly of a corresponding architecture of cognition and language in MR and NR people, is supportive of a similar mental structure hypothesis. Our position is that the empirical evidence favours the view that MR subjects develop through sequences of steps similar to normals. Also this is qualitatively the same development as NR subjects, which means constructing mental structures of the same kind as NR subjects, even if differences exist in the construction processes as well as in the resulting products (e.g. considerable underdevelopment, more primitive, incomplete or missing mental substructures).

Zigler's traditional view has been influential in motivating years of intensive research on cognitive development in mental retardation. While recognizing that the information gathered was still incomplete, Zigler (1973) claimed that his point of view had received empirical support. Our intention here is not to discuss Zigler's cognitive-motivational theory of mental retardation in itself, nor the data presented in support of this account (see Rondal, 1980a, for a critical analysis from a theoretical and an empirical point of view). We are using Zigler's traditional stand as a case in point illustrating the notion of a cognitive dichotomy between mildly MR individuals on the one hand, and moderately and severely (and profoundly) MR individuals on the other.

Other authors have classically entertained dichotomies between levels of mental retardation corresponding to that of Zigler, but for other reasons. Inhelder (1944, 1968) and Woodward (1959, 1963; Woodward and Stern, 1963) claimed that only mildly MR subjects reach the stage of concrete logical operations, as defined by Piaget. Lower IQ retarded are confined to preoperational stages. Abstract reasoning is out of reach of MR individuals (see Klein and Safford (1977) for a review of other studies relevant to this view). To the extent that Piaget's theory of cognitive development is a genuine stage theory (Flavell, 1963), therefore postulating major discontinuities in development, Inhelder's suggestion also amounts to dividing MR subjects into mildly retarded and others. Corresponding suggestions were made by Luria and the Russian defectologists (Luria, 1963) on the basis of vague considerations of the relative integrity of the central nervous system in non-organic retardates versus 'genuine' oligophrenes, the former being categorized as paedagogical retardates and assumed to be the exception in the Soviet Union at the time.

Theoretical points of view insisting on the *cognitive continuity* between categories of MR subjects have been proposed too. Milgram (1973), for example, stated:

> I am not convinced that aetiology in and of itself relates to behavioural differences or requires formulating different theories to account for the behaviour of retardates in aetiological categories. Aetiology may dictate, in some instances, the rate of retarded development and the severity of retardation that obtains at maturity without excluding the possibility – or desirability – of conceptualizing within one theory cognitive competence and performance and their relationships with other variables. (p. 171)

The same question as above may be asked more particularly for language development and functioning. Are there good reasons to postulate *qualitatively different* language organizations in mildly, moderately, severely and profoundly MR persons, respectively? Our belief is that there are *none*. We think that there is fundamental continuity in language at the various psychometric levels of mental retardation. Of course, the language problems of moderately and severely MR people are more pervasive and more important than those of mildly MR subjects, particularly in some areas (e.g. articulation, morpho-syntax, written language), but no profound dissociations are warranted in language functioning according to IQ levels. We would even venture the hypothesis that what profoundly MR subjects have left in language capacity, no matter how little this may be in absolute value, represents the very first steps in communicative and semiotic functioning.

3.2 Sex differences

3.2.1 The idea that girls enjoy linguistic abilities superior to boys is ancient and well spread. It seems to have found a basis in a limited number of descriptive studies conducted in the first half of the twentieth century. The results of these studies have been only partially confirmed in more recent years. Weiss (1925) reported higher frequencies of vocalization in NR female neonates in comparison with males. This observation was confirmed in babies aged 0–3 months by Lewis and Freedle (1973), but not in other studies (e.g. Rheingold, Gewirtz and Moss, 1967; Jones and Moss, 1971). It has been suggested that between approximately 1 and 3 years, at least, girls are more talkative than boys (e.g. Halverson and Waldrop, 1970; Brownell and Smith, 1973; Tauber, 1979). Other studies, however, failed to find significant differences in the amount of vocalizations or verbalizations produced by young girls and boys (e.g. Roberts and Black, 1972; Clarke-Stewart, 1973).

Young girls' syntax has sometimes been judged to be more advanced than boys' at corresponding CAs, particularly in early development (e.g. McCarthy, 1930; Young, 1941; see McCarthy, 1954, for a review). Fuchs-

Schachter et al. (1978) reported larger MLUs and upper bounds (i.e. length of longest utterance observed) in girls as compared to boys between 15 and 30 months-CA. However, Golinkoff and Ames (1979) did not confirm such a difference at 20 months-CA.

During school age, older studies generally tended to attribute slightly better reading abilities to girls (e.g. Benett, 1938). Dykstra and Tunney (1969) reported the existence of such a trend for children aged 6–7 years. But again, other studies failed to confirm a significant girls' advantage in learning to read (Parsley et al., 1963; Davis, 1967).

Numerous studies have dealt with the differential oral language capacity in school-aged children according to sex. Many studies used language tests (e.g. the verbal scale of the WISC, vocabulary tasks, verbal association tasks, tasks assessing verbal fluency, story comprehension, etc.). Maccoby and Jacklin (1974) have reviewed this literature. They conclude that there exist about as many studies finding no significant difference in language development between boys and girls as studies pointing towards a development advantage for girls. However, studies reporting a significant advantage in boys are relatively infrequent. It is interesting to add that the language differences according to the sex of the child seem to more marked (in favour of girls) at lower social class levels, attesting to a possible negative interaction between sex, social class and some aspects of language development, for example lexicon (Davis, 1937; Young, 1941). Reviewing these data, contemporary analysts (e.g. Reuchlin, 1979; Reuchlin and Bacher, 1989; Esperet, 1990) caution that the magnitude of individual differences according to sex should not be overrated. What emerges from the studies is simply a majority trend favouring girls.

Psychobiological explanations have been proposed for this trend. It has been suggested (Kimura, 1992; Hampson and Kimura, 1992; Crews, 1994) that the effects of sex hormones (oestrogens and androgens) on brain organization occur very early in life (during a critical period) leading to differential wiring of the brain in girls and boys; such differences rendering it impossible to evaluate the effects of experience independently of physiological predispositions. In other words, there may be definite sex differences in the physical structure of the human brain. Maturational influences are also involved. It is known that the male brain matures slightly slower than the female one, and also that the left hemisphere matures slower than the right one (Taylor, 1969; Scheibel, 1984). The left hemisphere controls speech and language in 96 per cent of right-handed individuals. The same is true of 70 per cent of left-handed people, while in 15 per cent of these individuals speech is controllled by the right hemisphere, and in the remaining 15 per cent control is bilateral (Bresson, 1991). The right hemisphere is more concerned with activities of a spatial nature. Estimates now suggest that approximately 10 per cent of the population is left-handed.

Men, on average, perform better than women on certain spatial tasks (e.g. object rotation and manipulation, mathematical reasoning, and navigating one's way through a route). Men are more accurate in tasks of target-directed motor skills (e.g. guiding or intercepting projectiles). Women, by contrast, tend to be better than men at rapidly identifying matching items, arithmetic calculation, as well as on certain precision manual tasks. Developmental language differences in favour of girls as well as the greater verbal fluency often reported for women may be other aspects of differential physiological predispositions (Kimura, 1992). Sex hormones can have lasting effects on the neural template. Such an influence affects particular abilities but has little influence on general IQ (almost by definition, as the IQs computed by the major scales of intellectual development are composite measures). This is consistent with the fact that there is no sex difference in the general population in global IQ.

Evidence from the menstrual cycle (when plasma concentrations of several hormones vary systematically) suggest that sex hormones might exert an activational influence on the brain and behaviour (Hampson and Kimura, 1992). For instance, in the studies conducted by Hampson (1990a, 1990b), significant variations in cognitive and motor performance were observed in women during the menstrual cycle suggesting that higher levels of oestrogen, and perhaps progesterone, can have a detrimental effect on spatial ability, an ability at which males typically excel. Conversely, higher levels of these hormones may be associated with better performance on certain tasks such as speech and speeded motor performance, at which women typically excel.

Sociorelational explanatory suggestions have been made regarding the verbal superiority of girls over boys. For example, Gunnar and Donahue (1980) proposed that female babies are more responsive to verbal stimulation than boys, hence an increase in the frequency of social contacts, vocal exchanges with the adults and a slightly better verbal development. Along the same lines, several studies have reported that mothers tend to address more questions, repeat more, and stimulate more their daughters' verbal productions (Clarke-Stewart, 1973; Lewis and Freedle, 1973; Maccoby and Jacklin, 1974; Cherry and Lewis, 1975). It is likely that the physiological predispositions favouring early language development in girls are what triggers mothers' and other adults' more stimulative verbal treatment of young girls.

To be added to this review is the well-established observation that some language disorders (e.g. congenital aphasia or lack of speech and language, acquired aphasia, stuttering and other speech defects) are more prevalent in men than in women (Ley, 1929; Azoy, 1935; Garai and Scheinfeld, 1968; Kramer, 1974; Taylor, 1974; Berko-Gleason, 1979). This has often been explained by pointing to the fact that speech and language seem to be statistically more bilaterally organized in females' brains (Hiscock and Decter, 1988; Geschwind and Galaburda, 1985). This puts them at a lesser risk in case something goes wrong with the left hemisphere. But there is more to it. The critical areas for speech and language are probably localized more anteriorily in women than in men (Kimura, 1992). Women, therefore, are more likely than men to suffer aphasia when the front part of the brain is damaged. Statistics show that restricted damage within one cerebral hemisphere more frequently affects the posterior than the anterior area in both men and women. This differential dependence may contribute to explain why women suffer acquired aphasia less often than men. According to Kimura (1992), a corresponding pattern exists for the control of hand movements, also programmed by the left hemisphere. Studies of apraxia (i.e. acquired difficulty in selecting appropriate hand movements) reveal that motor selection relies on anterior cortical systems in women and posterior systems in men. The proximity of women's anterior motor selection system to the motor cortex, located in the precentral gyrus in both men and women, may enhance fine motor skills, particularly manual ones. Conversely, men's posterior motor selection system, that is closer to the visual cortex, may facilitate motor skills involving movements directed towards external space.

The above summary makes it clear that sex differences in speech and language, as well as in a number of other domains, are under the control of genetically determined neurophysiological variables on which environmental influences may operate from early development. If this conclusion is correct, the same basic organization should be expected in MR individuals.

3.2.2 Published studies comparing MR males and females from a language point of view are rare. The relevant studies that we could locate (Roberts, 1967; Ogland, 1972; Evans, 1977; Wiegel-Crump, 1981; Shriberg and Widder, 1990; Rondal et al., 1981; Rondal and Lambert, 1983) reveal little significant sex variation in a long list of speech and language aspects in MR children, adolescents and adults (see Table 3.2). Parents' opinion sometimes has it to the contrary. For instance, the parents interviewed by Buckley and Sacks (1987) rated the speech of their DS adolescent boys more often as unintelligible to strangers than DS girls. One may signal also the report by Melyn and White (1973) indicating sex differences in speaking the first word (as well as in sitting, standing and walking), with females developing earlier than males (about 5 months in average value).

To be added to the above review is Stansfield's (1990) survey of 793 English-speaking moderately and severely MR adults (involving questionnaire, screening and assessment procedures). This survey shows more stuttering and cluttering in males than in females. But a rigorous comparison is impossible to make because there were more males included in the sample than females, and because the sex statistics that can be computed from Stansfield's data are in absolute rather than in proportional terms.

Table 3.2 Sex differences in the speech and language of mentally retarded children, adolescents and adults

Speech and language aspects	Studies						
	Roberts (1967)	Ogland (1972)	Evans (1977)	Shriberg and Widder (1990)	Wiegel-Crump (1981)	Rondal et al. (1981)	Rondal and Lambert (1983)
	100 mild MR children and adolescents (CA 9–14 years; MA 6–9 years; IQ 55–79 points)	182 mildly MR children (CA 6–12 years; IQ 50–69 points)	101 DS subjects – 48 females, 53 males (CA 8–31 years; MA 2 years 5 months–7 years 8 months)	40 non-institutionalized mildly and moderately MR adults, half females, half males (CA 20–50 years)	18 DS subjects (CA 2–7 years; MA 6–12 years)	24 French-speaking moderately MR adolescents, half females, half males (CA 12–18 years; IQ 35–55)	22 non-institutionalized French-speaking MR adults (DS and non-DS) (DS group: mean CA and IQ: 26, 45, respectively; non-DS group: 28, 46 respectively).
1. Articulatory test (designed after Templin, 1957)		—					
2. Dysfluency counts[1]			M>F				
3. Intelligibility score							
4. Rate of speech			—				
5. Loudness of speech				—			
6. Phonemic (natural) processes[2]				—			
7. Other (i.e. non-natural) deletions and substitutions[3]				—			
8. Allophonic modifications[4]				—			
9. Peabody Picture Vocabulary Test (PPVT)		M>F	—				
10. English Picture Vocabulary Test (EPVT; Brimer and Dunn, 1966)							

Table 3.2 Contd

Speech and language aspects	Studies						
	Roberts (1967)	Ogland (1972)	Evans (1977)	Shriberg and Widder (1990)	Wiegel-Crump (1981)	Rondal et al. (1981)	Rondal and Lambert (1983)
	100 mild MR children and adolescents (CA 9–14 years; MA 6–9 years; IQ 55–79 points)	182 mildly MR children (CA 6–12 years; IQ 50–69 points)	101 DS subjects – 48 females, 53 males (CA 8–31 years; MA 2 years 5 months–7 years 8 months)	40 non-institutionalized mildy and moderately MR adults, half females, half males (CA 20–50 years)	18 DS subjects (CA 2–7 years; MA 6–12 years)	24 French-speaking moderately MR adolescents, half females, half males (CA 12–18 years; IQ 35–55)	22 non-institutionalized French-speaking MR adults (DS and non-DS) (DS group: mean CA and IQ: 26, 45, respectively; non-DS group: 28, 46 respectively).
11. Type-token ratio (TTR)[5]							
12. Word understanding[6]							
13. ITPA global and subtest scores	M>F	M>F	Except in the Visual Motor Association subtest, where F>M			—	—
14. Noun proportion			—				
15. Verb proportion			—				
16. Proportions of other parts of speech			—				
17. Berko's test of grammatical morphology (Berko, 1958).		—					
18. Proportion of correct articles[7]						—	—
19. Proportion of correct verbal inflections[8]						—	—

Studies

Speech and language aspects	Roberts (1967)	Ogland (1972)	Evans (1977)	Shriberg and Widder (1990)	Wiegel-Crump (1981)	Rondal et al. (1981)	Rondal and Lambert (1983)
20. Correct marking of number and gender on noun phrase[9]							—
21. Proportion of correct pronouns[10]							—
22. Proportion of sentences[11]	—						—
23. Mean length of utterance (MLU)			—			—	—
24. Mean length of the ten longest utterances						—	—
25. Sentence structure score[12]			—				
26. Sentence complexity[13]						—	—
27. Syntactic usage on the Developmental Sentence Scoring (DSS) procedure (Lee, 1975).					—		
28. Proportion of information[14]						—	—
29. Proportion of new information[15]						—	—
30. Conversational continuity[16]							—

Notes: CA: chronological age; MA: mental age; IQ: intellectual quotient; DS: Down's syndrome; - : no significant sex difference; M > F: significant difference favouring males; F > M: significant difference favouring females; 1: repetitions, prolongations and broken speech (these measures of 'quality of speech' were derived from Johnson, Darley and Spriesterbach, 1963; and Beech and Fransella, 1968); 2: cluster reduction, liquid simplification, final consonant deletion, stopping, unstressed syllable, velar fronting, palatal fronting and assimilation; 3: singletons, clusters; 4: involving velopharynx, lip, stop release, juncture, stress-timing, tongue configuration, tongue position, larynx, strength, epenthetics/ties; 5: ratio of the number of different words (types) – all grammatical categories – to the number of words sampled (tokens); 6: Richards' Test of Understanding of the Spoken Word (Richards, 1967); 7: ratio of the number of correct articles to the total number of utterances; 8: ratio of the number of times a verb used was properly inflected to the total number of utterances; 9: ratio of the number of correct morphological markers for plurality (singular–plural) and for gender (masculine–feminine) on the noun phrases to the total number of utterances; 10: ratio of the number of correct personal and other pronouns to the total number of utterances; 11: ratio of the number of sentences to the total number of utterances; 12: obtained by the application of the Sentence Structure Test of Gulliford, Smith, and Philips (1971) to individual samples of 50 utterances recorded in a free-conversational dyadic situation, involving the MR subject and the investigator; 13: ratio of the number of compound verbs (e.g. *is going, have made*) plus subordinate clauses to the total number of utterances; 14: ratio of the quantity of information supplied verbally to the total number of utterances (by information is meant a complete relational meaning – i.e. a predicate with its obligatory arguments – in the sense of Chafe (1970)); 15: ratio of the quantity of information not previously stated in the conversation to the total quantity of information given verbally; 16: ratio of the number of times the MR individual correctly followed on the topic introduced or developed by the conversational partner.

Of passing interest is Evans' (1977) indication that no significant sex difference could be found between 48 DS females and 53 DS males, aged between 8 and 31 years-CA, on the Stanford-Binet Test of Intelligence (Terman and Merrill, 1960), as well as on the Harris–Goodenough Test of Mental Maturity (Harris, 1963). La Veck and La Veck (1977) found no significant difference in the mental quotients of 20 DS boys and 20 DS girls aged 12–36 months-CA on the Bayley Scales of Infant Development (but a significant difference existed between the motor quotients of DS boys and girls, favouring girls). Similarly, Gibson's studies (Gibson and Frank, 1961; Gibson, Pozsonyi and Zarfas, 1964) of institutional DS cases failed to expose any significant sex-IQ difference. Other studies, however, reported differences in modal intelligence between sexes, favouring females (e.g. Carr, 1970). One may recall that prevalence studies find more MR boys than girls. The exception is in Down's syndrome. This occurs regardless of time and place (Farber, 1968). The males constitute the majority of MR subjects at all IQ levels despite variations. Moreover MR males outnumber females about two times more at lower levels of intelligence than at higher levels. The only explanation advanced so far is in terms of a greater probability for recessive genotypes in males to affect brain development. This may have to do with the observation that at the population level the Gaussian curve for the IQs is slightly flatter for men than it is for women (meaning that the former are more represented at both ends of the distribution) (Terman, 1952; Piret, 1973; Larmat, 1979).

But, as analysed by Gibson (1981), estimates of modal intelligence in the sexes are difficult to interpret because there is seldom adequate control for CA and environment effects. Additionally, a number of caveats are potentially involved in issues that have not been properly dealt with so far. For example, the questions of possible differential mortality rates by sex, differential age stability of IQ for MR males and females, and possible differential variability of intellectual capacity by sex, have been little addressed. For DS, prevalence is higher among males up to adulthood. In subsequent age bands, the difference decreases and tends to vanish (Steele and Stratford, 1995). As there is no known difference in birth rate according to sex in DS, the above variations are consistent with increased mortality among young females (Forsman and Akesson, 1965) with male mortality taking the lead with advancing age as in the normal population. Regarding differential age stability for developmental measures, Carr (1970) reported that developmental quotients for DS infants constituted a larger range for DS girls than for DS boys.

Regarding language, and with the possible exceptions of dysfluencies and stuttering (the latter being more prevalent in MR males than in females, as it is in NR people), little difference exists according to sex. When there is a difference, for example on the PPVT and the ITPA in mildly MR subjects, it favours MR males over females.

Given the above indications, we see two possible explanations. First, it is conceivable that brain development being delayed and disturbed in several respects in MR subjects, the effects of sex hormones on brain organization occurring early in life, and thought by some to lead to differential brain wiring in NR people, are less pronounced in MR subjects. The consequence is that fewer and less important sex differences would be expected in MR than in NR subjects. Or, second, and not mutually exclusive of the first hypothesis, language is noticeably underdeveloped in MR subjects. This leaves less possibility for sex differences to appear. One should keep in mind, however, that sex differences in the language of NR children and adults do not concern basic structural dimensions but only particular aspects such as verbal fluency, length of utterance and lexical use.

3.3 Social class differences

3.3.1 Differences in language development and functioning according to social class have long been reported in NR subjects (see Rondal, 1978d, and Esperet, 1987, for reviews of this literature). A number of studies conducted in the midwest of the United States in the 1940s, and coordinated by researchers at the University of Chicago (Schulman and Havighurst, 1947; Eels et al., 1951) showed that social class differences between children and adolescents were most marked on the verbal subtests of the standard intelligence scales. Also quite noticeable differences were shown to exist, particularly between upper middle-class and lower working-class subjects, in verbal comprehension, word definition, verbal fluency, size of receptive vocabulary (estimations ranged from 45 600 words around 12 years for children in the upper middle class to 28 000 words in the lower working class), as well as in written language. Social class differences in receptive vocabulary and word definition, favouring middle-class children, were also reported by McCarthy (1952a, 1952b). More recent studies confirm and extend these findings (Wooster, 1970; Dowing, Ollila and Oliver, 1977). Other studies are suggestive of social class differences in favour of middle-class children, regarding morphosyntactic aspects of language: for example, morphological marking of number (Osser, Wang and Zaid, 1969; Parisi, 1971), imitation, production and comprehension of sentences (Nurss and Day, 1971) and comprehension of reversible passive sentences (Dewart, 1972). Social class differences going in the same direction have also been reported in children's oral text organization and free or elicited text recalls (Cession et al., 1987).

Some language-related social class differences may appear early in development. For example, Golden and Birns (1976) observed a greater ability to localize sounds as early as the first year of life in middle-class infants. According to these authors, middle-class children as a group tend to do significantly better on word imitation tasks than working-class children. Earlier, McCarthy (1930) reported a developmental advance of middle-class over working-class children in the production of two- and three-word utterances. Such variations in language development may have to do with differences in parent-child verbal interactions. Tulkin and Kagan (1972) reported similar frequencies for various maternal non-verbal behaviours to 10-month-old girls from contrasted social backgrounds, but the amount of verbal interaction between mothers and daughters was significantly lower in the lower social classes. These authors suggested that lower social-class mothers tend to underestimate the communicative capabilities of their young children. Clarke-Stewart (1973) also signalled less frequent verbal interactions in working-class families. Positive correlations were found in Clarke-Stewart's study between quantity of mothers' verbal stimulations of children aged between 9 and 17 months and the children's level of language development at 17 months. Several studies confirm the existence of a quantitative reduction in the language input addressed by lower social-class parents to their children (Cohen and Beckwith, 1976; Snow et al., 1976; Snow, 1977; Deblauw et al., 1979). The same general tendencies (see Rondal, 1985b, for a full analysis) are found in mother-child interactions across social classes. But differences exist regarding the syntactic and the pragmatic aspects of the speech to children. Lower social-class mothers tend to use more imperatives and to model out fewer deictics than middle-class mothers when addressing their language-learning children. They expand and repeat only half as many children's utterances as middle-class mothers. Such differences are not found invariably, however. Tizard and Hughes (1984) reported no evidence of social class differences in nursery-school-aged children interacting with their mothers or their teachers.

It is possible, therefore, that at least a part of the delays and differences usually reported in the language acquisition of lower-class children (none of them concerning basic structural aspects of the language system, however), finds its roots in parental interactive practices (see also Bernstein, 1975; Esperet, 1990). But this causal hypothesis could also be reversed. It could be considered that lower social-class parents actually adapt their language and interactive practices to an otherwise slower linguistic development demonstrated by their children (Rondal, 1978d, 1985b). If this is so, the primary source of the relative language delays in lower social-class children has to be looked for outside parental practices, perhaps in maturational aspects of development. It is known, in this respect, that a whole series of parameters (size, etc.) already differentiate *infants* according to social origin (see Reuchlin and Bacher, 1989; Tourrette, 1991, for reviews of this literature). The delays in prelinguistic and early linguistic development in lower social-class children could be another aspect of this evolution. These delays may contribute to setting the pace for quantitatively less stimulating environments for language development, which in turn slows down further development in these children.

3.3.2 Are these trends reflected in the MR population? Social class differences in intellectual development and functioning could be expected for nurtural reasons, such as the educational effects on the MR child of better educated parents. This seems indeed to be the case (see Gibson, 1981). Could there also be hereditary influences involved? From correlational studies of IQ between parents and their NR offsprings, some authors have proposed estimates of the heritability of (IQ or 'standard psychometric') intelligence varying between 0.45 and 0.80 (Vernon, 1979; Plomin and Defries, 1980). It could be (as Stickland, 1954, remarked) that pathological effects (including aberrant cytogenetic action in the genetic syndromes) responsible for the brain damage leading to mental retardation, might not entirely mask the familial transmission of intellectual characteristics. Gibson (1981) has reviewed a small number of studies relevant to the 'familial residuals' issue regarding intelligence in Down's syndrome. He concluded, unlike Gibson (1967), that there is no clear empirical indication that intelligence in DS depends, even in part, on heritable intellectual competency from the parents. Hodapp and Zigler (1990), however, propose another opinion. They state that the question of 'familial resemblance' in IQ between parents and their DS children is suggested even if (as they acknowledge) it is not clearly demonstrated. They review evidence from several studies (Fraser and Sadovnick, 1976; Golden and Pashayan, 1976) supporting their position. Fraser and Sadovnick (1976), for example, indicate that the distribution of IQ scores of DS children raised at home is similar in form to that of unaffected parents and siblings, and that the correlation of IQ scores between DS children and their parents or siblings is 'about where it would be in the absence of trisomy' (p. 181). However, in another study, Bennett, Sells and Brandt (1979) found no IQ difference between DS offsprings of parents with varying numbers of years of education (from 12 or less to more than 16 years). In spite of these findings, Hodapp and Zigler (1990) maintain that there is a probable familial resemblance between the intelligence level of DS children and their parents. Obviously, more research is needed on this question.

Social class comparisons in language development and functioning of MR subjects are very rare indeed. Ogland (1972) reported no significant difference as a function of socioeconomic status in a number of speech and language aspects (articulatory test, MLU, ITPA, PPVT and Berko's Test of grammatical morphology) with a sample of 182 mildly MR children (CA range 6–12 years). Similarly, Rondal et al. (1981) observed no significant difference on a variety of language aspects (the same list of lexical, morphosyntactic, and information aspects, as in Table 3.2) with a sample of 24 French-speaking adolescents from contrasted social classes (CA 12–18 years; IQ 35–55). These empirical data are only suggestive. Assuming, for the sake of discussion, that they reveal tendencies which will be confirmed in further work, what would be the proper interpretation? Given that the language input from parents to language-learning MR children is basically normal (see Chapter 5), it might be supposed that the same variations observed in the linguistic environment of NR children according to the social milieu (i.e. similar simplifying and adaptive parental modelling and feedback, but quantitatively reduced in lower social classes) also apply to MR children. A finding of no significant social class difference in language development of MR children might mean that the language ability of these children does not develop enough to incorporate variations pertaining to social class registers.

3.4 Syndrome considerations

Mental retardation has been, and still is sometimes, viewed as a nonspecific pervasive disorder resulting in general cognitive, linguistic and other deficits. Given the relatively high incidence of Down's syndrome and the long period of time since this syndrome was described scientifically, it is no surprise that it has served as the major reference for moderate and severe mental retardation. Between 1985 and 1990, Hodapp (in press, a) cites 73 behavioural studies published on Down's syndrome, compared to 40 on Fragile-X syndrome (see below for a definition), 7 on Prader-Willi syndrome, 8 on Rett syndrome, 5 on Williams syndrome (see below) and 3 on Turner syndrome.

The present work is no exception to this trend. In a sense, this is a natural move as data on the language associated with DS are much more numerous and systematic than the information available on other MR entities. However, there is no good reason to consider that DS is the prototypical entity for moderate and severe mental retardation. The delays and deficiencies in the language development of DS subjects probably have much in common with corresponding problems in other MR syndromes. The alternative hypothesis that the language problems of DS subjects are unique is untenable on the scant comparative basis available today. But there is no reason to believe that the language (and other) problems of DS people constitute precise templates for other categories of mental retardation, nor that mental retardation is a homogeneous category. It is possible to show that there are substantial syndrome differences in language development and functioning, resulting in uneven profiles, which may reflect varying mental and brain organizations. Such differences are interesting and may lead to a better understanding of the exact reasons why particular linguistic handicaps exist in the degree that they do in mental retardation. Genetic syndrome differences, when systematically compared and analysed, will illuminate some important aspects of the species-specific constraints on language development. This is good news for the fields of developmental language pathology and mental retardation. Indeed, many workers in these fields have tended to de-emphasize aetiology, favouring purely functional ways of describing affected individuals (Dykens, 1995). Instead of dismissing aetiology, researchers need to use it to promote advances in mental retardation.

The Manual on Classification of the American Association on Mental Retardation (1983 revision) lists approximately sixty aetiological entities of mental retardation regrouped into six major categories: *infections and intoxications, trauma or physical agent, metabolism or nutrition, gross brain disease-postnatal, unknown prenatal influence, chromosomal anomalies* and *other conditions originating in the perinatal period*. The number of known genetic causes of mental retardation has expanded dramatically in recent years. Dykens (1995) cites about 1000 causes, relatively few of these having received detailed phenotypic work. There is no a priori reason to believe that any one of these entities should yield symptoms of language disorders exactly similar to those of any other MR entity. This is an empirical question. An essential research task is to document the language problems of MR subjects in each aetiological category. Only on such an empirical basis will one be in a position to conceive of optimally suited therapies for MR subjects.

Besides DS, language problems of which will be analysed in Chapter 5, there exists an emerging knowledge of the language development in

MR children with other types of pathologies, particularly chromosomal anomalies. The remaining part of this section summarizes these data.

One of the first cross-aetiological studies of speech disorders was conducted by Blanchard (1964). She compared several MR aetiological groups for sequences of consonant development. Subjects were taken from the following groups: mild retardation, congenital cerebral defects, Down's syndrome, metabolic disorders, postnatal brain injury, asphyxia at birth, mechanical birth injury, prenatal infections, postnatal infections, and Rhesus (Rh) incompatibility. The total sample comprised 350 institutionalized subjects (222 males and 128 females), with CAs between 8 and 15 years, MAs between 17 months and 10 years, and IQs between 27 and 68 points. Articulation was measured by counting errors on an object-naming task. Misarticulations included sound omission and substitutions. Articulation status was poorest for the groups suffering from Down's syndrome, mechanical birth injury and, to a lesser extent, congenital cerebral defects and mild mental retardation. Blanchard (1964) concluded that speech disorders in mental retardation are associated as much with clinical category as with general physical and mental growth measures.

3.4.1 *Williams syndrome* (WS) also called *Beuren syndrome* and previously – particularly in Great Britain - *Infantile hypercalcemia*, has been the object of much research interest in recent years. This is a rare congenital metabolic disorder. Its occurrence is estimated to be 1 in 20 000 livebirths, with a higher prevalence in boys (63 per cent) than girls (37 per cent) (Vernant et al., 1980). However, Galaburda et al. (1994) indicate 1 in 50 000 livebirths with no sex variation. WS is characterized by a distinctive 'elfin-like' facial appearance, in some subjects a star-like pattern in the iris, medial eyebrow flare, depressed nasal bridge with anteverted nares, cardiac defects (e.g. supravalvular aortic stenosis, a narrowing of the aorta and/or pulmonary stenosis) in about 80 per cent of the cases, and infantile hypercalcaemia. Hyperacusis is frequent (94 per cent of the cases), together with normal threshold auditory acuity (Williams, Barrett-Boyes and Lowe, 1961; Beuren, Apitz and Harmjanz, 1962; Jones and Smith, 1975; Preus, 1984; Martin, Snodgrass and Cohen, 1984; Meyerson and Frank, 1987). Full-scale IQ may vary between approximately 40 and 70 points (Arnold, Yule and Martin, 1985). The exact aetiological mechanism is uncertain. It has been suggested that there is an underlying genetic disturbance in WS which results in the abnormal production of calcitonin and of calcitonin gene-related peptide. This peptide may play a role in the normal development and functioning of the central nervous system (see Bellugi et al., 1990; Jones, 1990; Bellugi et al., 1992). Molecular geneticists are pursuing identification of the chromosomal locus of this rare autosomal dominant disease (Morris, Thomas and Greenberg, in press). Recent reports (Ewart, Morris and Atkinson, 1993, quoted by Galaburda et al., 1994) suggest that WS is associated with hemizygous deletion, including the elastin locus at chromosome 7q11.23. This deletion is thought to involve several genes contiguous to the gene for elastin (e.g. the genes for laminin and for acetylcholinesterase).

Bennett, La Veck and Sells (1978), Bellugi et al. (1988) and Bellugi, Sabo and Vaid (1988) have suggested that individuals with WS present specific psychological and neuropsychological profiles. These profiles are characterized by marked dissociations between language and cognitive skills, severe spatial deficits and marked gross and fine motor problems. It is interesting to use the results of recent studies by Bellugi and her team at the Salk Institute, as well as complementary data, to illustrate a number of language differences (also mentioning non-language differences) between WS and DS individuals. Bellugi et al. (1990) made systematic comparisons of six WS and DS adolescents matched for CA and IQ. The mean CA of the WS group was 14 years 4 months with a range from 10 to 17 years. Mean full-scale IQ was 50.8 (SD 5.8). The mean CA of the DS (all regular trisomy 21) was 15 years 4 months with a range from 12 to 18 years. Mean full-scale IQ for this group was 48.8 (SD 8.7). WS diagnosis was independently confirmed by both medical and metabolic markers. Distinct profiling of the two groups of subjects was attempted from the comparison of results of a battery of language and visuospatial functions, a neurological examination and the results of neuroanatomical investigations involving magnetic resonance imaging. The six WS individuals were found to exhibit a fractionation of higher cortical functioning, with marked cognitive deficits but selective language preservation. At comparable levels of cognitive functioning, lexical and grammatical abilities were relatively spared in WS compared with DS adolescents. Responses of WS adolescents on the WISC-Vocabulary subtest as well as their production of unusual words in spontaneous speech, together with their ability to provide commentary responses upon request, showed a correct common understanding of those words (for example, given the word *non-toxic* in spontaneous speech, the comment 'It's non-toxic. That means it's not dangerous'). Such examples demonstrated that they had a better use and understanding of the words than CA- and IQ-matched DS subjects. This indication for WS subjects was confirmed on the Peabody Picture Vocabulary Test (PPVT). The scores of the six DS adolescents were at their MA equivalent (mean receptive vocabulary age 5 years 3 months, SD 1 year 5 months), whereas 5 of the 6 WS adolescents performed above MA expectation (mean receptive vocabulary age 8 years 4 months, SD 1 year 8 months). These findings indicate that referential lexical knowledge may be considerably better than MA expectation in WS.

On a test of *semantic fluency*, the WS and the DS groups also performed differently. The subjects were asked to generate as many examples as possible of given semantic categories (e.g. foods, animals) within 60 seconds. The WS adolescents produced significantly more words over trials (mean 26.8, SD 6.7) than the DS adolescents (mean 15.8, SD 3.9). The WS adolescents have less difficulty accessing and verbalizing members of given semantic categories than CA- and IQ-matched DS subjects. For some of the WS subjects, the number of words produced corresponded to the CA-norms (Semmel, Wiig, and Secord, 1980). This suggests near normal semantic categorial organization of the mental lexicon. Consistent with their observed tendency to produce unusual words in spontaneous speech, WS subjects frequently produced not just typical category members (e.g. *cat, dog* or *horse*, for animals) as did DS subjects, but also low-frequency, non-prototypical lexical category members (e.g. *brontosaurus, sealion, sabre-toothed tiger*). Such a capacity and 'taste' for correct use of unusual vocabulary is a curious facet of WS subjects' language. It may turn out, as Bellugi et al. (1990) suggest, that it is a feature that distinguishes their language performance from that of DS and possibly of other MR subjects. It may even separate them from matched normals (Bellugi, Wang and Jernigan, 1993, p. 32).

However, we are not eager to follow Bellugi and collaborators (1990, pp. 116–17) when they advocate a deviant rather than a delayed status for the lexical semantic abilities of their WS subjects (and, possibly, of WS subjects in general). It is better to speak of a preserved island of referential and semantic ability in the midst of a retarded general cognitive and conceptual functioning, corresponding to a sort of internal 'fractionability' of specific subcomponents within a given system of mind (see Marshall, 1984).

Syntactic abilities were also considered. Bellugi et al. (1990) have documented a clear difference between their WS and DS subjects' expressive language. The WS adolescents demonstrate larger MLUs and more complex noun and verb phrases than the DS subjects. Their spontaneous speech contain full passives, embedded relative clauses and conditionals, which are largely missing in the speech of DS adolescents. Unfortunately, Bellugi et al.'s (1990) report on this point is expeditious. They refer the reader to Bellugi et al. (1988) and to an unpublished abstract by Bellugi et al. (1987). The report of Bellugi et al. (1988) mentions only three WS adolescents (identified under the names of Van, Crystal and Ben). Their MLU in morphemes was estimated to be 8.6, 13.1 and 10, respectively. Bellugi et al. (1988) compared these measures with MLU data supplied by Gleitman (1983) for a group of three DS adolescents with MLU between 3.0 and 3.5, which is about or slightly below what should be expected for DS subjects in terms of MLU values at those ages (Rondal, 1985b; Fowler, 1988).

The WS and DS subjects' comprehension of linguistic structures was assessed using several grammatical probes including tests of semantically reversible passives, negation, conditionals, sentence completion, as well as correction of ungrammatical sentences. Many, but not all, of the six WS subjects performed better than the DS subjects who often performed at chance level or below (e.g. on reversible passives). Additionally, the WS adolescents were able to monitor sentences for grammatical correction and correct ungrammatical sentences, while the DS adolescents failed on these tasks. This suggests a superiority of meta- or epigrammatical functioning where epigrammatical functions include those activities belonging to the metalinguistic domain but not entailing a 'truly conscious' monitoring, such as creating tag questions, self-correction or error detection (Gombert, 1990).

Regarding prosody (intonation, stress and timing) and discursive ability (e.g. narration structuration and cohesion), preliminary studies (Reilly, Klima and Bellugi, 1991; Wang and Bellugi, 1993) indicate that WS adolescents have relative preservation of these skills. On a narration task, WS subjects were found to use prosody significantly more often than the DS group. The WS adolescents structured their narration much more cohesively than their DS counterparts. They were far more likely than the DS subjects to establish a clear orientation, state the problem correctly, introduce time and characters appropriately, and clarify the resolution.

Bellugi et al. (1988, 1990) did not assess the *pragmatic skills* of their subjects. There are other reports in the literature (admittedly, more anecdotal) concerning this aspect of the language of WS subjects. Arnold, Yule and Martin (1985), Frank (cited in Meyerson and Frank, 1987), Crisco, Dobbs and Mulhern (1988), Kelley (1990), and Udwin and Yule (undated) have reported weaknesses with pragmatic skills in the language and communication of WS children and adolescents. These include difficulties with conversational discourse skills, such as topic introduction, topic maintenance, turn taking and maintaining appropriate eye contact. WS individuals sometimes appear to be talking nonsense and will mimic others. Their speech may be socially inappropriate and repetitive, with irrelevant questions and much chattering in company ('cocktail party manners'). These limitations in the social area of language contrast with their strength in the lexical and morphosyntactic domains. Also, the expressive language skills of WS children and adolescents are reported to be superior to their verbal comprehension. They sometimes echo phrases and sentences spoken by the interlocutor, with limited understanding of what the person is saying. This echoing may be caused by poor comprehension (Udwin and Yule, undated). The articulation and fluency of most WS subjects is good, although occasional hoarse voice and hypernasality not associated with structural or functional velopharyngeal problems have been noted (Meyerson and Frank, 1987).

Returning to Bellugi et al. (1990), the comparison between WS and DS adolescents was extended to cover *non-verbal cognition*, particularly spatial cognition. Previous studies by Bellugi and her team (Bellugi et al., 1988; Bihrle et al., 1989) revealed marked spatial deficits in WS individuals. In Bellugi et al. (1990), the WS and the DS subjects were given a battery of probes of visuospatial, visuoconstructive and visuoperceptual tasks. The two groups performed equally poorly on a standardized visuoconstructive measure, the Developmental Test of Motor Integration (Beery and Buktenica, 1967). However, the WS subjects demonstrated a selective disability on items requiring integration of component parts (e.g. a triangle made out of circles). The same tendency to global processing of hierarchical visual stimuli was also apparent on a drawing task adapted from the Boston Diagnostic Aphasia Examination (Goodglass and Kaplan, 1972). Subjects were required to draw common objects, such as a bicycle. As a rule, the drawings of the DS children were simplified (exhibiting the usual DS problems in local analysis) but retained basic spatial organization and integration of parts. In contrast, the WS drawings lacked spatial organization and integration, and they were completely unrecognizable. Both WS and DS proved grossly impaired on a range of visuospatial tasks (block design, copying geometrical shapes, spatial transformations and line orientation using the Benton Line Orientation Test (Benton, Hannary and Varney 1975). Despite their severe spatial dysfunctions, the WS subjects (but not the DS subjects) demonstrated a surprisingly good ability to discriminate unfamiliar faces and recognize them under conditions of spatial transformation (using the Benton Test of Facial Recognition; Benton et al., 1983). Performance was at the level of normal 13-year-olds and the approached level of normal adults. Bellugi et al. (1990) suggested that preserved performance on a facial discrimination task in the context of generally impaired spatial cognition may be a unique neuropsychological marker of Williams syndrome. Interestingly, Bellugi et al. (1990), nor anyone else in the Williams syndrome literature (admittedly limited), have reported particular weaknesses in the spatial lexicon of the WS subjects related to their severe limitation in spatial cognition.

Bellugi et al.'s (1990) WS and DS subjects were given a *neurological examination*. Such studies offer an opportunity for linking brain findings to focal cognitive deficits. WS subjects demonstrated deficits including generalized hypotonia, tremor, midline balance problems and oral-motor and motoric abnormalities suggestive of cerebellar dysfunction. DS subjects showed minimal hypotonia, little evidence of cerebellar signs and better performance on oromotor functions. Neuroanatomical profiles from magnetic resonance imaging (MRI) were established. Both groups of WS and DS (compared to 14 normal controls aged 8–32 years; mean 19 years) demonstrated an equal degree of microcephaly, cerebral hypoplasia, reduced cerebral volume and decreased myelination, but overall brain shapes of each group proved distinct. The DS brains exhibited an important degree of hypofrontality whereas the WS subjects appeared to have relatively decreased posterior width with reduction in size of the forebrain posterior to the rolandic sulcus, i.e. the parietal, posterior temporal and occipital cortical regions, and narrowing of the corpus callosum anterior to the splenium. They exhibited elongated posterior to anterior length compared to normal brains. The characteristic of hypofrontality of neocortex in DS subjects together with an important reduction in frontal lobe projections from the corpus callosum was further attested in a magnetic resonance imagery study by Wang et al. (1992). These authors relate this neuroanatomical indication to a profile of frontal lobe dysfunction in DS corresponding to such deficits as poor verbal fluency, perseverative tendencies on various tasks and greater difficulty on tasks requiring flexible problem-solving strategies. DS subjects, however, seem to have relatively preserved basal ganglia and diencephalic structures. In contrast, WS subjects seem to have better frontal and temporal limbic structures (Jernigan, 1992; Wang, 1992; Jernigan et al., 1993). There is also evidence in WS of a dysregulation of the control of neuronal and glial numbers, as illustrated by increased cell packing density appearing at the cytoarchitectonic level (Galaburda et al., 1994). This may reflect an interference with naturally occurring cell death and the presence of neurotrophic factors (possibly linked to abnormal extracellular calcium levels).

Lastly, results of volume analyses suggest that the cerebellar volume in DS subjects is approximately 77 per cent of the equivalent volume in young normal controls, versus 99 per cent in WS subjects. This indication is surprising given the various signs of cerebellar dysfunction exhibited by WS subjects. Although cerebellar size is intact and neocerebellum largely preserved in WS (Wang, 1992), some other neurological findings are suggestive of cerebellar dysfunction, but, unlike in DS subjects, they occur without reduction in cerebellar volume. The posterior fossa structures of the 6 WS subjects and 2 DS subjects were further examined by Bellugi et al. (1990), leading to the identification in WS subject of an anomalous pattern, with neocerebellar vermal lobules showing hyperplasia in the context of low-normal paleocerebellar vermal development and significantly reduced forebrain size. Such an aberrant cerebrum/cerebellum volume ratio could serve to distinguish WS syndrome neurologically from other syndromes, such as DS or autism (Courchesne et al. 1988). Bellugi et al. (1990) speculate (following suggestions by Leiner, Leiner and Dow, 1986, on the possible role of human neocerebellar structures in mental and linguistic functions) that the observed hyperplasia of specific vermal lobules in the context of cerebral maldevelopment may be related to the specific language profile of WS subjects. A further study by Wang et al. (1992), using MRI with 11 WS subjects, 7 DS subjects, aged between 10 and 20 years (matched for CA, IQ and cerebral volume), and 18 normal controls (aged-matched with the WS and the DS subjects), confirmed that the neocerebellar tonsils of WS subjects are equal in size to control tonsils and larger than DS tonsils.

In summary, Bellugi et al.'s (1990) study reveals that the WS adolescents differ in their psychological, neurological and neuroanatomical profiles from DS adolescents matched for age and full-scale IQ. Additionally, the WS subjects demonstrate atypical characteristics distinct from the flatter profile (i.e. more homogeneous across the board of psychological functions) exhibited by DS subjects.

However, all WS individuals may not conform exactly to Bellugi et al.'s characterization of their six WS adolescents. There are observations suggesting that the language functioning of WS subjects may not always be as favourable as the picture suggested by Bellugi et al. (1990). For example, Kelley (1990) reports on a case of WS in a child, named John, aged 4 years and 8 months at the time of the observation, presenting a developmental age of 3 years 10 months on the PPVT-Revised, 3 years 8 months on the Expressive Word Picture Vocabulary Test (origin not identified), and 2 years 8 months on the Reynell Developmental Language Scales, Verbal Comprehension Scale A (Reynell, 1977). This points to language developmental ages well below his CA. His age levels on the ITPA subscales were also below his CA (2 years 6 months for Auditory Association – proposing sentences to be completed on an analogical basis; 3 years 7 months for Grammatical Closure – assessing knowledge of morphosyntactic regularities; and 3 years 6 months for Auditory Sequential Memory – repeating digits). John's MLU was 2.75 (Brown's stage III), which is below normal expectation (the expected range for this stage of language development is 24–41 months). Arnold, Yule and Martin (1985) signalled similar discrepancies between CA expectations and language developmental attainments. For example, on the Reynell Developmental Language Scales, 3 of their 23 WS subjects, aged between CA 7 and 12 years, exceeded the 7-year ceiling of the test, while the language skills of the remaining subjects ranged from 3 to 7 years. The mean group score was 5 years 9 months for expressive language and 5 years 5 months for verbal comprehension. Thal, Bates and Bellugi (1989) analysed the language of two young girls with WS (Becky: CA 5 years 6 months and Rachel: CA 23 months, at the date of testing). The two children had an MLU of 1.0 and were credited with 142 and 34 words in their productive lexicon, respectively. They understood 281 and 314 words, respectively, as reported by the parents. Comprehension (percentage correct on a picture identification task) was 66 per cent for Rachel and 32 per cent for Becky. Rachel's early language development seemed roughly similar to that of most NR children. Becky's language development was quite delayed. This latter case documents the possibility of a marked discrepancy between CA and language development in WS. It confirms the existence of a considerable variability in the language development of these subjects (Becky and Rachel were both at the one-word stage despite a 3-year CA gap). Thal et al. (1989) were not in a position to answer the question whether the two WS children would demonstrate the unusual skilled language compared to other areas of cognition by the time they reach adolescence. Nor does one find indications as to the language capacity of the WS adolescents studied by Bellugi et al. (1988 and 1990), when they were in their younger years.

A major problem for those studying Williams syndrome is to establish to what extent general psychological, and particularly psycholinguistic patterns, such as those illustrated by Bellugi et al. (1990), are truly representative of people with WS, and specify the range of individual variation within the syndrome.

But despite some likely interindividual intrasyndromic variation, WS individuals seem to present remarkable psychological, neurological and neuroanatomical profiles. Comparative studies of the type conducted by Bellugi et al. (1990) are well suited to illuminate the particular and common aspects of the various syndromes associated with mental retardation. Not every type of comparison is equally interesting, however. For example, Bennett, La Veck and Sells' (1978), and Crisco et al.'s (1988) comparisons of groups of children with WS and 'control' groups of children with *non-specific* developmental disabilities proved less informative. Similarly, MacDonald and Roy (1988) compared a group of WS children and a group of children referred for evaluation of developmental problems (unspecified except that children with obvious neuromuscular disorders or sensory impairment were excluded). They concluded that their results support the view that WS children suffer from a severe impairment in visual-motor integration. The use of a more narrowly defined control group could have helped to specify better the visual-motor impairment of the WS children. Regarding language skills (basically, PPVT scores and a Sentence Memory Test from Benton, 1965), MacDonald and Roy (1988) found no significant difference between the WS and their developmentally-delayed control subjects. But because the language profile and course of development of the latter subjects were not otherwise specified, the comparison was hardly instructive.

As indicated, a striking difference emerges from Bellugi et al.'s (1990) comparison of spatial cognitive and language functions in WS and DS subjects. The WS subjects' visuospatial construction is characterized by selective attention to details of the configuration at the expense of the whole whereas the DS subjects exhibit the opposite pattern (see Bihrle et al., 1989, for a discussion). The considerable impairment of DS subjects in analysis of local features as compared to global features points to problems related to the inferotemporal cortex (see Horel, 1994, for an analysis of the role of this area in local vs global perception). Conversely, the hypothesis of a preserved inferotemporal cortex in WS is compatible with the above indication that these subjects have good facial recognition, a function known to be associated with that part of the neocortex and its 'face neurons' (Perrett et al., 1988).

In the language domain, Bellugi et al.'s WS subjects demonstrate relatively preserved syntax and fairly advanced referential lexical abilities, whereas the DS subjects' language profiles, as expected, are 'flatter'. Bellugi et al. (1990) suggest that WS subjects are behaviourally grossly similar to unilateral right hemisphere-damaged (normal) adults whereas DS subjects are more like left hemisphere-damaged aphasics, demonstrating language impairment and a marked tendency to a global processing of the information. This is intriguing from a neuropsychological point of view given that in WS as well as in DS no focal brain damage is considered to exist. The curtailment of the dorsal parietal regions and posterior temporal areas of the brain in WS subjects, together with the thinning of the relevant portions of the corpus callosum, may be directly relevant to their visuo-spatial deficits (Galaburda et al., 1994), and indirectly perhaps to the dissociation between auditory-verbal (AV) and visuo-spatial (VS) short-term memory (STM). WS subjects indeed seem to have better preserved AV- than VS-STM, whereas the converse is true for many DS subjects (Wang and Bellugi, in press). Similarly, the relatively preserved size of the frontal lobes and most of the temporal lobes in WS is consistent with the relative preservation of formal linguistic capacity in many of these subjects.

According to Galaburda et al. (1994), several features of cortical architectonic differentiation in WS (e.g. increased cell packing density, horizontal disposition of neurons, immature vascular development, weak myelination) suggest arrest in neuronal development between the end of the second trimester and the second year of life. Incompleteness of neuronal development is suggested by a series of cytoarchitectonic features (e.g. incomplete connectivity reflected by the horizontal disposition of neurons as opposed to the normal columnar arrangement, migrational abnormalities illustrated by excessive numbers of subcortical neurons, anomalous layering of the cortex). It is interesting to signal that for Down's syndrome the estimated time of neuronal developmental arrest or marked slowing down is earlier, i.e. around birth (Nadel, 1986). It is tempting to speculate that this 6-month to 1-year difference in neural epigenesis is related to the better preservation of the formal organization of language in WS as opposed to DS. It does not relate to general level of cognitive development as this level is roughly similar in the two syndromes. This could constitute an indication that brain epigenetic development during the first six months or the first year affects the species-specific structures responsible for (later) grammatical development. Investigating fractionations of higher cortical functions in well-defined genetically based syndromes should shed light on the neural systems subserving language and cognitive functions.

Another interesting point to be discussed in relation to the data on WS subjects, concerns articulatory skills and speech fluency. According to Bellugi et al. (1990), the generalized hypotonia characteristic of children affected with WS is more pronounced than the one exhibited by young DS children. It is not uncommon to find in accounts of the marked articulatory problems of many DS subjects, generalized hypotonia advocated as one of the major causal factors (e.g. Zisk and Bialer, 1967). Judging from the data on generalized hypotonia and early oral-motor impairments combined with later normal or normal-like articulatory ability in WS subjects, it would seem that the 'hypotonia and motor-impairment' argument is not sufficient as an explanation for the articulation difficulties encountered by DS subjects.

Lastly, although they observed only older children, adolescents and adults with WS, Bellugi and collaborators (e.g. Bellugi, Wang, and Jernigan, 1993) suggest that the language of WS and DS subjects is equivalent at young ages. This suggestion is based on a preliminary study by Singer and Goodman (1992) with 30 WS and 30 DS children ranging from 12 to 55 months-CA. Communicative abilities were assessed through the Infant version of the MacArthur Communicative Development Inventory, parental reports, language production measures and communicative gestures. Results showed similar language trajectories in WS and DS children up to 55 months of age, with marked delays in the onset of vocabulary comprehension and production in both groups, falling far below the 10th per centile of NR infants. The results displayed by younger WS subjects, therefore, are in contrast with the phenotypes found in adolescents. Longitudinal studies should be conducted to define when, in what manner and why the linguistic abilities of WS subjects begin diverging from their cognitive underpinnings. As a rough preliminary to this longitudinal orientation, Galaburda et al. (1994) supply the clinical history of A.O., a male WS subject who died at 31 years of heart failure. He exhibited important delays regarding motor and cognitive milestones. As he developed, however, major characteristics of WS emerged, i.e. severe cognitive deficits with remarkable preservation of formal aspects of language.

3.4.2 The syndrome termed '*Fragile X*' (F-XS), an X-linked disorder (see Mulley et al., 1992, for a nomenclature of X-linked mental retardation), has also motivated a number of research works in recent years. Unlike DS, the genetic anomalies occuring in F-XS are passed on through generations. As such, F-XS is the most common *hereditary* cause of moderate and severe MR. Of particular interest is the demonstration in this syndrome of a direct link between molecular genetic pathology and symptoms of psychopathology. Yu et al. (1991) have described the molecular pathology of the gene responsible for the F-X syndrome. Hagerman (1992) has supplied a comprehensive account of genetics, physical phenotype, and a limited assessment of cognitive behavioural aspects in the F-X syndrome. Individuals with F-XS have a null mutation of the FMR-1 gene in which the levels of protein in mRNA (messenger ribonucleic acid) are greatly reduced. This is characterized at the DNA (desoxyribonucleic acid) level by an abnormal repetition of a trinucleotide sequence, either CCG (cytosine-cytosine-guanine) or CGG (cytosine-guanine-guanine). Normally, this is repeated about 30 times in mean value (range 6–54) at the site of the FMR-1 gene on the X chromosome (position q27). Individuals affected with F-XS have from 200 to more than 1000 trinucleotide sequence repeats. Such extreme amplifications of the sequence repeats are considered to constitute the full mutation at the Xq27 site. There seems to be a correlation between the length of the trinucleotide sequence and the severity of the clinical manifestations. In addition to the abnormal trinucleotide sequence repetitions, affected F-XS males have abnormalities in nearby regions called CpG 'islands', which are thought to play a role in gene regulation (see Oberlé et al., 1991). These islands are abnormally methylated in affected F-XS males (i.e. the DNA structure is the object of a chemical change that alters its activity). This corresponds to the loss of expression of the FMR-1 mRNA, ultimately leading to the null mutation seen in these subjects.

Although a common hereditary disorder, many cases of F-XS are not currently identified, making the exact prevalence of this disorder somewhat unclear (Warren, 1992). Unidentified cases are due, in part, to the genetic peculiarities of this syndrome. These peculiarities include a genetic vulnerability which is amplified as it is passed down through generations of families until it yields an individual who is fully affected with the F-XS. Recent estimates of the prevalence of F-XS in the general population suggest 0.73 to 0.92 per 1000 males (Herbst and Miller, 1980; Webb et al., 1986). Surveys of retarded populations indicate that F-XS may account for 2–7 per cent of all cases of mental retardation among males (Webb et al., 1986). Approximately one third of the females who carry and transmit Fragile-X are actually affected with a variant of the syndrome. They exhibit learning difficulties. Some are impaired with mild to moderate MR. The rest of the carrier females are unaffected, yet they may transmit the disorder to their children. The fact that one third or more of the carrier females of F-XS are affected with some degree of mental impairment is at variance with other X-linked disorders (such as haemophilia or colour-blindness). Most males are MR (from moderate to severe retardation; Chundley, 1984; Miezejeski et al., 1986). However, approximately one-fifth are of average intelligence. These latter males are called 'non-penetrant'. They necessarily transmit the X vulnerability to their daughters, who become carriers themselves (see Dykens, Hodapp and Leckman, 1994, and the references therein for more details). It could be that affected females receive the FMR-1 gene from their mothers. In contrast, carrier females who inherit the gene from their fathers are cognitively unaffected.

In humans, the FMR-1 gene is known to be expressed in a variety of tissues, with high levels in the brain and testes. This distribution corresponds to the salient features of affected F-XS males, i.e. mental retardation, slight enlargement of the head and marked enlargement of the testes (macro-orchidism), particularly in postpubertal males.

Klinefelter's syndrome (a genetic disorder found exclusively in males with an extra X chromosome, XXY) has been reported to co-occur in some very rare cases with F-XS (Pecile and Filippi, 1991). Klinefelter's syndrome is characterized by a tall stature, average intelligence (in a minority of cases, mild MR may exist) and small testes. When Klinefelter's syndrome co-occurs with F-XS, it seems that the subjects are more severely affected than when each pathological entity occurs alone. It could be that the Fragile-X mutation predisposes to the non-disjunction of the X chromosome in some rare cases (see Watson et al., 1988).

Dykens and Leckman (1990) and Einfeld (1993) have reviewed a number of studies on the cognitive functions of persons with F-X syndrome. There is little consensus regarding the cognitive profile in F-XS, apart from diminished intelligence. A number of studies exist, sometimes claiming to have identified differences in cognitive functions between F-XS subjects and controls. However, the small number of subjects used in many studies makes it highly possible that detected differences are merely a result of chance. Among more solid contributions, Fisch (1992) and Fisch et al. (1992) have documented IQ scores in males with F-XS. They found evidence of two groups of subjects, one with stable IQ scores over time and the other with declining scores, and speculated that their data might constitute evidence for two types of mutation. They also argued that the association sometimes suggested between F-XS and autism (as much as 10–12 per cent of the population diagnosed with infantile autism – often on the basis of 'poor eye contact' – according to Brown et al., 1986), is not confirmed when level of mental retardation is controlled (see also Cohen et al., 1991, on this question). Inattention and hyperactivity in F-XS males as well as females are often reported. They do not seem to be correlated with IQ. Hyperactivity may diminish with age in many subjects (see Dykens et al., 1994, for a discussion). Difficulties with verbal memory, attention deficits and impulsiveness have been reported for adult females with F-XS on the Complex Figure of Rey (Rey, 1967). Hinton et al. (1992) found defects of attention and visual memory in F-XS subjects with more than 500 CGG base pairs at the FMR-1 gene. This finding is probably the first one demonstrating a clear association between cognitive dysfunction and specific abnormalities of DNA. Preliminary suggestions (see Dykens et al., 1994) link the cognitive problems in affected male and female F-XS subjects to prefrontal functions involving planning, attention, short-term memory, problem-solving strategies, control of cognitive networks and selective inhibition. (See Benson, 1994, for a comprehensive account of the neuroanatomical foundations of higher cortical functions.)

Hodapp et al. (1992) compared cognitive processes in males subjects with F-XS, DS and 'non-specific' mental retardation (i.e. no known genetic or medical aetiology). Subjects were matched for CA and MA (about 9 years-CA and 4½ years-MA). They used the Kaufman Assessment Battery for Children (K-ABC; Kaufman and Kaufman, 1983), a psychometric instrument designed to tap different styles of information-processing. The test divides intellectual processing into sequential processing (relying on short-term memory and involving the temporal ordering of information) and simultaneous processing (involving the synthesis of separate elements in a holistic manner). Across all three aetiological groups, sequential processing proved less efficient than simultaneous processing. A general effect of MR, therefore, seems to be a deficit in the sequential processing domain. Aetiology-characteristic effects were apparent too. For example, the weakness in sequential processing was pronounced in the F-XS group and, to a lesser extent, in the non-specific group. When the subjects' performance on individual subtests was examined, patterns of aetiology-characteristic strengths and weaknesses appeared. Particularly, items in the Hand Movement subtest were much better performed by DS subjects. In contrast, the Hand Movement subtest was the weakest area for all F-XS subjects. Hodapp et al.'s study is in agreement with the results of a number of other studies: e.g. Bilovsky and Share (1965) with the ITPA; and Pueschel et al. (1987), who demonstrated a proficiency in DS children in reproducing sequences of hand movements. These data suggest that interventions which emphasize manual sign language can be helpful in the language training of DS children (see Abramsen, Cavallo and McCluer, 1985; and Chapter 6) and/or in facilitating communication in older DS subjects with major articulatory difficulties and high rates of dysfluencies. The same recommendation should probably be avoided in the case of F-XS subjects (Dykens et al., 1944).

Only a limited number of studies have reported on the speech and language functions in F-XS. Some time ago, Lehrke (1974), observing that X-linked forms of mental retardation seemed to be associated with particular speech difficulties (e.g. perseverative and staccato speech), hypothesized that several genes on the X chromosome might play a role in language functioning. More recent research seem to confirm and extend Lehrke's initial suggestion. F-XS male subjects indeed have difficulties involving *rate of speech*. Hanson, Jackson and Hagerman (1986) signal repetitions, fluctuating rates of speech and cluttering in MR F-XS males. Other studies (e.g. Levitas, McBogg and Hagerman, 1983; Newell, Sanborn and Hagerman, 1983) report unusual voice effects, dysrythmia (i.e. uneven rate of speaking), echolalia and poor intelligibility of speech, in males with F-XS. Borghgraef et al.(1987) found high rates of rapid speech rhythm and speech impulsiveness among F-XS boys aged 7–11 years, but not in younger subjects. It could be that problems in rate of speech in F-XS males become more pronounced with age. Wolf-Schein et al. (1987) compared groups of DS subjects and MR F-XS subjects matched for level of adaptative behaviour on the Vineland Adaptive Behavior Scales (Sparrow, Balla, and Cicchetti, 1984). They reported that F-XS subjects present significantly more jargon, perseveration and echolalia than DS subjects. The language of the F-XS subjects was pragmatically less appropriate. Their answers did not always match the questions they were asked, even if on the whole they spoke more than the DS subjects. Also the referential gestures and the facial and head movements of the F-XS subjects were globally less appropriate than those of the DS controls. It would seem that some speech and language aspects of F-XS subjects are particular to this syndrome and cannot be attributed to general level of retardation.

Another speech problem frequent in F-XS concerns omission or substitution of vocalic and consonant phonemes (e.g. *b* for *v*, or *d* for *g*) (Newell et al., 1983; Vilkman, Niemi and Ikonen, 1988). F-XS boys have difficulties in repeating close but non-reduplicative syllables (e.g. *pa – ta – ka*, or words such as *linoleum*) (Paul et al., 1984). The difficulties of F-XS males in rate of speech, impulsiveness, repetition and coarticulation could be related to an inability to sequence syllables appropriately, as is observed in developmental apraxia of speech (Paul et al., 1984). Attentional and short-term memory deficits may be involved too, particularly in the cluttering symptoms (Hanson et al., 1986).

Very few studies are available on the lexical ability of F-XS subjects. It would seem that the receptive as well as the expressive vocabulary skills are well developed in F-XS males (Marans, Paul and Leckman, 1987; Paul et al., 1987; Turk et al., 1994).

Less is known about the syntactic skills of F-XS males. Fryns et al. (1984) suggested that levels of grammatical skills in F-XS males are consistent with their overall levels of intellectual functioning. However, the measures made in this study were approximate. Grammatical level, for example, was determined from simple measures taken from naturalistic speech samples. Paul et al. (1984) and Marans et al. (1987), in contrast, signalled deficits in expressive syntax (e.g. MLU) in F-XS males. Sudhalter, Scarborough and Cohen (1991) assessed F-XS males' language across two grammatical measures: MLU and a locally devised measure of grammatical complexity, labelled Index of Productive Syntax (IPS). They reported that performance on these two measures correlated with MA. However, when the subjects' grammar scores were compared with their communication age scores (on the Vineland Adaptive Behaviour Scales), they fell below the latter, revealing syntax as an area of possible deficit. Further study is needed on the syntax of F-XS males to clarify the picture.

As F-XS boys (as well as many carrier females) are sometimes described as exhibiting autistic-like behaviours (e.g. shyness, withdrawal, social avoidance, poor eye contact), it is worth analysing the pragmatic aspects of their language functioning. Compared with autistic subjects, it turns out that males with F-XS have much better capacities regarding conversational turn-taking and conversational roles, e.g. eliciting utterances from the interlocutor, questioning, requesting for action and producing verbalizations that respond to previous utterances by the interlocutor (Ferrier et al., 1991). Autistic subjects provide a much greater number of inappropriate communications (i.e. instances when the subject is truly off topic) than CA- and IQ- matched F-XS males. However, this does not mean that F-XS males have no problems with conversation and the pragmatic regulations of language. Sudhalter et al. (1990) concentrated on a systematic analysis of conversational language in 12 MR F-XS males, whom they compared to 9 DS male subjects and 12 male subjects diagnosed as autistic, all matched for CA, communication age, and adaptive behaviour score on the Vineland Adaptive Behaviour Scales. The primary measure used was the proportion of deviant language acts for each subject. Deviant repetitive language was defined as perseveration, which could be phrasal, sentential or topic (i.e. talking incessantly about one topic). F-XS subjects produced significantly more deviant repetitive language than DS subjects in the three conversational contexts investigated: direct responses to questions, initiation of a new material and topic maintenance. DS subjects manifested little to no deviant repetitive language. It seems clear that the deviant repetitive language behaviours observed in F-XS subjects cannot simply be considered to be a reflection of their intellectual deficit. The autistic group produced significantly more deviant language acts than the F-XS group, when answering questions and initiating communication. In addition, the autistic subjects produced significantly more echolalia than the F-XS subjects and were not or much less capable of adding new information to a given topic. As a possible explanation for the high amounts of deviant repetitive language in males with F-XS, Sudhalter et al. (1990) suggest that this behaviour may reflect difficulties in processing the utterance and, particularly, in the lexical access of these subjects while they proceed the utterance or search for the correct word. Alternatively, these verbal characteristics may arise from difficulties with auditory reception, auditory sequential memory, hyperactivity and concentration, as indicated above (see also Hagerman, Kemper and Hudson, 1985; Wisniewski et al 1985).

Only minimal information is available on the speech and language of females with F-XS. Madison, George and Moeschler (1986) examined the speech and language characteristics of six F-XS females aged 6–63 years. Two of the five adult women were of low average intelligence; the remaining three showed moderate, mild and borderline intellectual level, respectively; there was also a 6-year-old girl who was severely MR. Madison et al. noted that the receptive and expressive vocabularies of the six subjects were equally developed. Their speech was clear and intelligible, but it included high percentages of self-corrections (up to 20 per cent of their phrases). The adults frequently repeated fillers such as 'well' or terms used idiosyncratically such as 'special'. Meanings were often inconsistent. These findings are in need of replication and further analysis.

In conclusion, male F-XS subjects seem to present a particular profile of language functioning with deviant repetitions, speech impulsiveness and sometimes an inability to sequence syllables appropriately. Lexical and grammatical functioning may be relatively spared, but more data are needed. It is doubtful whether the prevalence of autistic disorders in F-XS males is greater than expected, given their level of mental retardation. Their language characteristics seem to differentiate them from most autistic subjects. The extent of interindividual variation in language within the F-XS is not known, nor is it known whether females with F-XS are affected in the same way and to the same extent as F-XS males, independently of their less severe intellectual impairment. No extended developmental framework has been used yet to examine the language of individuals with F-XS. The reasons for the particular language profile of F-XS subjects are not known either. Future research in this domain needs to investigate possible reasons probably starting with the attentional and memory problems and to determine whether aspects of conversational contexts may be causally involved.

3.4.3 A number of *other syndromes leading to mental retardation*, both genetic and metabolic, have been or are currently the object of much research interest from a medical, physiological or cytogenetic point of view. They are *Prader-Willi syndrome* (Hall and Smith, 1972; Pettigrew et al., 1987; Smith, Volato and Trent, 1988), *phenylketonuria* (population incidence about 1/10 000 livebirths) (Guthrie, Whitney and Stuckey, 1963), the prenatal effects of *maternal hyperphenylalani-naemia* (Berry et al., 1988; Cohen et al., 1988), and the *Cri-du-chat syndrome* (Carlin, 1988a, 1988b). To date, there have been few studies on psychological, cognitive and language development aspects. However, there are suggestions (Seckel, 1960) that individuals with severe short stature, microcephaly and prominent nose (Seckel syndrome) have an exceptionally good command of language in spite of a moderate degree of mental retardation.

3.4.4 Some recent information on an improved prognosis in Cri-du-chat (cat cry) syndrome (CDC-S) has appeared (Carlin, 1988b). CDC-S is a rare syndrome caused by a loss of chromosomal material from the distal portion of 5p. It presents a recognizable phenotype with a characteristic (monochromatic) cry, certain dysmorphic craniofacial features with microcephaly, psychomotor retardation, slowed rate of growth, frequent respiratory and ear infections, and frequent orthopaedic malalignment. Standard reference sources list severe to profound mental retardation, lack of ambulation, lack of speech and a reduced life as almost inevitable for these individuals. Longitudinal data gathered by some researchers (e.g. Wilkins, Brown and Wolf, 1981; Wilkins et al., 1982; Carlin, 1988a, 1988b) show, however, that the prognosis today for most parameters of health, development and longevity in CDC-S are much more optimistic than those presented in common sources of medical information. For example, the risks of major organ anomalies and decreased survival are low. Home-rearing and early intervention seem to be the keys to the improved outlook. Data gathered by Wilkins et al. (1982) on 86 home-reared individuals with 5-p indicate average mental and social ages of 2 years 5 months and 2 years 6 months, respectively, at CAs of 6 and 7 years, with mental and social quotients inversely proportional to the age at which early intervention began. Carlin (1988b) reported on 31 individuals with CDC-S seen longitudinally, some of them for 10 years or more, and cross-sectional data from 31 other cases. Taken together, the sample contained 36 females and 26 males, both caucasians and black. Cytogenetically, the sample included a majority of terminal deletions, some interstitial deletions, mosaicisms and translocations, some of the latter cases resulting from parental translocations. Carlin confirms previous observations by Wilkins and associates (1981, 1982) and notes that in spite of large variations in the size and location of the chromosome deletions in the CDC-S subjects, remarkable phenotypic consistency exists. Early growth failure, microcephaly, significant psychomotor retardation and respiratory and ear infections, have been noted in all CDC-S individuals. Almost 100 per cent of CDC-S subjects have hypotonia, at least in the early months. In later years, about 50 per cent retain some degree of hypotonia and experience limitation in their range of motion at certain joints. Attention deficits seem general. Most individuals are friendly and enjoy interacting with other people. All CDC-S subjects seem to demonstrate cognitive, language and behavioural deficits, but these deficits have been little studied so far. Lack of speech and severe language problems have been noted. However, according to Carlin (1988b), home-rearing and early stimulation have resulted in the development of speech in 50 per cent of the subjects and the early introduction of sign language has promoted the use of signs in 75 per cent of the subjects studied. Limited speech and language development occurs in a large proportion of CDC-S individuals, providing that they are correctly stimulated. As verbalizations develop, there is usually a decrease in signing and the use of non-verbal features. Detailed and systematic studies of these developments are still lacking. It would seem, however, that the ultimate levels of communication skills reached by CDC-S subjects always fall short of exclusive speech and language (Carlin, 1988b). In Carlin's (1988b) sample, half the non-institutionalized CDC-S subjects above 10 years of age were in vocational settings, but none of the institutionalized individuals had developed vocational skills. More research is needed to optimalize educational intervention (particularly cognitive and language intervention) with CDC-S subjects and take advantage of their residual capacities. Such studies may also yield precious information on the constraining role of portions of chromosome 5 in mental development.

3.4.5 Linguistic abilities associated with other perinatal organic syndromes leading to MR are currently being studied. For instance, the early language and communicative abilities of cognitively delayed children with *periventricular leukomalacia* have been scrutinized by Feldman et al. (1992). Periventricular leukomalacia (PVL) is a brain injury which damages the deep cerebral white matter around the cerebral ventricules. It is associated with prematurity (the highest rates are known to occur in premature babies weighing less than 1000 g at birth). PVL remains the major cause of neurodevelopmental impairment of the premature infant. The incidence of PVL varies across studies from 8 to 26 per cent preterm infants, particularly under the age of 30 gestational weeks (Valleur-Masson and Vaivre-Douret, 1994). In some studies, only approximately 50 per cent of the infants with the PVL lesion survived (Rushton, Preston and Durbin, 1985). PVL is associated with both visual and hearing impairments (Sinha et al., 1990). Affected children are also at risk of mental retardation (prevalence rates 40–100 per cent; Devries and Dubowitz, 1985). Feldman et al. (1992) assessed several aspects of spontaneous language samples from five PVL children aged 2 years who were cognitively delayed, and five PVL children with normal cognitive developmental scores (delay was defined as a score of less than 80 points on the Mental Development Index of the Bayley Scales of Infant Development (Bayley, 1969)) Normally developing children were matched with the PVL children on CA and developmental level. No significant differences were observed between the delayed PVL group and either comparison group on a range of measures. These included a measure of morpho-syntax (MLU), amount of intentional communication (communicative acts) and number of different words used. In contrast, the delayed group produced significantly fewer lexical tokens and spontaneous verbal utterances than the CA-matched non-delayed group. Picard (1994) assessed various speech and language functions (phonetic discrimination, receptive lexicon, conversational speech) in a group of 50 French-speaking children with sequelae of PVL. All the children were born before 35 weeks' gestation, and were aged between 5 and 15 years at the time of the study. Ten children demonstrated diminished verbal spontaneity and lexical productivity, lower phonetic discriminative ability and reduced lexical kowledge. The author does not supply the CA of the children with language difficulties, which is unfortunate given the large range of CAs in the sample studied allowing for the causative intervention of variables extraneous to PVL, the more likely so with time passing. He reports, however, that three of the PVL children with language delays had IQ below 80 points on the intellectual test administered (WPPSI, WISC or WAIS). Two other PVL subjects with language difficulties had damage in the deep white cerebral matter underlying the left-temporal area of the brain. These preliminary data suggest a relation between cognitive abilities and measures of verbal productivity in children with PVL.

Related language disorders can be observed in low birthweight children having sustained *intraventricular haemorrhage* (IVH) with or without hypoxic-ischaemic damage. Sequential scanning of preterm infants during the first few months of life have placed the incidence of IVH between 35 and 55 per cent for infants less than or equal to 1500 g birthweight (Papile et al., 1978; Partridge, et al., 1983), with an even higher rate (67 per cent reported for infants weighing less than 1000 g (Partridge et al., 1983). Frisk and Whyte (1994) have studied the language and verbal memory of 68 children with IVL, at 6 years of age. Their performance was compared to that of 20 children, born at term, who were matched to the preterm children for CA and socio-economic status. Deficits in sentence comprehension and working memory were associated with IVH. In addition, a reduced receptive vocabulary and naming difficulties were observed in subjects in whom the IVM included ventricular dilatation or in whom there was associated widespread periventricular leukomalacia. Damage to the caudate nucleus could be the critical determinant of the deficits associated with early periventricular damage. Of interest is the indication that extreme prematurity, in and of itself, does not lead to slower development of language or memory skill (Frisk and Whyte, 1994). The performance of preterm children without damage to the periventricular region of the brain is indistinguishable on all the language and memory tasks from that of age-matched peers born at term.

3.4.6 Some other syndromes leading to mental retardation have begun to be studied systematically, but little to nothing is known about the language development of children with these syndromes. For example, Venita, Chan and Becker (1990) reported on the results of quantitative Golgi analyses indicating definitive dendritic abnormalities in human foetuses and 0–6 month-old infants with trisomy 18 (T18) or Edwards syndrome. The possibility of establishing simple operant eyelid conditioning in surviving children with trisomy 18 was demonstrated some time ago (e.g. Brownfield and Keehn, 1966; Lloyd, Russel and Garmize, 1970), proving the possibility of at least minimal learning in these children. However, a recent literature search has yielded no reference relating to further work along this or other learning alleys in T18 syndrome. Singh (1990) has documented a rare case of survival into adulthood of a person with trisomy 13 (T13 or Patau syndrome), but no cognitive or language information was presented.

3.4.7 Let us return to *Down's syndrome* to specify that in approximately 97 per cent of the cases (standard trisomy 21), the genetic error takes place in the ovula or in the spermatozoid before syngamy or during the first cell division. All the living cells of the embryo receive three chromosomes 21. In 1 per cent (Hamerton, Giannelli, and Polani, 1965) or 2 per cent of the cases (Richard, 1969), the genetic error occurs during the second or the third cell division. In those cases (labelled mosaicism), the embryo develops with a mosaic of normal cells containing the regular number of 46 chromosomes and cells with three chromosomes 21. In the remaining 2 per cent (or 1 per cent) of the DS cases (translocations), the excess chromosomic material is a triplicate of chromosome 21 plus a part of another chromosome.[3] It is known that standard trisomy 21 (T21), DS mosaicism and translocation subtypes of DS display differences in dermatoglyphic, physical, clinical and mental status (e.g. Gibson and Pozsonyi, 1965; Baumeister and Williams, 1967; Fishler, 1975). Possible variations in cognitive and language development could be expected, therefore, depending on the aetiological subtype of DS. Gibson (1973) reviewed a number of studies in this area starting with Clarke, Edwards and Smallpiece (1961), in which the 'karyotype question' regarding mental development in DS was raised. Overall findings suggest that mosaic subjects are less retarded intellectually than translocation subjects who themselves exhibit less intellectual deficit than subjects, with standard T21. Judging from some of the studies reviewed by Gibson (1973), the mean global IQs of mosaic subjects could be situated around 60 or 65 points (67 points, according to Fishler, 1975), and around 50 or 55 for the translocation subjects. Modal IQ for standard T21 is considered to be approximately 45. One has to keep in mind that measurement error for most standard intelligence tests is 3 or 4 points. Gibson (1981; also Gibson, 1973) cautions, however, that 'The extent of agreement – between studies – is by no means perfect and methodological faults abound' (p. 79). A more economical explanatory suggestion according to Gibson (1973), is that 'any departure from the standard or classical trisomy-21 karyotype might contribute to increased somatic and behavioral variability for the syndrome, but little else. Since small and biased samples are common, nonauthentic directional differences (among the cytological variations of Down's syndrome) might easily emerge' (p. 132).

Few specific data exist on the same problem regarding language abilities. Finley et al. (1965) and Rosecrans (1971) reported a 5-year longitudinal study of a DS child aged 5 years 2 months at the time of first examination. This child had [46, XY, t(Dp+)] and came from a family with a 13–15/partial 21 translocation. Verbal IQ (WISC) was 86, in contrast with performance IQ which was 68. Low scores were gained in

---

[3] Partial trisomies 21 also exist (Pueschel, Padre-Mendoza and Ellenbogen, 1980). Jenkins et al. (1983) reported a case of partial trisomy 21 presenting a reduced number of physical stigmata.

Picture arrangement, Block design and Object assembly. The subject's pronunciation and verbal comprehension were reported as 'rather good' (p. 292). Good abilities were also noted on the Vocabulary subtest of the Stanford-Binet Intelligence Test. The boy's reading ability was estimated to be equivalent to grade 3 on the Gray Oral Reading Test. The existence of serious problems in spatial perception and cognition was confirmed on the Bender-Gestalt Visual-Motor Test.

Fishler and Koch (1991) reported a mean IQ difference of 12 points on Wechsler's scales between a group of 30 subjects with regular T21 (mean IQ 52, SD 14.6) and a group of 30 mosaic DS subjects (mean IQ 64, SD 13.8). The two groups were matched on CA (between 2 and 18 years), sex and parental socio-economic background. Results also suggest that many DS subjects with mosaicism show better lexical abilities than standard T21 subjects. In a previous report (Fishler, 1975) – apparently involving 15 mosaic DS children among the ones studied by Fishler and Koch (1991) –, one finds anecdotal observations regarding 'unusually good quality of speech ... well-modulated speech and normal intonation' (p. 93) in mosaic children contrasting with the usual speech of T-21 subjects. According to Fishler and Koch (1991), the mosaic subjects also demonstrated advanced visuo-spatial perceptual skills in paper-and-pencil tasks. Contrary to the conclusion of the authors, however, there is no objective basis in this study for the claim that mosaic DS subjects have 'relatively normal speech' (p. 345). Language normality or quasi-normality in mosaic DS subjects remains to be shown. It could be that some of them have better referential and semantic abilities keeping up with their usually more advanced intellectual capacities. In a recent work, Ponthier (1995) found no significant difference between regular trisomy 21, DS translocation and DS mosaic subjects, in intellectual functions (assessed by means of the Wechsler scales) and a series of language tests involving expressive and receptive phonological, lexical and morphosyntactic tasks).

On the above (preliminary and contradictory) empirical basis, one could propose tentatively that if (regular) T-21 DS subjects usually have major speech and language problems together with difficulties in spatial cognition, translocation DS subjects could have better language abilities but nevertheless have serious problems in spatial cognition, whereas mosaic DS subjects could have both better language and spatial abilities. This being the result of a (genetically based) neurological heterogeneity between the aetiological subtypes of Down's syndrome. This hypothesis is based on the possibility (borrowing from Slater and Cowie, 1971 and extending it to language) that an admixture of normal cells at certain 'chromosomal locations' with trisomy 21 may ameliorate the mental status of DS persons.

3.4.8 In concluding this section, it is important to stress that the very notion of mental retardation is becoming too general and perhaps obsolete, except for global classificatory purposes. Various syndromes (and possibly, subsyndromes) related to mental retardation may have specific profiles. This is an important indication. From a therapeutic point of view, it makes it all the more necessary to implement syndrome-specific intervention procedures in order to optimalize the treatment effects with MR subjects.

A second concluding point is that syndrome comparison is an important task. Such a task, however, is fraught with methodological difficulties. Researchers need to be attuned to the limitations imposed by various groups. It is not sufficient in a number of comparative cases to match subjects on CA, MA and other developmental variables. Control of aetiology-specific profiles or variations in samples requires matching subjects carefully across groups on certain speech-language variables. No matter how delicate to implement, this comparative orientation will make it possible to define the extent to which problems are unique to some groups or are shared by various groups of subjects. In addition, such comparisons will favour observations of the relationships between neuropsychological, neurophysiological and neuroanatomical features of brain development and functioning.

Thirdly, this section shows that important linguistic variations may exist across syndromes at similar levels of cognitive retardation. Apart from Down's syndrome, only a few syndromes have been studied thoroughly from a language point of view. It is possible that additional studies will reveal further and more extensive syndrome variation. The available comparative data point towards the existence of clear dissociations between cognition and language and between major aspects of the language system.

Fourthly, some of the studies reviewed suggest that the label *specific* may be attached to some aspects of the language functioning or the cognitive organization of subjects with a particular MR syndrome. This is the case in Bellugi and her collaborators' publications regarding Williams syndrome. This is also the case in Dykens, Hodapp and Leckman's (1994) work concerning Fragile-X syndrome. Gibson (1981) asserted that 'The Down's syndrome group is evidently different from normal children and other categories of mental retardation in respect to language use. Among the differences are a prevalence of certain parts of speech over others, a better verbal understanding than word use, a tendency to emphasise the first consonant and vowel sounds of words and a propensity to communicate with a minimum verbal complexity' (p. 243). We need to evaluate such specificity claims carefully. This is the topic of the next section.

3.5 The question of specificity

3.5.1 The question whether specific organic and/or behavioural features characterize some syndromes has been touched upon in the preceding section. However, as usually posed, the specificity question is ambiguous. Strictly speaking, 'particular' or 'specific' implies that some symptoms or aspects of the organic and/or the behavioural organization of DS (or other MR syndromes) are *pathognomonic*, i.e. 'characteristic or indicative of a disease; denoting especially one or more typical symptoms, findings, or patterns of abnormalities specific for a given disease and not found in any other condition' (*Stedman's Medical Dictionary*, 1990). This is clearly unsubstantiated on the evidence to date. There is no diagnostic linguistic or behavioural feature that would independently separate or isolate persons with DS, WS, F-XS, CDC-S, PVL, T18, T3, etc., from other moderately or severely MR individuals (also Dykens, 1995). For example, it is known that articulatory problems are frequent in DS persons. This could be considered specific or typical of Down's syndrome. However, clearly, this is not a diagnostic feature. Articulatory difficulties are commonly found in many other MR syndromes and pathological entities, and, importantly, they may be absent in a small proportion of DS cases. Bellugi et al. (1990) suggest that preserved performance in facial discrimination may be a specific neuropsychological marker of Williams syndrome, but this is only a hypothesis relative to other aspects of the syndrome. This is the good performance on facial discrimination *in the context of* impaired spatial cognition which may constitute a unique character of WS.

Do we have indications that pathognomonic features of DS, WS or other MR entities exist in 'more organic' aspects of these conditions, for example, in the biological bases of the cognitive functions, cerebral pathologies, or the organization of the brain? Probably not, but see the contributions to the 1993 Palma Symposium on 'Specificity in Down's syndrome' (Perera, 1995). What about the aetiologies of trisomy 13, 18, 21, and other genetic conditions? By definition, these aetiologies are specific in the strict sense. However, the pathological mechanisms involved are not. For example, non-disjunction before syngamy or during the first cell division(s), a phenomenon responsible for approximately 98 per cent of the DS cases (standard T21 and mosaic cases) is also found in T13 and T18. The same is true *mutatis mutandis* of other pathological mechanisms such as (partial) chromosome loss in CDC-S.

Summarising the indications so far, the search for pathognomonic symptoms for DS or other MR entities at any level of organization of the organism is not promising. Should this be taken to mean that nothing specific to any MR entity exists? The answer is also a negative one. Specificity does exist (see Rondal, 1995b) not at the level of separate symptoms, but at a systemic (i.e. more comprehensive) level of analysis. In many syndromes, there is a particular set or system of characteristics justifying the specificity claim, and demanding therapeutic, educational and social measures, tailored to persons with particular MR syndromes. In some rare cases, there could be juxtaposition of two or several sets of features pertaining to different nosological entities. For example,

Collacot et al., (1990) have reported on the case of a single patient (a 21-year-old female with the karyotype 47, X, fra (X) (q27), + 21) demonstrating phenotypical features of both DS and F-XS. There could be a small proportion of F-XS cases in whom sets of autistic features can be identified for reason of a partial recovery or association between the two syndromes. Similarly, some authors have suggested that in some DS patients there is coexisting autism (e.g. Ghazinddin, Tsai and Ghazinddin, 1992).

In what follows, focusing exclusively on language, and based on the data summarized in Section 3.3, we shall illustrate the systemic (syndromic) claim. Table 3-3 summarizes basic information relative to DS, WS and affected males with F-XS. No other syndrome has been sufficiently studied so far from a language point of view to justify the type of formalization attempted here.

Table 3.3 Three MR syndromic profiles for speech and language

Language aspect	Syndromes		
	Down's	Williams	Fragile-X (affected males)
Phonetico-phonological	– –	+	– –
Lexical	–	+ +	+
Thematic semantic	+	+	?
Morphosyntactic	– –	+	–
		(comprehension?)	
Pragmatic	+	– –	–
Discursive	– –	+	–

Key: +(+): relative strength; –(–): relative weakness; ?: insufficient data available.

As Table 3.3 shows, the language profiles of DS, WS and F-XS subjects differ substantially in ways that have nothing to do with the psychometric levels of retardation in each syndrome. Additional research is needed, of course, to examine these comparisons in more detail and to extend the 'syndromic profile search' to a larger number of MR aetiological categories.

It may be too early to discuss possible explanations for the language syndrome specificity. Some informed speculation may be in order, however. One possibility is that language syndrome differences correspond to syndrome differences in brain anatomy and physiology, and perhaps to syndrome differences in the interaction between (1) the calendar of neuropsychological development, and (2) the calendar of the 'attacks' against target sites and functions of the developing brain and the damages caused therein by pathological factors associated with each aetiological condition and coming into action during prenatal and/or early natal periods of development. There is overwhelming evidence of anatomical, physiological and neurochemical abnormalities in the brain of DS children (see Chapter 4). An interesting point, as stressed by Nadel (in press), is that the neural dysfunctions observed in DS, WS and, probably, other genetic syndromes, are not spread evenly throughout the brain. They affect some regions of the brain more than others. It is essential to determine which brain regions are compromised in the various syndromes. Such brain differences have not yet been specifically related to differences in language functioning. A start has been made in this direction in Bellugi et al.'s work, as illustrated earlier. Much additional research work is needed employing a multidisciplinary approach involving psycholinguists, geneticists, neuroanatomists, neurophysiologists, and brain imagery specialists.

3.5.2 A recurrent claim in the literature on Down's syndrome is that DS subjects 'differ' from other MR categories with respect to speech and language particularly (e.g. Gibson, 1981), or even that DS *qua* DS is more detrimental to language development than other syndromes leading to corresponding cognitive impairment (e.g. Zisk and Bialer, 1967). It is worth recalling that DS subjects have not been found to differ from unselected MR subjects of similar MAs, IQs and CAs, on behavioural characteristics other than speech and language, with the exceptions of sensory acuity (audition and vision), which tends to be more impaired, and perceptual speed tending to be reduced (Clausen, 1966, 1968). Reasons for the language claim regarding DS have not been provided and there have been opposing views (Evans and Hampson, 1968; Bloom and Lahey, 1978; Rosenberg, 1982; and Barrett and Diniz, 1989, regarding lexical development). A differential point of view was echoed again in recent contributions by Fowler (1990) and Kernan (1990). Fowler (1990) suggested the existence of a specific syntactic deficit in DS. Kernan (1990), substantiating previous studies, stated 'the linguistic ability of persons with Down's syndrome ... is even more impaired than is that of persons with mental retardation of other etiologies ...' (p. 169).

As a first argument, Fowler (1990) cites punctual discrepancies between measured language skills and expectations based on MA assessments (Thompson, 1963; Evans and Hampson, 1968; Gibson, 1981; Wisniewski, Miezejiski and Hill, 1988), and there are developmental discrepancies in childhood between language measures and motor or personal-social skills in favour of the latter aspects of development (Share, 1975). Fowler (1990) also signals the results of more recent studies suggesting that the deficiencies in language and language-related skills may extend back to the earliest stages of development (Dameron, 1963; Share et al., 1963; Greenwald and Leonard, 1979; Mahoney, Glover and Finger, 1981; Mervis, 1990). Observations of this sort are not sufficient to support the notion of a specific syntactic deficit in DS. Important discrepancies between language measures and MA expectations are found in most MR individuals, not only in DS subjects (see Chapter 4 for the data pertaining to the so-called delay-difference question and particularly the outcome of the studies using an MA-matched paradigm). Similarly, developmental discrepancies between language measures and motor and/or personal skills or other aspects of development, presenting either in the early years or later, are not valid argument in favour of a specific syntactic deficit in DS. Such discrepancies are found in most MR individuals (see, for example, Woodward and Stern, 1963).

As a second argument in favour of her thesis, Fowler (1990) proposes the results of comparison studies of DS with other MR groups matched for CA or IQ. On the basis of such studies, typically involving heterogeneous contrast groups of MR individuals, it has been claimed that individuals with DS show a consistent disadvantage in language tasks (Johnson and Abelson, 1969; Evans, 1977; Burr and Rohr, 1978; Marcell and Armstrong, 1982). Kernan (1990) quotes studies by Lyle (1959, 1961a, 1961b), Mein (1961), Blanchard (1964), Rohr and Burr (1978), Ashman (1982), Hartley (1982, 1985), and Smith and von Tetzchner (1986), in support of a similar argument. Some of the studies cited do not actually supply data relevant to the comparative issue evoked. For example, Johnson and Abelson (1969) compared 254 standard T21, 21 translocation and 18 mosaic DS subjects, all institutionalized adults, on a number of measures. These were: intelligence test scores, number of physical stigmata and behaviour rated for activity aggressiveness, sexual activity, and psychosis. No language data were actually analysed. Some studies claiming specific linguistic deficiencies in DS children did not measure lexical or syntactic skills but focused on processing skills supposed to underlie language abilities. For example, in the ITPA literature (e.g. Evans, 1977; Burr and Rohr, 1978; Rohr and Burr, 1978), DS children exhibit disadvantages in auditory tasks relative to visual tasks. This auditory disadvantage is often of a larger magnitude in DS than in groups of MR subjects of undiagnosed aetiologies. Spreen (1965) and Kirk and Kirk (1974) claimed that a distinctive DS profile had been established, in which motor encoding (the expression of ideas in terms of meaningful gestures) was superior to verbal encoding and other psycholinguistic abilities. These data are indicative of a relative visuo-motor superiority over the auditory-vocal channel in DS subjects (a superiority already mentioned). They do not prove that DS subjects are necessarily always inferior to non-DS subjects in auditory-vocal tasks or in language tasks in general. The relative advantage of DS persons in visuo-motor functioning may have to do, at least in part, with short-term memory. It is known that immediate memory span in NR people is larger for auditory than for visual input (modality effect; see Conrad, 1964; Penney, 1975). DS subjects do not seem to present the same modality pattern, having either similarly reduced auditory-verbal (AV) and visuospatial (VS) STM spans or a VS-STM span that is actually larger than their AV-STM span (Marcell and Armstrong, 1982; Marcell and Weeks, 1988). According to Marcell and Weeks (1988), non-DS MR subjects, on the contrary, exhibit a reliable modality effect (in the same sense as NR subjects, albeit inferior in magnitude due to lower scores in the AV modality). As indicated earlier in this chapter, WS subjects also exhibit a clear modality effect in the same sense as NR subjects.

One may relate to the above literature the reported inferiority of DS subjects in serial or sequential cognitive processing (as opposed to parallel or simultaneous processing) (see Ashman, 1982; Hartley, 1982, 1985). Again, some interpretive reservations must be voiced. First, in many MR subjects sequential cognitive processing (i.e. the subjects' ability to deal with stimuli presented in temporal or serial order – e.g. hand movements, number recall, word order) is lower than simultaneous processing (the integration of stimuli in a spatial, gestalt-like manner – e.g. face recognition, gestalt closure and matrix analogies). For example, Hodapp et al. (1992) reported sequential cognitive processing significantly lower than simultaneous processing in 30 DS, F-XS and children with 'non-specific' mental retardation, using the Kaufman Assessment Battery for Children. Actually, Hodapp et al. (1992) signalled a tendency toward a greater weakness in sequential processing in their F-XS and non-specific MR groups than in their DS subjects. Second, despite suggestions that sequential processing is related to syntactic structure (Caramazza et al., 1976; Cummins and Das, 1978), equating serial processing with language tasks and simultaneous processing with non-language ones is questionable. Linguistic processing may be as much parallel as serial, and processing of non-linguistic information may involve similar or different, but equally complex processing parameters.

However, if one takes into account a series of other comparative data, perhaps more convincing, it is possible to accept the hypothesis that some persistent speech and language differences may indeed exist between DS and non-DS MR persons. Such data are supplied by Kernan (1990), observing that DS adults have significantly more comprehension difficulties with compound and complex temporal sentences where temporal sequence is indicated by syntax with no supporting pragmatic or extralinguistic context, than adults with comparable mental retardation of 'no specific' aetiology. Rondal and Lambert (1983) reported shorter MLU values, lower proportion of (complete) sentences, lower sentence complexity, reduced use of articles, verbal inflexions, and personal pronouns (but similar type-token ratios -TTR), in the conversational speech of a group of French-speaking DS adults in comparison to non-DS MR adults of similar CA and MA (see Table 5-3, Chapter 5, for a summary of Rondal and Lambert's (1983) data. It should be noted, however, that none of the differences in group means between DS and non-DS MR adults proved significant in this study due to the relatively large interindividual variability in the two groups of subjects); Rondal, Lambert and Sohier (1980a, 1981), and Lambert, Rondal and Sohier (1980) showed shorter MLU values and lower articulatory scores (but similar types of articulatory errors) in groups of French-speaking DS and non-DS MR children matched for CA and MA, and Ryan (1975) reported lower intelligibility of speech in DS children with CAs between 5 and 9 years in comparison to CA-matched non-DS MR children of various aetiologies and MA-matched NR children.

It should be noted that only *quantitative* variations have been identified between DS and other MR subjects for *some* language aspects. No qualitative differential pattern has emerged. Nevertheless, a combination of voice, articulatory, morphosyntactic and, to a lesser extent, lexical delay and limitation may be said to be specific to DS in the sense of 'systemic specificity' defined earlier.

Chapter 4
Exceptionality and Language Modularity

It might appear slightly strange to the reader that we plan to consider exceptionality in language development and functioning in MR subjects before dealing with 'typical' development (so to speak) in these subjects. This calls for a justification. But let us first specify what we mean by exceptional language in MR subjects. At the present time, approximately a dozen case studies have documented (sometimes in great detail) language development in moderately and severely MR subjects which is much better than what is usually expected from these subjects. Exceptional language and exceptionality, in this context, are relative. They correspond to levels of development and language functioning that are exceptional for moderately and severely MR people, although usual for NR persons. Actually, the language levels reached by the exceptional MR subjects are not generally fully comparable to normal functioning, and, very importantly, they vary from language component to language component (for example, semantics and morpho–syntax). This second observation brings us to the second half of the heading given to the present chapter, that is, language modularity. The dissociations just mentioned in conjunction with a series of dissociative evidence coming from other studies in language pathology, including neurolinguistic analyses, attest to the modular organization of language. These indications will be related to theoretical proposals regarding language modularity and the question of the modularity of mind.

With the above considerations, the reader should now begin to understand why the notions of language modularity and language exceptionality in MR subjects have been included in the book and how they will be dealt with. The modularity scheme also supplies a theoretical validation for analysing separately the major language components, which we will do in Chapter 5. The existence of exceptional language in mental retardation reminds us that nature has not excluded more advanced language functioning in MR subjects.

In this respect, language development in exceptional MR subjects can be conceived of as a theoretical 'possibility'. Language development in typical MR subjects, by the same token, can be viewed as a less than satisfactory evolution even given the series of problems that characterize the condition of these subjects.

In this chapter, we shall first review the evidence available regarding language exceptionality in MR subjects and establish exceptionality beyond reasonable doubt in comparing these data with corresponding data representative of typical MR subjects. In so doing, the delay vs. difference issue in language development of MR children will arise. Modular accounts of language functioning will be discussed with particular attention to the question of the relationship between language and cognition. At this stage, additional observations from studies in neurolinguistics and clinical neuropsychology will be called upon. Lastly, reasons for explaining the exceptional cases of language development documented in MR subjects will be explored.

4.1 Exceptional language development in mental retardation

A number of exceptional cases of language development in MR subjects (mostly and most impressively in moderately and severely mentally retarded) have been reported in the recent literature (with the exception of an earlier case reported by Seagoe (1965), They are abstracted in Table 4.1.

4.1.1 Bellugi et al. (1988) have documented the cases of three adolescents with Williams syndrome (2 girls, Van and Crystal; 1 boy, Ben) exhibiting unusual linguistic capabilities for their level of mental retardation. They were aged 11, 15 and 16 years, respectively, at the time of the study. Their (full–scale) IQ scores (WISC) varied between 49 and 54. On tasks assumed to measure cognitive growth, as viewed within a Piagetian framework (e.g. seriation, classification, conservation), they demonstrated preoperative functioning. The three adolescents revealed impressive productive and receptive linguistic abilities, although not quite at chronological age levels. Their MLUs (computed according to Brown's rules, 1973) varied from 8.6. to 13.1. Their speech included full passives, embedded relative clauses, conditionals and multiple embeddings. Grammatical morphology was mostly correct. The subjects demonstrated comprehension of full reversible passives, affirmative and negative comparative, equative relational expressions and other complex linguistic structures. Receptive vocabulary was evaluated at the 9– to 12–year level depending on the particular subject. The three WS subjects were able to judge and correct sentences that were ungrammatical due to violations of subcategorization features, phrase structure rules or errors in reflexive pronoun usage (for example, violations of coreferential agreement in number, gender, and/or person), thus confirming quite a sophisticated grammatical capacity.

Table 4.1 Exceptional cases of language development in MR subjects. Studies and keypoints

Study	Subjects	CA[1]	IQ[2]	Operational level[3]	MA[4]	MLU[5]	Other language aspects
1. Bellugi et al. (1988)	Van Crystal Ben	11 15 16	50 49 54	Preoperative Preoperative Preoperative		8.60 13.10 10.00	Correct articulation and phoneme discrimination Receptive vocabulary at the 9–12 year level Advanced expressive and receptive morphosyntactic abilities
2. Curtiss and associates (Curtiss, 1989 for a summary; Yamada, 1990)	Antony Rick Laura	6-7 15 16	50 41	Preoperative Preoperative Preoperative	2 years 9 months		Correct articulation and phoneme discrimination Receptive vocabulary at the 6-year level and lower Advanced expressive and receptive morphosyntactic abilities, except for Laura who exhibited receptive morphosyntactic limitations Semantic, pragmatic and discursive deficiencies
3. Rondal (1994a, 1994b)	Françoise	32	64	Late preoperative to early operative	7 years 4 months	12.24	Correct articulation and phoneme discrimination Moderately retarded lexical development Advanced expressive and receptive morpho-syntax (virtually normal) Moderate problems with discourse organization (e.g., text cohesion)

4. Seagoe (1965)	Paul	11-43	60		Good command of written language expression and reading (average number of words per written sentence varying from 7.14 to 12.50 between 15 and 33 years)
5. Hadenius et al. (1962), Anderson and Spain, (1977), Tew (1979)	Series of hydrocephalic children	3-8		Severely impaired cognitive development	Good ability to articulate, learn words, and use complex syntax. Semantic deficiencies
6. Cromer (1991)	DH	Adolescent	Performance IQ below 35		Correct articulation. Use of extensive vocabulary. Use of complex morpho-syntax. Use of standard pragmatic devices in conversation
7. O'Connor & Hermelin (1991)	Christopher	29	Performance IQ 67		Good level ability in translating in English from French, German and Spanish, and satisfactory levels of lexical and morphosyntactic comprehension in the four languages. Score on the English Peabody Picture Vocabulary Test (EPPVT): 121. German PPVT 114. French PPVT 110. Spanish PPVT 89

Notes:
1. Chronological age in years at beginning of study
2. Intellectual quotient according to major standard intellectual scales (e.g., WISC)
3. According to Piagettian criteria
4. Mental age in years
5. Mean length of utterance (computed in a number of words plus grammatical morphemes)

N.B. Empty boxes in table correspond to pieces of information not supplied by the authors in the original sources

4.1.2 Curtiss and associates (Curtiss, 1981, 1982, 1988, 1989; Curtiss, Fromkin and Yamada, 1979; Curtiss and Yamada, 1981; Curtiss, Kempler and Yamada, 1981; Yamada, 1981, 1983, 1990) have reported on the study of three language–exceptional MR subjects (one child, a boy named Antony; two adolescents: one girl, Marta (real name Laura, as she is referred to in Yamada's monograph, 1990; in what follows, following Yamada, we shall call her Laura), and one boy, Rick). Rick suffered severe anoxia at birth. In the other two cases, mental retardation is of unknown aetiology .

Antony was 6–7 years at the time of the study. His IQ estimate was about 50. At CA 5 years 6 months, the MA was 2 years 9 months. His logical sequencing (ordering pictures) was at the 2–year–old level. His logical conservation level could not be assessed. Antony's language is described by Curtiss as 'well formed phonologically and syntactically and [was] structurally rich... fully elaborated with inflectional and derivational bound morphology and "free" grammatical morphemes, and it included syntactic structures involving movement, embedding, and complementation' (Curtiss, 1988, p. 374). In contrast to this remarkable morphosyntactic ability, Antony's language was semantically deficient. He tended to use words incorrectly and, when requested, defined them incompletely and sometimes inaccurately. This, at times, resulted in miscommunications with others. None of Antony's lexical errors involved violations of syntactic class, subcategorization features, grammatical case, or word order. Almost all his errors were errors in semantic feature specification. Errors with lexical substantives involved confusions or inadequate differentiation between words within a particular semantic area (e.g. 'birthday' for 'cake', 'cutting' for 'pasting'). Errors with prepositions involved errors in marking direction, location or semantic case, or function (e.g. 'to' for 'from', 'in' for 'with'). Pronoun errors involved errors in gender or animacy (e.g. 'who' for 'what', 'that' for 'he'). Antony's language was also deficient in terms of contents. He frequently failed to grasp the full meaning of his own and others' utterances. On the pragmatic and discursive sides, Curtiss (1981, 1982, 1988) reports that Anthony had mastered a range of pragmatic functions and communicative intentions (e.g. turn-taking, requesting, commenting, responding to requests and questions), using language to these effects. However, he had poorly developed topic–maintenance skills, was only moderately sensitive to the interest of his interlocutors, and was little concerned with the need to be relevant or informative in conversation.

Rick was 15–years–old at the time of the study. His language was parallel to that of Antony. He had well–developed phonological, morphological and syntactic abilities, alongside poorly developed lexical and semantic abilities. Rick was extremely social. He made appropriate use of social routines and other conventionalized conversational forms.

However, his semantic deficiencies reduced the efficiency of his proposi-tional communications. He had difficulties in correctly understanding the meaning of the utterances addressed to him, and often made mistakes in the meaning aspects of his propositional realizations. Rick's non-language performance profile was similar to Antony's. His classifica-tion and seriation abilities were those of a child aged 2–3 years. Laura's case is documented in several publications by Curtiss (e.g. 1988). She was studied for several years since she was 16. In addition, the parents supplied written documentation on her earlier development. At 14 years 9 months, her (full–scale) IQ estimate was 41; performance IQ 32, verbal IQ 52.

Overall Laura's linguistic profile was similar to Antony's and Rick's, with the proviso that her lexicon was richer, containing more quantifiers and adverbs. Laura's level on the Peabody Picture Vocabulary Test (PPVT) was 6 years 1 month. But despite her larger vocabulary, Laura presented semantic, pragmatic and discursive deficiencies akin to those of Antony and Rick. Her language, however, was phonologically correct, fully elab-orated morphologically, and it contained complex and well–formed syntactic structures. For example, she used agentless and full passives, sentences with coordinated and subordinated clauses, including WH–relatives, multiple embeddings, infinitival complements and complements containing participal forms. Laura also correctly used elliptical utterances. Receptively, however, the picture was different. In addition to her semantic deficiencies, Laura demonstrated genuine grammatical difficulties in comprehension. She was given the Curtiss–Yamada Comprehensive Language Evaluation (CYCLE, 1992). Her receptive performance on the syntactic subtest was poor. She performed at or below the 2–year–old level on most subtests, including the object manipulation version of various items (e.g. active voice word order, passive voice word order, WH–questioning of grammatical subject and object, relativization tests). Laura performed poorly on the Token Test (De Renzi and Vignolo, 1962), scoring 17 out of a total of 39, which is below the mean score of normal children at 3 years 6 months (i.e. 19.55). It is of interest to note that in her spontaneous speech, Laura produced many of the structures that she failed to understand on the comprehension tests. In some cases, she proved able to understand syntactic structures in conversational context, but did poorly on the corresponding formal receptive test. Laura's comprehension of gram-matical morphemes likewise was reduced. On the CYCLE battery of morphology, she demonstrated mastery over two grammatical morphemes only (i.e. tense/aspect marker –ing and comparative –er). Again, it is remarkable that she spontaneously and correctly used some of the same forms in her speech. Moreover, she could detect and correct surface syntactic and morphological errors in imitation tasks; therefore, demonstrating at least minimal capacity for grammatically judging forms that she could be proved not to (completely) understand. As with Antony and Rick, Laura's non-linguistic performance showed marked dissociations between grammar and general knowledge. She lacked the concept of number and could not correctly apply basic counting principles to concrete objects. Her reasoning in seriation, classification and conservation tasks was at the preoperational level.

4.1.3 A few years ago, one of us had the good fortune to discover another case of exceptional language development, this time in a young Down's syndrome woman (regular trisomy 21) – one of the most astonishing cases documented so far (see Rondal, 1994b, 1995b). Her name is Françoise. She was 32 years at the beginning of the study. Françoise's MLU count yields an index of 12.24 (standard deviation 9.65). Sound articulation is normal. Speech is fluent and normally intonated. Tonic and stress accents are correctly distributed. As to syntax, the sentences are mostly complete (except for regular ellipses) and conventional French word order is followed. Declarative, interrogative (WH– and Yes–No subtypes), imperative, emphatic, and exclamative sentences are used either affirmatively or negatively, and in the latter case with the negative elements properly located in the sentence's sequential structure. Reflexive constructions are not infrequent and they are correctly formed (e.g. *Je me suis dit*...). Full syntactic passives are used at times. Lexical passives are more common (e.g. *Quelqu'un est venu, être marié, être coiffé comme tout le monde*). Coordinated as well as subordinated clauses are used. Among the latter are observed: nominal subordinates (subject and object completives), relatives and circumstantial subordinates (temporal, comparative, causal, consequential and conditional ones). Simple and at times multiple embedding are observed. Tense agreement between main and subordinate clauses is properly marked. The various phrases (noun phrase, verb phrase, prepositional phrase, adjectival and adverbial phrases) are correctly formed. Some are quite complex with the use of coordination, determiners, modifiers and embedded or chained relative clauses.

The grammatically obligatory free and bound morphemes are correctly used without exception. Articles are properly marked for number, gender, and for the contrast between specific and non-specific reference (e.g. *The bike I have vs A bike I saw*). Pre-articles (absolute and relative quantifiers are correctly placed before articles, preceded by the preposition *de* in the case of the relative quantifiers (e.g. *tous les hommes, beaucoup de romanichels*). Post-articles (cardinal and numeral) are properly located following articles (e.g. *On a été tous les deux*). Personal pronouns are correctly marked for number, gender, person and case, and they are regularly positioned with respect to the verbs. Pronominal coreference is usually clear. Possessive pronouns and adjectives are correctly marked for person, gender (of things possessed), number (of thing–s possessed and of possessor–s). Epithets are correctly marked for number and gender where applicable. Demonstrative pronouns and adjectives are correctly used with respect to number, gender and the proximal–distal contrast. This, together with the proper use of personal and possessive pronouns, attests to Françoise's mastery over the deixis function of language. Relative and interrogative pronouns and adjectives are correctly marked for number, gender and case (where applicable). The presence of some of the most usual indefinite pronouns and adjectives (either expressing absolute or relative quantitative value – e.g. *chaque, quelque,* – or qualitative value – e.g. *même, autre*) is attested in the corpus. Lastly, verbs are correctly inflected for mood, tense, aspect, number and person including the French polite plurals. Auxiliaries and modals are properly used.

Françoise's normal (productive) grammatical functioning is confirmed by her results on a number of specific psycholinguistic receptive tasks. Reversible as well as nonreversible relative clauses introduced by the relative pronouns *qui* or *que* are correctly understood, whether embedded or derived on the right side of the main clause. Causal subordinate clauses introduced by the conjunctive locution *parce que* are correctly understood whether the subordinate clause precedes or follows the main clause. Temporal subordinate clauses are correctly understood whether the clause order matches the order in which the events referred to happened, are happening, will happen, or not. The mechanism of coreference in the case of anaphoric personal pronouns also proved to be mastered. Françoise appears to make systematic use of the number and gender correspondence between pronoun and noun to establish anaphoric coreference in paragraphs (e.g. *La secrétaire joue au tennis avec le professeur. Il vous téléphonera demain*).

Comprehension of declarative affirmative active and passive sentences varying in plausibility and plausible reversibility was also experimentally investigated. Active and passive designating requests were used to elicit interpretive responses (see Rondal, Thibaut and Cession, 1990 for more detail on the procedure as well as normative data relating to French). Françoise correctly interpreted 61 out of 64 sentences; the 3 errors could be attributed to distraction. Most remarkably, she could correctly identify the underlying grammatical subject or the underlying grammatical object in irrealis sentences with low–transitivity verbs – see Hopper and Thompson(1980) (e.g. *Le livre est imaginé par la boîte*), therefore with no pragmatic and semantic help, and even irrealis sentences that would turn realis were they reversed (e.g. *Le monsieur est imaginé par le livre*), therefore going against possible pragmatic interpretive tendency. (See Rondal (1995a) for a full report on the evaluation procedures applied to Françoise, the complete results and their analysis, as well as for a large amount of additional information on the case.)

4.1.4 Françoise's truly remarkable phonological and grammatical capacity is in sharp contrast with what is known of regular moderately and severely MR persons including other DS subjects (see Chapter 5).

4.1.5 Turning now to Françoise's lexicon. Although lexical usage seems to be generally correct, there are occasional mistakes: incomplete locutions, for example *y a, y avait*, instead of the correct form *il y a, il y avait*; incorrect adverbial derivations *drol' dement* instead of *drôle-ment*; incorrect expressions, for example *habillé comme l'as de pique* and *Il m'faut déjà toutes les plumes pour voler* instead of *habillé à l'as de pique* and *Il m'faut déjà toutes mes plumes pour voler*, incorrect word forms, for example *décrapitude* instead of *décrépitude*. Françoise was given the TVAP (Test de Vocabulaire Actif et Passif) – form F 5 to 8 years; the TRT (Test des Relations Topologiques); the vocabulary task of the Test Battery used at the University of Liège for the assessment of aphasia; and the vocabulary subtest of the WAIS. The picture denomination and pointing scores indicate delayed lexical development, particularly concerning the locative expressions. On the word definition tasks, Françoise scored one standard deviation below the population mean (WAIS Vocabulary subtest standard score: 7; population mean: 10). She supplied incorrect definitions for such terms as *grouper, réparer, portion, clôture, empoigner, aumône, tanière, instruire, fade, persévérant, monopole.*

4.1.6. The most striking limitation in Françoise's conversational speech is at the level of discourse organization. A basic theme–rheme distinction is respected throughout the clauses and the usual given/new information structure is applied with no exception. But although discourse taken at the level of the speech turn and the paragraph is coherent, the larger text often lacks cohesion. According to Halliday (1985), text cohesion, a characteristic distinct from the thematic and the information structures of the clause, depends on making explicit the external relationships between individual clauses or groups of clauses. This realization is considered not to depend on grammatical structure. Textual competence is thought to have the following major components: *reference* (an element introduced at one place in text can be taken as a reference point for something that follows); *ellipsis; conjunction* (marking the semantic relation holding between clauses or groups of clauses); and *lexical cohesion* (choice of words and repetition of the same words or use of related words to insure semantic continuity). The conjunction process is defective in Françoise's speech. She uses a number of conjunctive forms (e.g. *et, alors, mais, donc*), often located at the beginning of the utterances; but these forms do not really denote relationships between clauses or utterances. They are loose sequential connectors. Many utterances contain several repetitions of the same word, locution or phrase. Stereotyped (idiomatic) expressions are placed here and there in the utterances (*comme vous voyez, si j'peux* *dire, pour vous l'dire honnêtement*, etc.). These hold for speech a turn. When she starts using one such stereotyped expression, she continues using it for the rest of the speech turn, as if the first use had a self–priming effect. Also she has a tendency to alternate ideas, that is, she expresses one idea, turns to a connected one, then returns to the first idea and the second one. The above characteristics attest to a difficulty with text planning. In this respect, the stereotyped fillers that she uses may be the functional equivalent of the hesitation pauses identified by Goldman–Eisler (1968, 1972) and assumed to correspond to moments of planning for the discourse ahead.

4.1.7 Françoise's *non-linguistic capacities* are in marked contrast with her grammatical achievement. As she was 32 years old at the beginning of the study and as the whole evaluation procedure was spread over a period of almost four years, it was necessary to have her general mental functioning retested towards the end period of the study, in order to rule out (or document) a possible age–related cognitive decline. Such a decline, often tied to Alzheimer–like neuropathological changes, affects a proportion of Down's syndrome people over the age of 40 years (see Chapter 5 for more details). The WAIS given at the beginning and towards the end of the study yielded similar results (final non-verbal IQ: 64, verbal IQ: 70; Global IQ 65). There was no ground for suspecting cognitive decline over the 4–year evaluation period. Her non-verbal IQ at the beginning of the study at the WAIS was 60 (verbal IQ: 71; global IQ: 64) with low to very low standard scores in spatial subtests (object assembly, completing images, cubes), arithmetic and memory for numbers (she recalls 4 digits forward as well as backward). Françoise was also given the Epreuves Differentielles d'Efficience Intellectuelle (Perron–Borelli and Misès, 1974), an intelligence test made of 8 subtests (verbal and nonverbal). She obtained a verbal MA of 9 years and 10 months and a non-verbal MA of 5 years and 8 months, which gave a global MA of 7 years and 4 months. Without exception, Françoise's performance on the non-linguistic tests (computational capacity, Rendement Mnésique de Rey, Bushke's Test of Cued Recall and Selective Reminding, Figure Complexe de Rey, Figures Enchevêtrées de Poppelreuter, and many others) is compatible with the average performance of typical DS subjects (see Gibson, 1981, for example), which means that it is quite underdeveloped.

Françoise was also given the Piagetian tasks of seriation, classification and conservation. She is able to classify correctly 18 tokens (varying as to shape, colour and size) and 27 pictures of familiar objects (varying as to nature, colour and size), according to one criterion at a time. She can juxtapose two classifications each one organized according to one criterion, but she is unable to integrate or relate two classifications (i.e. double–entry tables or 'matrices'). On a seriation task with a material composed of 5, and then 10 sticks of different colours, Françoise can seriate without difficulty, including the insertion of an additional stick in the series upon request and placing it immediately in the correct location. A number of conservation tasks were administered: number and term-to-term correspondence, length (comparison of a straight line with another line that was first straight, then broken), surface (by displacement of elements), liquids, solid substance, discontinuous quantities and weight. Françoise could correctly solve all the conservation problems presented. However, she used only one argument in order to justify her conservation judgements and resist counter-suggestions, i.e. the simple identity argument (for instance, as to the conservation of liquids, 'It is still the same water', 'It simply has been poured' and 'Nothing has been taken away or added'). She never referred to any other operative arguments. Françoise spontaneously acknowledged that years ago, she had been trained by her father (a mathematics professor aware of some of Piaget's work) to disregard the physical appearance of the objects following transformation and keep in mind that the same quantity always remained because nothing had been added or taken away. It is not clear, therefore, whether Françoise's cognitive functioning really demonstrates decentration from action or physical appearance, and a capacity to subordinate concrete states to reversible transformations, or whether she expresses learned stereotyped answers and exhibits only pseudo–operative cognitive structuration. On the whole, she seems to have reached operative seriation. She is close to operative classification, but fails spontaneously to use matrix–like arrangements of elements. As to the conservation tasks, she is no longer functioning at the preoperative level (fully preoperative children usually refuse the suggestion according to which transformations do not falsify the initial equality). We classify Françoise as being cognitively between late preoperative and early concrete operative levels, but closer to the latter stage. This level is compatible with her mental age, as measured at the EDEI test.

4.1.8 Other remarkable cases of exceptional language in MR subjects have been published. They include Paul, a Down's syndrome male with an IQ of 60 and exceptional written language (no information was made available on his oral language), who was studied by Seagoe (1965), and a number of hydrocephalic MR subjects with exceptional language abilities (Hadenius et al., 1962; Anderson and Spain, 1977; Tew, 1979). The latter subjects present a severely impaired general cognitive development together with a good ability to learn words, articulate and talk using a quite complex syntax but often semantically inaccurately. Expressions such as 'cocktail party syndrome' or 'chatterbox syndrome' were coined to express the major language aspects of the condition (e.g. Hadenius et al., 1962). Cromer (1991) reports on his personal study with D.H., a spina–bifida adolescent girl with arrested hydrocephalus, exhibiting chatterbox syndrome. D.H. performs at the severely retarded level on standardized tests of intellectual ability. She cannot handle money properly and has been unable to learn to read and write. In contrast, her speech is fluent and correctly articulated. Her language is meaningful with extensive vocabulary. It incorporates the normal use of standard pragmatic devices. D.H.'s language contains complex syntactic forms, such as elaborated noun and verb phrases, conditionals, complex subordinate and embedded clauses. Judging from the limited excerpt of conversational speech supplied by Cromer (1991), D.H.'s use of grammatical morphemes appears correct. Also, she gave evidence of understanding conversation contents and of being able to monitor conversation properly and follow its course in dyadic contexts. This would seem to indicate that, contrary to previous reports with other hydrocephalic MR subjects, D.H. understands what she is talking about as well as what is conveyed to her by the others in conversations. Unfortunately, Cromer does not supply the outcome of any formal test of language comprehension that would have been administered to D.H., in order to objectify the impression gathered from free conversation.

Another exceptional case of brain damage with mental retardation was reported by O'Connor and Hermelin (1991). The subject, Christopher, a 29-year-old, had a performance IQ of 67. He exhibited a good level ability in translating into English from three languages (French, German and Spanish), and in expressing himself in these languages (although to a different degree depending on the particular language). His comprehension of the lexicon and of the morphosyntactic structures of the three languages seemed quite satisfactory. The study of Christopher was taken further by Smith and Tsimpli (1995). It turned out, astonishingly, that he is able to translate from and communicate at least minimally in any of a number of languages: Danish, Dutch, Finnish, French, German, Greek, Hindi, Italian, Norwegian, Polish, Portuguese, Russian, Spanish, Turkish and Welsh. Little information is available on Christopher's personal history. He was late in walking and talking, but how late could not be ascertained. His fascination with foreign languages started when he was 6- or 7-years-old.

Christopher's case exemplifies the same dissociation between cognition and language as demonstrated in the other language exceptional cases. He has great linguistic ability in the presence of severe cognitive deficits. Smith and Tsimpli (1995) contend that his practice and knowledge of English is within the normal range, including complex metasyntactic judgements. However, Christopher's non-verbal cognition, particularly his visuospatial and computational abilities, are extremely poor. He fails on conservation of number tasks and is unable to match geometric shapes with representations of the same figures embedded in more complex designs. Christopher has a range of incompetencies that are sufficiently severe to necessitate his living in a sheltered community.

Christopher's case also illustrates some of the intralanguage dissociations observed in other cases of exceptional linguistic talent in MR subjects. On tests of production and judgement, he shows considerable direct transfer of specific structural principles from English. His multilingualism appears to be based primarily on a remarkable ability to acquire lexical entries in a number of languages, together with their morphological characteristics. This lexical ability is intriguing in view of Christopher's mental retardation and the relationship holding between lexical and cognitive functioning.

4.1.9 The cases reviewed in the preceding sections, including Françoise, reveal important dissociations between language components: phonology and morpho–syntax, on the one hand, semantics, lexicon, pragmatics and discourse organization, on the other. This dissociation corresponds to Chomsky's (1980) distinction between computational and conceptual aspects of language. It is also clear, in the exceptional cases presented, that the computational components function independently with respect to the severely limited non-verbal cognitive capacities exhibited.

4.2 Dissociative tendencies in typical mentally retarded subjects

A large number of data exist revealing delays in some aspects of language development in regular moderately and severely MR subjects that are greater than what can be predicted on the basis of MA. (See Fowler (1988) for a corresponding analysis concerned with DS subjects.) This has been referred to as the MA lag. It relates to the delay–difference problem in language development of MR subjects. A summary of a number of relevant data is found in Table 4.2.

As the data indicate, lexical, semantic structural and pragmatic developments in MR subjects follow with increased MA and/or MLU. The sole discrepancy reported between MA–matched MR and non-retarded (NR) subjects concerns word definition (a metalinguistic activity). But MR subjects lag behind MA– or MLU–matched NR subjects in aspects of phonological development and as to correct use of grammatical morphemes. Little difference appears in the simplest aspects of sentence comprehension and production. However, at corresponding MA or MLU levels, MR subjects present significant differences in more sophisticated aspects of syntax, such as the comprehension of function words; gender and number agreement; double object construction; passive comprehension; comprehension of temporal clauses and temporal relationship between clauses; reverse of order of subject and copula or auxiliary *be* in interrogative sentences; case and developmental level of personal and indefinite pronouns produced.

Table 4.2 Data on the delay-difference issue in moderately and severely mentally retarded children

Item	Linguistic aspect	Study	Matching variable	Subjects' CA in years (unless otherwise indicated)	Expression (E) or Comprehension (C)	Aetiology of retardation	Major result
			1. Babbling and phonological development				
1. Characteristic sounds of babbling; phonetic patterns and sequences of development.		Dodd (1972); Smith and Oller (1981)	CA CA	1 0–2	E E	V V	— —
2. Phonological aspects of (meaningful) speech (phoneme sub-stitutions and approximations in the articulation of *k*, *f* and θ).		Smith and Oller (1981)	CA	2–5	E	DS	—
3. Frequency of phonological errors made in picture naming and in elicited imitation.		Dodd (1976)	MA	6–15	E	V	NR > MR
4. Acoustical clarity and intelligibility of speech.		Ryan (1975); Rondal (1978a)	MLU MLU	5–19 3-12	E E	V DS	NR > MR NR > DS
			2. Lexical development				
5. Producing and understanding common object and action words.		Lyle (1961a)	MA	6–13	E; C	V	—
6. Understanding spatial words (e.g. *big, long, in, on, under*).		Cook (1977)	MA	3–6	C	DS	—
7. Understanding lexical items on the Carrow Auditory Test of Language Comprehension.		Bartel, Bryen and Keehn (1973)	MA	9–13	C	V	—
8. Basic vocabulary.		Mein and O'Connor (1960); Beier, Starkweather and	MA MA	10–30 11–24	E E	V V	— —

Table 4.2 (contd)

Item Linguistic aspect	Study	Matching variable	Subjects' CA in years (unless otherwise indicated)	Expression (E) or Comprehension (C)	Aetiology of retardation	Major result
	Lambert (1969); Lozar, Wepman and Hass (1972)	MA	5–15	E	V	—
9. Word definition.	Papania (1954)	MA	9–16	E	V	NR > MR
10. Responses on word association and word generalization tasks.	O'Connor and Hermelin (1959a);	MA	9–16	E	V	—
	O'Connor and Hermelin (1963);	MA	10–20	E	V	—
	Sersen et al. (1970)	MA	2–14	E	V	—
11. Type–token ratio (index of lexical diversity of speech).	Rondal (1978a);	MLU	3–12	E	DS	DS > NR
	Miller, Chapman and Mackensie (1981);	MA	1–7	E	V	MR > NR
	Harris (1983)	MLU	2–6	E	DS	DS > NR
12. Diversity of noun vocabulary.	Ryan (1975)	MLU	5–9	E	V	MR > NR
13. Beginning of word comprehension of familiar words of nursery rhymes.	Glenn and Cunningham (1982)	MA	9–15 months	C	DS ¿	—
14. Object name vocabularies.	Cardoso-Martins, Mervis and Mervis (1985)	MA	17–37 months	E; C	DS	—
15.Vocabulary size.	Dooley (1976)	MLU	3–5	E	DS	—
3. Semantic structural development						
16. Frequency and type of basic semantic relations.	Buium, Rynders and Turnure (1974a);	MLU	4	E	DS	—
	Coggins (1979);	MLU	1–6	E	DS	—
	Dooley (1976);	MLU	2–5	E	DS	—
	Rondal (1978a);	MLU	3–12	E	DS	—
	Layton and Sharifi (1979)	MLU	7–12	E	DS	—
17. Comprehension of basic semantic relations	Duchan and Erickson (1976)	MLU	4–8	C	V	—
4. Grammatical morphological development						
18. Use of familiar English inflections	Mueller and Weaver (1964);	MA	10–16	E	V	NR > MR

Item	Linguistic aspect	Study	Matching variable	Subjects' CA in years (unless otherwise indicated)	Expression (E) or Comprehension (C)	Aetiology of retardation	Major result
as assessed by the subtest Auditory-Vocal Automatic or Grammatical Closure of the Illinois Test of Psycholinguistic Abilities.		Bateman and Wetherell (1965); Bilovsky and Share (1965)	MA MA	6–12 9–16	E E	V DS	NR > MR NR > DS
19. Omission, substitution and incorrect generalization of grammatical inflections in free conversational speech.		Ryan (1975)	MLU	5–10	E	V	—

5. Syntactic development

Item	Linguistic aspect	Study	Matching variable	Subjects' CA in years	Expression (E) or Comprehension (C)	Aetiology of retardation	Major result
20. Change in relative proportions of types of words produced at early stages of language development.		Mein (1961)	CA	3–7	E	V	—
21. Progression through various stages of early language development (*mostly babble, mostly words, primitive phrases,* and *sentences*) with increasing CA.		Lenneberg, Nichols and Rosenberger (1964)	CA	3–22	E; C	DS	—
22. Progressive use of imperative, affirmative and negative active declarative, and interrogative sentences with increasing MA.		Lackner (1968); Gordon and Panagos (1976)	MA MA	2–9 3–5	E E	V DS	— —
23. Rank ordering of syntactic difficulties in a sentence comprehension task.		Mittler (1970b); Wheldall (1976)	MA EPPVT	8–12 9–15	C C	V V	— —
24. Comprehension of grammatical words, gender and number agreement, and double object construction.		Semmel and Dooley (1971); Bartel, Bryen, and Keehn (1973);	CA MA	6–14 9–13	C C	DS V	NR > DS NR > MR

Table 4.2 (contd)

Item	Linguistic aspect	Study	Matching variable	Subjects' CA in years (unless otherwise indicated)	Expression (E) or Comprehension (C)	Aetiology of retardation	Major result
25. Comprehension of affirmative active declarative sentences.		Semmel and Dooley (1971)	CA	6–14	C	DS	—
26. Comprehension of passive declarative sentences.		Semmel and Dooley (1971); Chipman (1979); Dewart (1979)	CA CA CA	6–14 8–15 7–18	C C C	DS O O	NR > DS — —
27. Comprehension of affirmative active declarative sentences including *ing* forms and possessive constructions.		Berry (1972)	EPPVT	10–16	C	V	—
28. Comprehension of temporal clauses and temporal relationships between clauses.		Barblan and Chipman (1978)	MA	6–10	C	V	NR>MR
29. Upper-bound (i.e. longest utterance in a corpus of speech).		Rondal (1978a)	MLU	3–12	E	DS	—
30. Number of modifiers per utterance.		Rondal (1978a)	MLU	3–12	E	DS	—
31. Incidence of utterances without verb.		Rondal (1978a)	MLU	3–12	E	DS	—
32. Productivity (number of words and utterances produced in a corpus of speech obtained in a given period of time).		Rondal (1978a)	MLU	3–12	E	DS	—
33. Proportions of imperative, declarative, WH-interrogative, and Yes–No interrogative sentences in a corpus of speech.		Rondal (1978c)	MLU	3–12	E	DS	—

Item	Linguistic aspect	Study	Matching variable	Subjects' CA in years (unless otherwise indicated)	Expression (E) or Comprehension (C)	Aetiology of retardation	Major result
34. Proportion of complete and incomplete sentences.		Ryan (1975)	MLU	5–9	E	V	—
35. Proportion of so-called *cliché* and *ready-made* utterances.		Ryan (1975)	MLU	5–9	E	V	—
36. Range and variety verb transformations.		Ryan (1975)	MLU	5–9	E	V	—
37. Word order.		Ryan (1975)	MLU	5–9	E	V	—
38. Word order in early combinatorial speech.		Dale (1977)	MLU	4–6	E	DS	—
39. Strategies used to identify agents and objects in basic strings received (chance performance, first, semantic-lexical strategies, second, and responses based on word order, third).		Dale (1977)	MLU	4–6	C	DS	—
40. Reversal of order of subject and copula or auxiliary verb *be* in interrogative sentences (Lee's Developmental Sentence Scoring Procedure, 1975).		Rondal (1978b)	MLU	5–12	E	DS	NR > DS
41. Frequency of use of elementary main verbs (i.e. uninflected verbs like *I see you*, copula like *it's red, is +* verb + *ing* like *He is coming, can, will may* + verb like *I can go*) (Developmental Sentence Scoring Procedure).		Rondal (1978b)	MLU	5–12	E	DS	DS > NR
42. Frequency of use of secondary verbs (i.e. complementing infinitives like *I wanna*		Rondal (1978b)	MLU	5–12	E	DS	NR > DS

Table 4.2 (contd)

Item	Linguistic aspect	Study	Matching variable	Subjects' CA in years (unless otherwise indicated)	Expression (E) or Comprehension (C)	Aetiology of retardation	Major result
	see, I'm gonna see, non-complementing infinitives like *I stopped to play*, complementing present and past participles like *I see a boy running, I found the toy broken*) (Developmental Sentence Scoring Procedure).						
43.	Proportion of sentences that are grammatically correct in every respect (Developmental Sentence Scoring Procedure).	Rondal (1978b)	MLU	5–12	E	DS	DS > NR
44.	Frequency and type of indefinite pronouns (Developmental Sentence Scoring Procedure).	Rondal (1978b)	MLU	5–12	E	DS	NR>DS
45.	Developmental level of personal pronouns used (Developmental Sentence Scoring Procedure).	Dale (1977)	MLU	4–6	E	DS	NR>DS
46.	Proportion of erroneous but progressive forms (e.g. *I want go*).	Dale (1977)	MLU	4–6	E	DS	NR>DS
	6. Pragmatic development						
47.	Illocutionary devices.	Rondal (1978a)	MLU	3–12	E	DS	—
48.	Conversational skills.	Leifer and Lewis (1983)	CA	18–23 months	DS	NR > DS	
			MLU	3–5	DS	DS > NR	
	- double matching procedure -						
49.	Non-verbal response to action requests	Scherer and Owings (1984)	MLU	5–7	DS	—	

Item	Linguistic aspect	Study	Matching variable	Subjects' CA in years (unless otherwise indicated)	Expression (E) or Comprehension (C)	Aetiology of retardation	Major result
50. Production of clarification requests in uninformative extralinguistic contexts.		Abbeduto et al. (1991)	MA	9-10	E	O	NR>MR

Notes: CA: chronological age; MA: mental age; MLU: mean length of utterances (in number of words plus grammatical morphemes); EPPVT: English Peabody Picture Vocabulary Test; V: mentally retarded subjects of various aetiologies including Down's syndrome; DS: Down's syndrome subjects; O: mentally retarded subjects of other aetiology(ies) than Down syndrome;–: no significant difference between MR and NR subjects; x > y: significant difference in favour of x, whereby x and y are NR, MR, or DS subjects; * indicates an utterance that is ungrammatical.

From the preceding data, it may be concluded that if the language problems of MR subjects reflect their cognitive limitations, general cognitive level per se (as captured in the MA measures, for example) is not a satisfactory explanation for language functioning in these subjects when it comes to advanced phonological, grammatical morphological and syntactic aspects of language. It is our opinion that these discrepancies between components of the language system, and between general cognitive level and the phonological and the grammatical aspects of language in the typical MR subjects, reveal the same dissociative trends as those exemplified in the exceptional cases of language development in MR subjects reviewed above. The interesting difference between the two sets of observation is that, with respect to the relationship between language and general cognition, the dissociations go in opposite directions for the typical and the exceptional MR subjects. The former subjects have lower phonological and grammatical levels from what can be expected on a MA and/or a MLU basis while the converse is true for the latter.

4.3 The delay–difference question

As said above, data regarding the existence of dissociative tendencies in typical mental retardates concerning components of the language organization also relate to the delay–difference question in language development of MR subjects. This question has enjoyed some popularity in the last three decades. Adapting from the problem set for mental retardation at large by Ellis (1963) and Zigler (1966), one has asked whether language development in MR children is 'simply' delayed and only quantitatively different from language development in NR children, or whether it is qualitatively different (see Yoder and Miller, 1972; Rosenberg, 1982; Rondal, 1984, 1985a, 1987b, 1988a, 1988b; and Cromer, 1988, 1991; for detailed analyses).

There are caveats in the way the question is usually set:

(1) No complete dichotomy exists between delay and difference. A simple answer to the question largely depends on whether one considers language as a whole, or separate components of it. Imagine an MR child who is acquiring one aspect of language, say lexicon, in the normal although moderately delayed sequence while another aspect of language, for example expressive syntax, is also being acquired in the normal sequence but is markedly delayed. The answer to the delay–difference question is delay for the two aspects considered separately. However, language development as a whole may be regarded as different. Indeed suppose our retarded child is a 7–year–old, and he is, say, at the 5–year level for lexicon and at the 3–year level for syntax. That does not make him equivalent to any younger NR child. Whenever there is varying degree of delay in several aspects of language, there is a difference with respect to language as a whole. It is essential, therefore, to establish for each language component considered separately whether development proceeds similarly in MR and NR individuals. 'Similarly' means that the development stages passed by the MR and NR subjects are the same and follow each other in the same order. If so, components of language in the retarded might rightly be said to be simply delayed.

(2) The delay position predicts that language development in the retarded will come to a stop before reaching its final stage. It is conceivable that one could distinguish between incomplete and different developments. However, no study known to us has addressed the issue. We are unable in practice to indicate whether some of the differences observed between NR and MR individuals should be better interpreted as evidence for a difference position or whether they demonstrate a development arrested at an earlier but normal stage.

(3) The label 'mental retardation' covers a number of aetiological categories. There is no guarantee that the linguistic problems are similar in all categories. In Chapter 3, we have documented a number of syndrome differences in language, based on a limited number of studies performed recently. The delay–difference issue must be raised separately for the various MR syndromes.

(4) The final answer to the delay–difference question will have to be based on extensive longitudinal data. There is still a marked lack of large–scale longitudinal studies on the language development of MR children.

Three types of matching procedures have been used in comparing speech and language in MR and NR children. (1) *The CA–match*: studies using a CA–match reveal large gaps between MR and NR children. They are helpful with respect to the delay–difference question only in so far as the data obtained with the MR subjects can be compared to corresponding data on younger NR children. Otherwise these studies will only confirm that the MR subjects are indeed retarded, but they will not suffice to document interesting questions regarding the developmental process (Cicchetti and Pogge–Hesse, 1982). (2) *The MA–match*: matching children for MA should guarantee that they function cognitively at similar levels. If it can be shown that MR children differ linguistically from MA–matched NR children, this is considered to be supportive for a difference hypothesis. If this is not the case, one considers that a delay hypothesis is supported. The assumption that matching subjects on MA guarantees that they are cognitively equivalent has been questioned (Baumeister, 1967; Milgram, 1973). There is no one–to–one correspondence between IQ, MA scores and response patterns to test items. The same IQ can be obtained in different ways. It follows that one can never be fully confident that MA–matched children function exactly at corresponding cognitive levels. (3) *The LL–match*: Another strategy is to match subjects for linguistic level. One may use mean length of utterance as the criterion variable and look at various characteristics of the language used by the subjects. With this type of matching, both the criterion and the dependent variable pertain to the language domain. The rationale behind this LL–procedure is as follows: if NR and MR individuals matched on linguistic aspect X (disregarding other parameters like CA or MA), can be shown to be similar with respect to aspects A, B, ..., of the language system, it may be assumed that this system is structured in the same way in the two groups of subjects. This is consistent with a delay position and antithetical to a difference position.

The resulting picture (see Table 4.2) is complex. A strict delay position only captures relatively trivial aspects of the language problem of MR individuals. Language development in the mentally retarded is not a slow motion picture of the same development in NR children, even if it is correct to say that referential lexical, semantic and pragmatic developments follow regularly with the evolution in MA, and that the sequences of acquisition as to basic aspects of phonological, grammatical morphological and syntactic developments are the same as in NR children. However, differences between MR and NR subjects are apparent with the gradual unfolding of the acquisition process, particularly as to phonology and morpho–syntax (but not in all syndromes and not to the same degree in all syndromes, as documented in Chapter 3). These differences tend to deepen along with the various developmental plateaux affecting the course of language acquisition in MR subjects (see Fowler, 1988, 1990), until this development, still incomplete in many respects, eventually comes to a stop. In view of the above, and as argued in more detail in Rondal (1988a), it may be suggested that the delay–difference framework is not fully appropriate for characterizing language development and functioning in MR. A strict delay–difference dichotomy is even likely to be misleading.

4.4 The cognition–language question

The above data, and particularly the data on the language exceptional MR subjects, have important implications for theories regarding the relationship between language and non-language cognition, for contemporary theorizing concerning modular and non-modular accounts of the higher mental functions and the functional architecture of mind, as well as for discussing the internal organization of the language system.

4.4.1 Piaget's position

Probably the boldest case for the existence of direct causal relationships between cognitive development and language development is found in the position of Piaget and followers. Piaget (1945, 1970, 1976, 1979a, 1979b; see also Furth, 1969) claims that the capacity to represent depends on the same knowledge structure permitting the construction of the known object. The representative capacity gradually emerges in the second half of the sensorimotor intellectual period (between approximately 12 and 18 months). It first manifests itself in the child's symbolic play and mental imagery. Language is just one product of this representational function. It follows that lexical and semantic developments depend on cognitive development. Most people agree that language encodes particular concepts, and this is not controversial. However, the Piagetian hypothesis stipulates not only that language is dependent on thought for its meaning contents, but also that particular (non-linguistic) cognitive structures and processes are causally involved in the acquisition of the grammatical system. In other words, Piaget insists that grammar is not autonomous and that the general conceptual system of mind underlies as much the morphosyntactic as the lexico–semantic aspects of language.

Empirical studies with normally developing children have yielded little clear support for Piaget's position on the cognition–language issue. General mental development precedes or is contemporaneous with early lexical and semantic developments. Children's holophrases, for example, entail meanings that correspond to what Piaget (1945) called 'action schemes'. Sinclair (1970, 1973) and Edwards (1973) showed that basic thematic categories in language present convergences with complex action schemes developed by children in the course of the later sensorimotor period. It may be indeed that the action schemes studied by the Piagetians constitute an important part of the common world knowledge on which basic semantic structures are constructed. Other researchers demonstrate that specific thought contents have to be mastered for the child to understand and use appropriately linguistic structures involving these contents. For example, Ferreiro's work (1971) shows that children make significant progress in the understanding of temporal clauses in proportion with their related cognitive evolution. In particular, they have difficulties decoding temporal clauses in which the verbalized order of the events does not match the order of events in reality (e.g. *Before having breakfast, he shaved* vs *He shaved before having breakfast*).

Bronckart (1976) observed that the first verbal inflections in children have an aspectual rather than a genuine temporal character. Related to this observation may be the fact that in cognitive development the child first concentrates on the states and results of the actions before being able to take into account physical transformations. Therefore, the content aspects of language are in relation to and may develop from non-language cognition. However, when it comes to specific relationships between cognitive structures and processes and particulars of grammatical development, things are different. On the basis of the observation that early semantic relations are related to sensorimotor schemes, Sinclair (1971) claimed, without empirical evidence, that action patterns are a *necessary* condition for the acquisition of syntax. This type of extrapolation does not follow. Moreover, it is contradicted by observations showing that children with severe congenital motor problems do not necessarily have difficulties in grammatical development, nor even in intellectual development, as was first observed by Lenneberg (1967). (See Mehler and Dupoux, 1990 for corresponding arguments along the same line of reasoning).

Inhelder (1968) suggested that children overcome their inversion difficulty with non-canonical temporal clauses around 7 years of age, the time at which they have access to the concrete operational level of thinking and, therefore, are able to reverse actions. This argument is highly doubtful. Ferreiro (1971) reports that until 8 or 9 years, that is well into the concrete operational stage, children do not correctly understand temporal clauses, the sequential order of which does not match the order of events.

A similar situation prevails with passive sentences. Sinclair and Ferreiro (1970) (see also Sinclair, Sinclair and de Marcellus, 1971) postulate the intervention of a general cognitive factor. This is logical decentration, or the ability to view an event from different perspectives, which is tied to reversibility and the concrete operational stage. This might explain children's evolution in passive sentence comprehension, which extends beyond the specific morphosyntactic and discursive–pragmatic characteristics of the passive forms. Again, the acquisition ages do not correspond. Non-reversible passives are correctly understood by children at 3 or 4 years of age (Beilin and Sack, 1975). But children do not need to analyse such sentences syntactically in order to extract their meaning. Lexical and semantic knowledge is sufficient. Full reversible passives are not correctly understood before approximately 9 years, again well into the postulated operational stage. See, Cromer (1988,

1991) for reviews of additional studies and discussions along similar lines.

Even assuming that one could find strong data showing convincingly the co–occurrence of grammatical and cognitive acquisitions, one would still be left with simple correlations allowing diverse causal hypotheses. Experimental analyses of factors involved in determining the course of human development are notoriously hard to come by and many experiments by design cannot be realized for ethical reasons. Pathological cases are instructive. In aphasic patients, for example, there is no clear relation between intellectual dysfunction and gravity of language disorder. Many subjects with grossly abnormal grammatical abilities exhibit little generalized intellectual difficulties (see Marshall, 1990). Mental retardation offers natural experimental situations for studying the relationship between cognitive and language development. In this respect, the available data do not support the Piagetian cognition hypothesis either. For example, in a study by Kahn (1975), several MR subjects with combinatorial language were functioning cognitively at the Piagetian sensorimotor stage VI (sometimes referred to as a 'prerequisite' for access at the level of syntax), but several other subjects were not and they could be shown to produce correctly patterned multi–word utterances. Several similar 'exceptions' had already been signalled by Woodward and Stern (1963); others have been documented by Smith and Von Tetzchner (1986). Data of this type constitute strong evidence against any theoretical position claiming that specific structural cognitive developments are necessary conditions for particular advances in grammatical development.

But, undoubtedly, the most damaging blow to the Piagetian cognition–language hypothesis is caused by the observations of exceptional cases of grammatical development in moderately and severely MR subjects, as summarized in the preceding sections. We do not see how the Piagetian position could account *in principle* for the facts uncovered in the language exceptional cases studied, as well as, although to a lesser extent, the corresponding dissociative tendencies exemplified in regular MR subjects. Given that the Piagetian position is not otherwise supported by strong unequivocal data on cognitive and language developments in NR children, one can conclude that it has been empirically falsified. Let us stress that what has been proved false is not the existence of a cognitive basis for some aspects of language (the conceptual aspects), there is convincing empirical litterature supporting this notion, *but the idea that grammatical regulations deductively follow from cognitive regulations*. It can be argued, however, that a minimal level of cognitive–semantic development is necessary to trigger an otherwise autonomous grammatical development. In other words, cognitive concepts underlying semantic entities may bear a trigger relation, perhaps indirectly through semantic categories, to grammatical entities

(Chomsky, 1981; Roeper, 1987; Finer and Roeper, 1989). Trigger is used here in a biological sense for releasing mechanism, i.e. a 'brute–causal' mechanism not bearing a deductive relation to the thing triggered. Such a proposal sails far beyond the Piagetian suggestion regarding the necessary relationship between grammatical and operatory developments.

There may be some interesting ground for the semantic triggering hypothesis if one considers the late onset of combinatorial language development reported for Françoise and Laura, two of the language–exceptional MR subjects referred to above. Unfortunately, no specific information is available on the other exceptional cases in this respect. Françoise's onset of grammatical language was about 41/2 years. Laura is reported by Yamada (1990) as having been linguistically delayed from early on. No further information is given, except that around 5 years, she had already developed her language substantially. The delays in the onset of grammatical development in Françoise and Laura may be related to the additional time that is necessary for MR subject due to their maturational and cognitive retardation, to build the semantic basis from which triggering of the grammatical system may take place (when there is something to be triggered, which is probably not the case, or much less for the regular MR subjects). As reported in Chapter 3, Bellugi, Wang, and Jernigan (1993; see also Neville, Mills and Bellugi, 1993) observed that the languages of WS and regular DS subjects are formally equivalent at younger ages. This is in contrast with the language levels exhibited by many WS adolescents. The above observations converge in suggesting that one has to reach a baseline in cognitive–semantic ability, roughly equivalent to that of an NR child of about 2 years, for a preserved morphosyntactic system to start functioning properly.

4.4.2 Other cognitive approaches

An interesting question is whether the MR data summarized above cast a sceptical slant on other theoretical frameworks also assuming that 'cognition drives language' or more precisely that 'cognition drives grammar'. A number of accounts of language development and functioning, other than Piagetian, may be regrouped under a loose 'cognitive' label. Langacker's (1987) so–called cognitive grammar incorporates some of Piaget's beliefs. For example, the ideas that grammar is not a separate mental function and that semantics, itself based on non-linguistic cognition, is the fundamental feature of language rather than syntax. A defining characteristics of several lines of work often grouped in the 'cognitive approach' category (Slobin, 1973; Karmiloff–Smith, 1979; Maratsos and Chalkley, 1981; Bates and MacWhinney, 1987; MacWhinney, 1987; Bates, Bretherton and Snyder, 1988) is an effort to explain language development in terms of underlying cognitive mechanisms shared with other cognitive domains.

Most of these approaches acknowledge linguistic categories as useful tools, but do not consider them as domain–specific and innate primitives determining the course of development. Rather, they support the possibility that cognitive abilities such as those underlying concept formation and information–processing skills, largely contribute to the development of language including the development of grammatical categories. Some cognitive models make the hypothesis that linguistic categories are acquired through learning processes which are probabilistic in nature. Maratsos and Chalkley (1981), for example, proposed 'correlational bootstrapping' as a solution to the question of how the child gets a proper start in forming the correct type of morphosyntactic rules for his language. They assumed that the child analyses distributional properties of the language input, such as serial position of the words, inflections, and, in so doing, constructs his grammatical categories. See Pinker, (1987), for major logical and empirical arguments against this suggestion; e.g. the impracticability given the number of noticeable distributional properties that the child could attend to and the existence of many linguistically relevant properties that are not perceptually marked in the input.

Bates and MacWhinney (1987), and MacWhinney (1987), in their competition model, also assume that distributional regularities (or 'cues') available in children's input play a major role in language learning. As this model has been more elaborated theoretically than other cognitive approaches to language development, let us consider it in some more detail. The model is presented as a 'neo–Tolmanian' functionalist approach to the acquisition of grammar; a model which refuses to separate form and function and avoids making innatist assumptions as far as possible. It has two major distinguishing features: (1) 'lexicality', i.e. it assumes that grammatical knowledge is represented by connections in the lexicon; (2) *competitiveness*, i.e. lexical items are viewed as competing with each other during comprehension and production (e.g. competition of nouns for grammatical roles). Learning is considered to take place through the shaping of connections between lexical items on the basis of positive instances from language input.

The competition model may be viewed from the language pathology perspective through the lexical, cognitive principles and the analyses involved. The insertion of grammatical knowledge in the lexicon of the language does not render the task of the regular MR child easier, nor does it help explain the remarkable grammatical levels reached by the exceptional MR subjects. As indicated previously, lexical development, on the whole, is not particularly outstanding in these subjects. It parallels their conceptual levels more closely than their morphosyntactic abilities. The competition model also uses a set of cognitive principles assumed to provide the learner with the tools necessary to achieve input–sensitive language learning. These principles are as follows: first, the *representational principles* emphasizing the importance of the lexicon as an organizer of language knowledge (syntactic as well as semantic), and corresponding to the lexical dimension of the model, as indicated above. Second, the *processing principles* emphasizing the ways in which lexical items compete with each other during language comprehension and production. Third, the *learning principles* working to isolate lexical items and shape connections between them and their properties. Equipped with such principles, the language–learner will attempt to map forms and functions (i.e. 'vertical correlations') in language comprehension and production.

Major predictive constructs in the competition model are cue validity and cue strength. Cue validity is defined as the product of cue availability (i.e. how often a piece of information is offered during a decision-making process) times cue reliability (i.e. how often a cue leads to a correct conclusion when used). For example, Italian (or Spanish), as opposed to English (or German), is a 'pro–drop' or a 'null–subject' language (i.e. a language in which it is accepted and common to omit lexical subjects). As a result, the most frequent form in Italian discourse (particularly in informal speech) is not Subject–Verb–Object (SVO), as is the case in English, but (S)VO or O(S)V. Given this combination of variation of word order plus pro–drop, the cue validity of word order or pre– and post–verbal position for identifying grammatical subject and object is not high in Italian, whereas it is very high in English. Cue validity is a property of the language. Cue strength is a subjective property of the learner and language user. It is 'the probability or weight that the organism attaches to a given piece of information relative to some goal' (Bates and MacWhinney, 1987, p. 164). Cue validity partially determines cue strength. Another important feature of cue strength has to do with task frequency. Bates and MacWhinney (1987) also consider so–called horizontal correlations in language, i.e. relationships between forms themselves and relationships between functions. In so doing, they seek to integrate the correlational type of grammatical learning proposed by Maratsos and Chalkley (1981)and Maratsos (1982) in their functionalist theory. In Bates and MacWhinney's view, however, the child does not have to consider all possible correlations between all items in all sentences in acquiring accurate sets of form–form correlations. Rather, the child is guided by semantic connections and positional patterning in acquiring these correlations.

The above presentation, no matter how sketchy, is sufficient to illustrate the ubiquity of the cognitive principles and cognitively–based analyses needed in grammar acquisition according to the competition model. This is the reverse of Lasnik's claim (1989, p. 102), that the less structure the language acquisition device of the developing organism has, the more data of all sorts and the more cognitive work to treat these data are needed. It is easy to understand why regular moderately and severely MR subjects fail to develop adequate grammar according to the competition model, as they have difficulties with the type of cognitive tasks demanded by such models (e.g. drastic limitation of working memory, attention problems, poor organization of semantic memory, retrieval difficulties, etc.). The language–exceptional MR subjects mentioned in preceding sections have the same cognitive limitations as regular MR subjects. However, they develop sophisticated, at times quasi–normal or normal language abilities, particularly grammatical abilities. The conclusion is that the competition model, inasmuch as it relies heavily on general cognitive principles, can account for the exceptional cases of language development documented in MR subjects no more than the Piagetian model, or any other cognition–drives–grammar model. Any model postulating too important a cognitive basis for grammatical development is seriously challenged by cases of exceptional development in these subjects.

4.4.3 Grammatical predispositions

As indicated above, the data on exceptional cases of grammatical development in MR subjects support the Chomskyan thesis of the autonomy of grammar. One of us has argued elsewhere (see Rondal, 1995a; also, for corresponding opinions, Curtiss, 1988; Yamada, 1990) that these data also constitute strong arguments in favour of the hypothesis of the existence in human beings *qua* human beings (including MR subjects) of innate predispositions towards developing sophisticated grammatical systems. It is reasonable to assume that the genetic programmes relevant to grammatical development have been realized, at least partially, in the cases of the language–exceptional MR subjects studied, whereas they have been prevented from being carried out in regular MR individuals for reasons unknown at the present time, but that probably concern the anomalies in early brain development characteristic of typical moderate and severe mental retardation.

One can only speculate about these reasons in the present state of knowledge regarding human genetics and brain development. For example, some of the serious problems affecting brain growth in DS have begun to be better known (Ross, Galaburda and Kemper, 1984; Wisniewski et al., 1986; Epstein, 1986, 1987; Nadel, 1986; Lott, 1986; Wisniewski, 1990; Becker et al., 1991; Wisniewski and Kida, 1994; see Wisniewski, Kida and Brown, in press, for a review), particularly, the existence of an abnormal morphogenesis of brain tissue early in gestation and a severe neuronal reduction focused on granule cells in several cortical areas (temporal, parietal and occipital lobes; cerebellum; hippocampal formation). Brain weight is significantly reduced (10–50 per cent lower than in individuals without DS) particularly in the cerebellum and brain stem (Crome and Stern, 1967). There is reduction in neuron density in a number of brain areas including the hypothalamus, decreased synaptic density, decreased presynaptic length, decreased average surface area per synaptic contact, and anomalies in synaptic morphology. Myelination of nerve fibres is delayed. Neurotransmitter abnormalities (e.g. serotonin, noradrenaline) have been signalled (e.g. Florez et al., 1990). Early structural alterations caused by biochemical imbalances at critical periods of brain maturation, associated with the overexpression of some genes in the band 21p22 of chromosome 21, and therefore excess gene product, have been noted. A convincing suggestion is that DS results in arrested maturation of neurons and synapses some time around birth. Rather than a uniform abnormality in all instances, differences may exist in terms of the proportion of DS individuals who show abnormal values. One may predict that a premature arrest or a marked slowing–down of brain development will affect more late–maturing neural subsystems (e.g. the hippocampus structures) (Sylvester, 1983; Scheibel, 1984; Nadel, 1986; see also Uecker et al., 1993; and Nadel, in press). Postnatal brain growth in NR individuals is quite remarkable and long-lasting (for example, the human brain more than triples its weight between birth and 18 years; Purves, 1994). Major psychobiological problems in DS could reflect primarily the distortions in relatively late developing mental systems, due to the premature arrest in neuron and synapse formation, the overall neural reduction, and the structural alterations and biological imbalances determined by excess gene product. At this stage, it could be suggested that genetically coded phonological and grammatical information, corresponding to 'late' developing mental systems (according to the time scale envisaged in this discussion), will not be realized phenotypically in typical MR cases because of early developmental anomalies in some brain areas. Speculating from suggestions by Damasio and Damasio (1989, 1992), these areas coud be the posterior perisylvian sector of the left cerebral hemisphere, including the basal ganglia, with particular respect to processing of speech sounds, phoneme assembly into words and selection of entire word forms; the anterior perisylvian sector of the left hemisphere, including the basal ganglia, with respect to receptive and expressive morpho–syntax. Stowe et al.'s (1994) review of PET scan (positron emission tomography) studies of language points to the involvement of the left cerebral hemisphere extrastriate cortex and superior temporal cortex in lexical access; Brodmann's areas 41, 42, and mid-Brodmann's 22, in phonological processing; superior temporal cortex in syntactic processing; and the inferior frontal gyrus, the mid and inferior temporal gyri, Brodmann's area 8 and the temporal poles, in story comprehension. These neuroanatomical indications are preliminary in the present state of knowledge. However, the imaging technologies currently developed promise rapid advances in this domain (see Posner and Raichle, 1994).

There have been relatively few functional studies of brain function in DS individuals so far. Devinsky et al. (1990) reported normal EEG activity in young DS adults, but McAlaster (1992) signalled abnormal development of EEG profiles in DS subjects. Schapiro, Haxby and Grady (1992), using positron emission tomography, reported a disruption of normal neuronal interactions between the frontal and parietal lobes, possibly including the language area of Broca.

A general mechanism for aberrant brain development has been suggested (see Wisniewski, Kida and Brown, in press). It has been found that genetic programming of development in vertebrates occurs under the control of master genes named homeobox. Some of the genes on chromosome 21 could be homeobox or homeobox modifier genes. Their imbalance could result in abnormal brain development.

4.5 Language modularity

4.5.1 The data presented in preceding sections are interesting dissociations between language and non-language cognition as well as within the language system itself. Theoretical as well as empirical work in linguistics, psycholinguistics and patholinguistics, over the last decades, has led to a reconceptualization of the very notion of language. It is being recognized that language is a system with a number of integrated parts. Current PET studies provide evidence for physiological modules in language processing (Stowe et al., 1994). It may be that language normality has the general effect, or is the result of the effect, of 'holding the various language components tightly together' with the consequence that 'from the outside' they appear more united than they really are. In other words, language components interact with each other in language functioning, but they are not intrinsically united, as the dissociations brought about by pathological processes demonstrate. It may be appropriate to call this 'federal'[1] system 'language'. The intricacies of functioning have to do with the particular nature of the individual components, their modus operandi, and the ways along which they interact with each other. Unfortunately, little is known about the functional interactions between language components.

The detailed nature of the language organization may be modular (Fodor, 1983) and the mind may be organized according to basic modularity principles (Chomsky, 1984). However, no generally accepted definition of modularity exists today. Examples of the debate may be found in Fodor (1983), numerous individual contributions to the *Précis of the modularity of mind* (collective, 1985), books edited by Garfield (1987) and Mattingly and Studdert–Kennedy (1991), and a chapter by Moscovitch and Umilta (1990).

One can probably define modularity as the characteristics of an

---

[1] Faced with the comparable task of defining basic brain organization, Charcot (1893, pp. 3–4) resorted to the French expression *'fédération'* of organs with distinct properties and functions.

organic system in which constitutive parts, although interacting with each other in several ways, are special–purpose devices dedicated to particular tasks. These devices retain a fair amount of autonomy, present differentiated developmental timetables, as well as particular lines along which deteriorations take place in pathological cases. Additional characteristics of modular systems have been proposed (e.g. Fodor, 1983; Moscovitch and Umilta, 1990) and discussed in the specialized literature, although no consensus has been reached so far as to their number, exact definition and field of application (such as innate specification, informational encapsulation, domain specificity, mandatory modus operandi, limited central access to the representations computed by the modules, hard–wired fixed neural architectures, and computational autonomy).

4.5.2. In Chomsky's writings (e.g. Chomsky, 1979, 1980, 1981, 1982, 1984), the notion of language modularity has two extensions. There is postulated modularity within grammatical theory itself (i.e. internal modularity) to the extent that the subtheories of universal grammar (the binding theory, the government theory, the case theory, etc.) are considered to be distinct but interacting subgrammars, each one with its particular principles and functional rules (see Rizzi, 1985 and Grodzinsky, 1984, 1986, 1990 for theoretical and empirical indications supporting such a hypothesis). There is also modularity in a second sense (external modularity). We are more particularly concerned with this second type of modularity here, i.e. the indication that components or processing levels of the linguistic system (i.e. phonology, lexicon, semantics, morpho–syntax and pragmatics) are relatively autonomous in terms of functional organization and, possibly, in terms of organic substratum and architecture. They are among the so–called vertical faculties with particular kinds of content or data types, discussed by Fodor (1983). These modularity considerations predict dissociations corresponding to the levels of analysis identified. Such dissociations can be documented in pathological cases.

4.5.3 Section 4.1 has supplied some empirical support for the notion of a fair degree of informational encapsulation holding true for phonological and morphosyntactic functioning in language–exceptional MR subjects. A corresponding dissociation between phonological and morphosyntactic abilities, on the one side, and cognitive functioning, on the other, exists in children with specific language impairment (SLI), although this type of child shows the reverse pattern to the MR child. For extensive studies of the phonological and morphosyntactic problems of SLI children, the reader is referred to the works of Leonard (1985, 1992), Leonard and Brown (1984), Leonard et al. (1987), Johnston (1988), Gopnik (1990a) and Clahsen, Rothweiler and Woest (1992). The incidence of unusual phonological characteristics in these children is significantly higher than in young normal children. The language errors typical of SLI children include inaccurate use of morphological and syntactic features such as the proper marking of number, gender, tense and aspect, and the frequent omission of pronouns, particularly subject pronouns before tensed verbs. These errors show up in spontaneous speech, writing, repetition and grammaticality judgement. As the deficits are apparent in all aspects of language, their roots most probably lie in the underlying grammatical system rather than in peripheral processing or in subsystems associated with language processing. Some of these problems appear to have an inherited component. They seem to follow the pattern of a dominant fully penetrant autosomal gene (see Tomblin, 1989; Gopnik, 1990a, 1990b; Hurst et al., 1990). This incidentally constitutes an interesting indication that some aspects of grammar acquisition are genetically based. The SLI children, by definition, have normal or normal–like non-verbal intellectual capacities. There is no reason, therefore, to believe that their grammatical impairment is secondary to conceptual deficit (Marshall, 1990).

If the data on language–exceptional MR subjects and SLI children are considered together, they demonstrate the existence of a double dissociation between morpho–syntax and general cognition: i.e. advanced morpho–syntax and restricted cognitive development, in the language–exceptional MR subjects; morphosyntactic difficulties and normal cognitive development, in SLI children. Such a double dissociation across syndromes constitutes a strong argument in support of the separability of the two functions with respect to each other (Shallice, 1988). It is fair to mention, however, that some authors are of the opinion that a double dissociation is not logically sufficient to demonstrate the independence of two functions (see Caramazza, 1986, for a discussion). The data gathered by Gopnik and others regarding a possible inheritance of some morphosyntactic difficulties in SLI subjects may suggest the existence of diverging evolutionary constraints on grammar and other cognitive functions, thus reinforcing the dissociation case.

4.5.4 Dissociations between particular components of the language system itself can be documented. Casual observation of NR children and adults show that articulatory and grammatical abilities are independent of each other. It is well known that some people, although exhibiting excellent grammatical capacities, have functional or organic articulatory difficulties. Stuttering coexists with intact morphosyntactic as well as lexical or pragmatic abilities. Anarthria in its pure form may occur without any other language pathology in people with particular cerebral lesions (Hecaen and Albert, 1978). Conversely, receptive aphasias exhibit comprehension and production difficulties, including grammatical problems, without (major) articulatory disorders. The alleged independence of articulation from other language components implies that the observation that all the language–exceptional MR individuals studied so far have normal articulatory skills is coincidental. There could be language–exceptional MR persons with impaired articulation. Actually, such cases have been described (see Lebrun and Van Borsel, 1991; Van Borsel, 1991). These authors report the case of a DS adolescent with marked articulatory deficiencies (e.g. slurred articulation, phoneme substitutions and deletions) and stuttering symptoms. This subject exhibited a non-trivial degree of grammatical competence as demonstrated in her spontaneous speech. She had the correct use of inflectional affixes on nouns and verbs, the production of grammatically correct declarative and interrogative sentences and she could produce some compound sentences.

The existence of dissociations between grammatical and pragmatic competence is attested in the cases of Antony, Rick and Laura (see above). John, a possible case of 'minimal cerebral dysfunction', reported by Blank, Gessner and Esposito (1978), illustrates the possibility of a dissociation between semantics and pragmatics. This subject demonstrated age–appropriate language functioning in terms of grammar and semantics, but he was restricted in the use of these systems in interpersonal communication. He could not answer questions with relevant statements nor follow on the interlocutor's discourse in regular conversations. His attempts at initiating verbal exchanges were bizarre and mostly devoid of the usual pragmatic conventions. Corresponding dissociations between grammatical and semantic/or pragmatic abilities have often been reported in young schizophrenic and autistic children. Features of 'non-communicative language' in these subjects were noted by Kanner (1943). Such children tend not to develop combinatorial language beyond the rudimentary stages (Leblanc and Page, 1989). Their language typically is characterized by a mixture of grammatical utterances, jargon with neologisms, non-grammatical fragments, and verbatim imitations or echolalia (Despert, 1968; Shapiro, Roberts and Fish, 1970). Their difficulties with the appropriate use of personal pronouns and, more generally, with deictics have often been noted (Fay and Schuler, 1980; Rosenbaum and Sonne, 1986). It is generally accepted that autism involves a primary deficit in pragmatics (see Tager–Flusberg, 1981, 1985a, b), which may be related to a corresponding inability in non-verbal communication (Fay and Schuler, 1980). Recent work by Tager–Flusberg (1994) confirms and extends previous indications that autistic children are not usually impaired in their grammatical development. There is no deviance in the order or in the process of development in the domains of syntax and grammatical morphology. But the social deficits characteristic of autism, particularly the paucity of joint attention, limited empathy and difficulties in reciprocal social interactions, have a marked impact on the development of communicative, pragmatic and functional aspects of language.

Cromer (1988) suggested the possibility of a dissociation between grammatical morphology and syntax in language–exceptional MR subjects. He seems to have based his suggestion on the case of Curtiss's

Rick (see above). Curtiss (1988, 1989) and Yamada (1990) have indeed reported occasional difficulties with grammatical morphemes (for example, errors in gender marking on pronouns), not only for Rick, but also for Antony and Laura. However, these problems were not major ones for Curtiss and Yamada's subjects, and they do not qualify as evidence for the generality of these features. Such dissociations between grammatical morphology (or aspects of it) and syntax have been documented in the aphasia literature, however. In cases of agrammatic aphasia (e.g. constructional agrammatism), phrase structure is considerably altered, but grammatical morphology is preserved (Tissot, Mounin and Lhermitte, 1973). In other types of agrammatic aphasia, grammatical morphology is seriously impaired or even largely missing, but basic word order and elementary syntactic constructions are preserved (Grodzinsky, 1990). SLI children most often exhibit serious and selective impairment in the use of grammatical morphemes, particularly verb inflections and such function words as auxiliaries and articles. But it would seem that they also regularly show a moderate deficit in a range of other language areas including syntax (Frome–Loeb and Leonard, 1988). Clahsen (1989), however, claims that SLI children have specific problems with the morphological categorization of verbal elements as well as with building up agreement paradigms, but not so much with the acquisition and use of syntactic rules. Along this line, some reported syntactic difficulties in SLI children (e.g. problems with verb–placement patterns in German) could perhaps be regarded as secondary to the SLI children's problems with morphological categorization.

4.5.5 The neuropsychological study of regular (i.e. non-progressive) aphasias and primary degenerative diseases also offers interesting hints as to the existence of possible modular entities in the organization of the higher mental functions, and particularly of the language system. In agrammatic aphasia, subjects are unable (to a variety of degrees depending on particular cases) to organize grammatically their verbal productions and to assign grammatical rules to lexical items in sentences. As alluded to above, agrammatism of the constructional type is characterized by minimal phrase structure with preserved grammatical morphology. (Standard) expressive agrammatism is defined as a disorder of speech planning in which syntactic structures are reduced in number and in complexity, function words and inflecional morphemes are frequently omitted, and there is a predominance of verbs in the infinitive form (Hecaen and Anglelergues, 1965; Berndt and Caramazza, 1980). However, in these forms of aphasia, lexical use and interpretation may be spared to an important degree. In contrast, in some forms of receptive aphasia, a kind of converse situation prevails. The subjects may be able to speak grammatically (although one may often observe the existence of jargon and of more or less subtle forms of 'dyssyntaxie' (Hecaen and Anglelergues, 1965), i.e. inappropriate use of some syntactic structures), but they have marked difficulties in consciously assigning meaning to lexical items. It would seem, judging from the above dissociations, that on–line syntactic processing (i.e. syntactic parsing and sentence meaning recovery) and receptive lexical analysis are effectuated by separate mechanisms and entities, which may be selectively impaired.

Primary degenerative diseases, such as progressive aphasias (see Mesulam, 1987), Pick's disease or Alzheimer's disease (AZ) seem to have a predilection for particular sites of the brain, and often result in isolating functional subsystems. Observations by Schwartz and Chawluk (1990) suggest that some subjects display a reduction in semantic elaboration. One patient, carefully studied by these authors over a period of four years, progressively lost her expressive spoken and written abilities as well as her knowledge of word meaning. For example, over a 14–month period her receptive vocabulary dropped from the 11–year level to the 5–year level on the PPVT. The same words tended to be misunderstood in the same way in spoken as well as in written presentations. It is likely, therefore, that the processing problem responsible for the observed state of affairs in this patient had to do with the meaning representations shared by the spoken and the written input modalities rather than with the access mechanisms to these stores. Additionally, the same subject had retained only some degree of sensibility to basic phrasal organization as realized in word order. This case is at variance with the literature on dementia where a common observation is the preservation of most if not all syntactic competence, although there are impairments in semantic processing (Irigaray, 1973; Whitaker, 1976; Schwartz, Marin and Saffran, 1979). Yet, despite serious impairments in semantics, syntax and phonology, this subject had retained a normal functioning of those subsystems assigning lexical status and grammatical category to language input. It seems likely, in summary, that Schwartz and Chawluk's subject benefited from a relative sparing of her lexical and phrasal 'input systems' in the face of devastating phonological, syntactic and semantic impairments. Kempler, Curtiss and Jackson (1987) observed a normal range and frequency of syntactic construction, but poor lexical use in the spontaneous speech and in the writing of a group of non-retarded ageing people with probable AZ (age range 62 to 87 years; mean age 75 years). These phenomena suggest that syntactic ability tends to be selectively preserved in AZ, perhaps due to its automatic nature resisting better cognitive dissolution and cortical degeneration. Appel, Kertesz and Fishman (1982) administered the Western Aphasia Battery (Kertesz, 1980) to categorize 25 AZ patients into classical aphasic syndromes. Results indicated that transcortical sensory and Wernicke's types of aphasia were frequent, while transcortical motor and Broca's aphasias were absent. The patients were impaired in cognitive and lexical operations, but exhibited preserved phonological and syntactic abilities. Along the same interpretive line, Bayles (1982) reported that failure to detect and correct semantic errors was the most obvious problem of AZ patients in a series of linguistic tests involving sentence judgement, disambiguation, verbal description and story retelling.

The empirical indications gathered in the preceding sections, as well as a number of other observations in the specialized literature (see Shallice, 1988, for example; and Schwartz, 1990), clearly argue in favour of an important degree of autonomy of the morphosyntactic component of language as well as for the relative mutual independence of various levels of organization of the language system. What exact type of modular organization is involved here is not clear at the present time. Moscovitch and Umilta (1990), on the basis of their review of the neuropsychological literature, proposed a definition of language as a type–II modular organization, i.e. a system consisting of 'a collection of modules whose organization is innately given and whose output is integrated or synthesized by a devoted, non-modular processor' (p. 15). By 'devoted' processor, they meant a processor that is able to deal with information coming only from a particular group of modules. Type–II modules are considered to be capable of modification through learning and not just by maturation. They may integrate Fodorian or type–I modules (mechanisms of speech perception, word recognition and syntactic parsing are good candidates here) in addition to other modular subsystems. Continuing research, particularly in language pathologies, neurolinguistics and cognitive neuropsychology, will permit the specification of a theory on these matters.

Chapter 5
Language Development and Functioning

This chapter summarizes data on language development and functioning in typical children, adolescents and adults with mental retardation. The componential approach defined in preceding chapters will be maintained throughout. Prelinguistic aspects relevant to further language development will be considered. Major components of the language system will be analysed with particular regard to development. The question of the existence of a critical period for language acquisition in MR subjects will also be considered. Adult–child interactions when the child is mentally retarded will be discussed and their possible role in language acquisition will be suggested. Lastly, the problems encountered by ageing people with mental retardation in the speech and language domains will be touched upon.

Some generalizations in this chapter are tentative as many relevant data are still missing. For example, it is possible that further comparative work on the language profile of various mental retardation syndromes could undermine some of the general statements proposed on issues related to the speech and language of MR children, adolescents or adults. We offer the analyses as provisional pieces of work which further research will have to complete, limit, reassess or reorient.

5.1 The critical period hypothesis

5.1.1 Recent research has supplied data on the critical period hypothesis for first language acquisition which are partially in agreement with Lenneberg's arguments (see Chapter 2). It seems likely that there exists a critical period for language acquisition, which ends short of puberty, or before for some language aspects. The very nature of the hypothesis implies that the most compelling evidence will necessarily come from cases of deprivation up to and beyond the end of the period. This means weak evidence, but there is no other way. Animal researchers feel that they are authorized to deafen sparrow chicks and prevent kittens from receiving significant amounts of daylight. Obviously, in humans, crucial experiments of that sort cannot be conducted. Only the outcome of unfortunate cases of so-called natural experiments can be used for scientific purpose but always within a helping and remediative perspective (Rondal, 1994b).

Important data are available in the observations of Curtiss and associates (see Curtiss, 1977, for a full report) with Genie, a modern-day 'wild child', who was kept away from social contact for most of the first 13 years of her life. When she was discovered, she could hardly walk, could not chew or bite, understood only a few individual words, and did not speak at all. From the time of her discovery, she developed relatively rapidly despite the fact that aside from some sign language instruction, she had very little overt language training. Genie mother's report that she had started to speak words before her confinement, at 20 months, constitutes evidence against a diagnosis of MR. It is known that delay of language onset is one of the most prevalent characteristics of MR. Four years later, she demonstrated most aspects of concrete operational intelligence, in the Piagetian sense. Her language progressed in terms of the enrichment of referential lexicon and semantics. However, the acquisition of grammatical rules and their use in more complex utterances never followed. Her expressive language has remained grammatically underdeveloped. Word order is globally appropriate but utterances lack almost all bound and free grammatical morphemes and advanced syntactic devices. Regarding Genie's phonology, it is necessary to distinguish between receptive and productive ability. Receptively, she can discriminate and recognize the sounds of English. Productively, however, Genie's system appears abnormal. Curtiss (1977) notes: 'Almost all of the rules are optional, and many of the substitutions and deletions distort the phonological structure to a degree which at times makes Genie's speech almost impossible to understand' (pp. 90–1). But there is a system underlying her phonetic output. This is not the phonology of normal English but rather the reflection of some idiosyncratic processes at work, although Curtiss speculates on the possibility that it reflects universal (i.e. natural) phonological processes. Genie's failure to develop appropriate phonology and morpho-syntax, the latter confirming additionally that operational intellectual development is not sufficient for promoting morphosyntactic development, was attributed to her having passed the estimated boundary of the critical period for language acquisition. Curtiss (1977) also remarks that Genie appears to be right-hemisphere dominant for language and thinking functions. This was assessed through dichotic listening measures and a series of other procedures such as tachistoscopic tests and evoked potentials. This fact could be a direct result of her not having acquired language during the critical period. 'It suggests that after the critical period the left hemisphere may no longer be able to function in language acquisition, leaving the right hemisphere to assume control' (Curtiss, 1977, p. 234).

It may seem that only the left hemisphere as a whole (or in large part) is functionally specialized for grammar acquisition, as indicated by data from hemispherectomy or hemidecortication in childhood (e.g. Day and Ulatowska, 1979; Dennis, 1980a; Dennis and Whitaker, 1976). Curtiss (1977) further quotes from reports by Dennis (1980b) of strokes in childhood and on (developmental) dyslexia (Galaburda et al., 1985) suggesting that certain areas within the left hemisphere are especially important for 'normal and complete' mastery of the grammar. This, of course, is congruent with the data on adult (acquired) aphasia (e.g. agrammatic aphasia and Wernicke's aphasia; Hecaen and Anglelergues, 1965) stressing the importance of certain areas of the left hemisphere for the maintenance of normal linguistic ability (see Chapter 4, for anatomical suggestions).

However, some authors claim that in case of early lesions of the left cerebral hemisphere, transfer of the control over the language functions to the right hemisphere may occur with no or little subsequent linguistic deficit (see, for example, Bishop, 1983, 1988a, 1988b, analysing the language evolution of children having undergone left hemidecortication for infantile hemiplegia). There is also the possibility in very early unilateral brain injuries (i.e. congenital or prior 1 month of age) that further language development proceeds normally under the continued control of the same hemisphere, suggesting that the neural substrate underlying language development may be partially redundant initially such that unilateral injuries do not severely distort the course of early language development (Feldman, 1994). Another explanation of the same phenomenon would be that language functions can remain in the same left hemisphere as long as some crucial areas have not been damaged. Milner (1974) suggested that this would usually be the case if the temporo-parietal area of the left hemisphere remained mostly intact. Later in life, however, lesions to the left hemisphere seem to determine irreversible damage to the language functions (Van Hout and Seron, 1983).

Directly related to the above, is the continuing discussion over the initial equipotentiality of the two cerebral hemispheres with respect to language development. 'Anti-equipotentiality' authors point to a number of indications running contrary to the equipotentiality hypothesis. Anatomically, a series of studies since the 1970s show a clear asymmetry between the two hemispheres at the level of the planum temporale (a portion of the language area located behind the primary auditory cortex in the upper surface of the temporal lobe) favouring the left hemisphere, in foetuses, premature babies and infants born normally from 1 day to 18 months (Tezner et al., 1972; Witelson and Pallie, 1973; Wada, Clark and Hamm, 1975; Chi, Dooling and Gilles, 1977). The degree of asymmetry between the two hemispheres increases between infancy and adulthood (Wada et al., 1975). Molfese, Freeman and Palermo (1975) observed hemispheric asymmetries in evoked potentials comparable to those existing in adults, in infants as young as 6 months of age. Gardiner and Walter (1977) analysed infants' EEGs and found evidence of hemispheric specialization as early as 6 months (i.e. a decrease of the alpha activity of the left hemisphere when verbal stimuli are presented vs a similar decrease in the right hemisphere for visuo-spatial stimuli). Studies using a dichotic listening technique adapted for young children have documented a right ear advantage, indicative of a left hemispheric dominance for receptive speech in NR children, as early as 2 or 3 years of age (e.g. Kimura, 1961; Knox and Kimura, 1970). Coupled with an experimental paradigm of habituation of the cardiac rhythm or non-nutritive sucking, the dichotic listening technique has made it possible to objectify reliable cerebral left-hemisphere superiority for syllables in babies as young as 1–3 months (e.g. Entus, 1977; Glanville, Best and Levenson, 1977; Mehler and Dupoux, 1990). Anti-equipotentiality authors also challenge the previous indication that there is a higher incidence of aphasia in children following a lesion located in the right cerebral hemisphere. They claim that the incidence of aphasia following a lesion to the right hemisphere is no more frequent in children at all ages than in adults (see Van Hout and Seron, 1983, for a review of relevant studies). Some authors also doubt that in case of early lesions to the left cerebral hemisphere, the right hemisphere can mediate language functions to the same extent that the left one can. The claim in this case is not simply that there is a delay in language development after left-hemisphere damage, but that the ultimate linguistic competence which the right hemisphere can achieve is less than that of the left hemisphere (Dennis and Kohn, 1975; Dennis and Whitaker, 1976; Dennis, 1980a).

A middle-of-the-road position with potential to accommodate these contrasting interpretations would be as follows. Although it is species-specifically predisposed towards dominance for the computational aspects of language, the left cerebral hemisphere needs both time and speech stimulation in order to establish its dominance firmly, whereas there is slightly more rapid maturation of the right hemisphere (Galaburda, 1984) which controls non-segmental phonological features such as intonation and stress. The two hemispheres are thought to be co-involved in the treatment of semantics and pragmatics. As the control of the left cerebral hemisphere over the language aspects it is devoted to is not complete for some time, early damage that cannot be compensated within that hemisphere may determine the transfer of the computational language functions to the right hemisphere at no functional cost. With the progressive establishment of the left hemisphere dominance, such a move is more and more costly in terms of loss of computational efficiency. Problems can wait several years to appear (particularly with respect to more advanced aspects of grammar) because regions of the left cerebral hemisphere not mediating language exclusively in the early stages of language acquisition may be recruited for higher levels of language function later in development.

A lesion to the left hemisphere is probably not the only possible determinant of a reorganization of the cerebral control over language functions. As suggested by Curtiss (1977), Genie's case may illustrate the possibility that lack of speech stimulation during the maturational period of brain structures devoted to language could render these structures unable to play their developmental role (also Hecaen and Albert, 1978). No restoration of the capacity linked to the left hemisphere would be possible beyond this period, the subject retaining a full right hemisphere dominance for language at great cost regarding phonological and morphosyntactic functioning.

Another case showing the same general pattern as Genie has been documented by Curtiss (1988). Chelsea is a hearing-impaired adult of normal intelligence who first attempted to acquire spoken language in her thirties, prompted by successful auditory amplification. Her lexical knowledge progressed regularly and became substantial. She scored above the 12th grade level on the Productive Word Association Subtest of the Clinical Evaluation of Language Functions (Semmel and Wiig, 1980). In contrast, her ability to combine vocabulary items into grammatical utterances has remained extremely limited, resulting in multiword utterances being, almost without exception, unacceptable grammatically at the levels of the phrase and the clause. Canonical phrasal and clause word order is not respected. Constituent structure, subcategorization constraints and agreement phenomena are usually violated. Chelsea's lexical knowledge is limited to the referential function and does not include either subcategorization information or logical structure constraints. As Curtiss summarized it, Chelsea's expressive language appears at best limited to the production of semantically relevant substantives (1988, p. 372). Along the same line of observation, the older case of Kaspar Hauser (in the nineteenth century) may also be called upon (see Curtiss, 1988). Kaspar was totally isolated from the age of 3 or 4 years until about 16. Reportedly, he never mastered the morphology or the syntax of German, his mother tongue. Kaspar, however, developed most remarkably in other areas, including the semantic aspects of language and various intellectual abilities (e.g. mathematics). Generally speaking, the evidence from cases of extreme deprivation in early childhood suggests that, in the absence of genetic or congenital anomalies or a history of gross malnourishment, victims have a good prognosis (see Skuse, 1993, for a review), except in the area of computational language where persistent deficits may exist.

Still other data suggest a critical period for the development or the first utilization of grammar-setting mechanisms. They relate to the age of acquisition of an esoteric sign language such as ASL (American Sign Language). Mayberry, Fisher and Hatfield (1983) showed that individuals who acquired ASL as adolescents perform worse on tasks testing grammatical knowledge in ASL than those who acquired ASL in childhood. In additional work by Mayberry (1984, quoted by Curtiss, 1988), there is already a marked difference in ASL proficiency between those who learned ASL from 8 years up and those who learned it before 8 years, in favour of the latter individuals. Ploog (1984) observed, 'children who learn ASL after, say, 7 years of age, will have a sort of foreign accent phenomenon, as Eric Lenneberg called it; they will not speak [sic] like native signers' (p. 88). Corresponding data are reported by Newport (1984, 1990, 1992). More than 30 years after first exposure to ASL and with daily practice of this language, 'native learners' (first exposed to ASL from birth by their deaf signing parents in the home and then from age 4–6 by deaf peers at special school) exhibit a superiority in comprehension and production of ASL morphology over 'early learners' (first exposed to ASL from age 4–6 by deaf peers), who themselves demonstrate a markedly better performance than 'late learners' (first exposed to ASL by deaf peers after age 12). In addition, those studies point to the possibility that the hypotheses entertained by late learners are actually *different* from those of native or early learners. For example, late learners show high frequencies of response patterns not found in native users of ASL, such as producing 'frozen' lexical items or whole-word signs lacking internal morphological structure (Newport, 1992). Another interesting characteristic of late learners involves highly inconsistent use of ASL morphology, with frequent substitution of ungrammatical forms for those required grammatically.

The above data argue in favour of the existence of specialized neuropsychological mechanisms for the computational aspects of language. These mechanisms are tied to the left cerebral hemisphere. They appear to develop with respect to strong maturational constraints. There is no clear indication that the development of lexical and pragmatic skills would also be characterized by critical periods. Vocabulary ability is maintained throughout adult life (Feifel, 1949; Ricks, 1958; Botwinick and Storandt, 1974).

5.1.2. It is likely, in our view, that the critical period for language development exhibits *modular characteristics*. The 'gross phenomenon' may be an aggregate of particular phenomena coinciding only partially in time. This idea was not alien to Eric Lenneberg. He wrote: 'there seems to be not just one but several types of critical periods. For example, control of voice and articulation may be tied to a much shorter period than the learning of languages as a whole' (Lenneberg, 1975, p. 1). It may be that the phonological critical period terminates at around 6 or 7 years. There could be an earlier critical period for voice setting and control, as suggested by the difference in vocal development between congenitally or early deaf individuals (i.e. before 2 years approximately) and individuals with deafness that occurrs later in life (Menyuk, 1977). Termination may not be the most appropriate term. A good deal if not the whole naturalness of phonological learning seems to disappear after the end of the critical period, leaving room to qualitatively different processes yielding non-native outcomes (e.g. foreign accents). But the end of the critical period does not rule out the possibility of some phonological learning. It is better probably to think of phonological plasticity showing a marked decline after 6 or 7 years of age, rather than a sudden drop-off. Generally, critical periods do not end abruptly (Atkinson and Braddick, 1989). But this means meagre benefits to be expected for phonological learning after the end of the critical period. The ending of the critical period for morpho-syntax may be around 10 or 12 years of age. Krashen (1973, 1975), having reanalysed Lenneberg's data and arguments, suggested 5 years for the closing time. This seems too early given that important linguistic developments, e.g. mastery over complex sentences and reversible passives, usually take place after that age. Like its phonological counterpart, the decline in natural grammar-learning ability takes the form of an asymptote relative to the coordinate symbolizing the age increase. The exact reason for this decline is not known. It is not related in any major way to the establishment of dominance of the left cerebral hemisphere for the grammatical function (as Lenneberg thought). Indeed this dominance is established considerably earlier. It is not related to the brain having set in definitive ways either (as Lenneberg also thought) for the two following reasons: first, there is a substantial completion of cortical maturation at about 8 years (e.g. synaptic density increases sharply between 2 and 8 years in many cortical areas, at which age it culminates before beginning to fall off significantly; see Purves and Lichtman (1985)); and second, myelinization in some cortical areas continues into the adult years (Menyuk, 1977). Hurford (1991) suggests that the main determinant for the ending time parameters of the critical periods are the evolutive consequences of the interplay of genetic factors influencing life-history characters in relation to language acquisition. He argues that possession of language is beneficial to an individual and the longer the period of one's life that one possesses the whole of one's native language the greater the benefit. Individuals with a capacity to acquire language relatively early in life tend to arise by natural selection. Hurford's evolutionary account is consistent with the modular characteristic of the critical period. As indicated above, only hard core aspects of the linguistic system, i.e. phonology and morpho-syntax, exhibit critical periods. They are also the ones for which the likelihood of the existence of species-specific predispositions and constraints are greater. The evolutionary thesis is also consistent with the fact that virtually only non-basic aspects of language, from a linguistic structural core point of view, may continue to be acquired beyond 10–12 years. Such aspects involve vocabulary growth, pragmatic skills, stylistic, rhetorical and discursive abilities, proficiency in writing the standard language and reading (Singleton, 1989).

Contrary to what Lenneberg thought, there may not be an onset of critical period in the strict sense. Roughly stated, phonological and morphosyntactic development begins whenever the organism is ready for it and has been properly stimulated. In NR children, this is usually around 1 year of age for phonology (somewhat earlier or later depending on how one defines this development), and around 18–20 months for morphosyntax (taking the appearance of multiword utterances as a reflection of this beginning). The notion of 'readiness' demands specification. According to the continuity assumption (Chomsky, 1981; Pinker, 1984; Finer and Roeper, 1989), basic grammatical mechanisms in children and adults are identical. In other words, children have the computational mechanisms they need to analyse language right from the start. However, these mechanisms, must be set in motion, so to speak, by other acquisitions: notional knowledge (thematic semantic) and linguistic material knowledge (words). As these acquisitions take time, the onset of computational language is delayed in proportion. For example, phonological rules need words and morphemes to apply. Grammatical mechanisms need semantic structures to assign thematic roles to syntactic configurations. Maturational accounts of morphosyntactic development (Borer and Wexler, 1987; Wexler, 1994), in (partial) opposition to the continuity assumption, assert that parts of a child's innate grammatical endowment may be unavailable at early stages of language development and become available for grammatical construction only later. However, continuity and maturational accounts predict that computational language development will proceed according to a specific time dimension. The establishment of the left cerebral hemisphere dominance over language functions is part of that developmental scheme. It is probably directly related to the maturation of the neural mechanisms underlying computational language development. In our opinion, however, the above developmental phenomena should not be considered as defining the onset of a critical period for language development.

As said, reported development beyond the critical period concern non-basic structural aspects of language. Genie and Chelsea, the subjects studied by Curtiss, developed valuable referential lexicons and semantic structures well beyond the end of the critical period, but not grammatical rules and other central aspects of grammar, including interrogative structures, relative and indefinite pronouns, the structure of the auxiliary verb, embedded clauses, complex subordinates, passives and grammatical morphology. Corresponding observations were made by Quigley and associates in several studies of deaf adolescents learning oral language (Power and Quigley, 1973; Quigley, Montanelli and Wilbur, 1974; Quigley, Smith and Wilbur, 1974). Despite years of oral language training in special schools, the severely and profoundly deaf adolescents with normal IQs studied up to 19 years of age (having had hearing impairment prior to 1, 2 or 3 years) showed only limited improvement over time in comprehension and production of the passive voice, and grammaticality judgement of negative and relative sentences.

5.1.3 Assuming that the evolutionary constraints advocated by Hurford (1991) apply similarly to MR individuals, and there is no reason why they should not, it could be predicted that no spontaneous basic computational language development will be observed in these subjects beyond approximatively 12 years. However, some systematic training effect probably can still be induced. Continued development in the conceptual aspects of language should be possible during adolescence and beyond in correspondence with the growth in mental age reported in those years for many MR subjects. For example, Fisher and Zeaman (1970) showed in a semi-longitudinal study that most MR subjects of mixed aetiologies have MA scores increasing until 30 or 40 years-CA, even if the rate of growth is modest. Berry et al. (1984) confirmed Fisher and Zeaman's indication in a five-year longitudinal study with DS adolescents and adults. (For a recent review of other indications of continued cognitive growth well beyond adolescence in DS, see Carr, 1994.)

An alternative explanation to the critical period theory would be that MR subjects cannot develop further in computational language because of intrinsic grammatical and/or cognitive limitation. The exceptional cases of grammatical development in otherwise cognitively average MR individuals documented in Chapter 4, are sufficient to reject this counterargument. Additionally, it is interesting to note that all the language-exceptional MR subjects in question had developed linguistically the way they did before 10 years of age despite the fact that an important delay in the onset of language was attested for each one of those subjects for whom early information was available.

Regular MR subjects have considerably less grammatical ability. They develop very slowly linguistically. The closing of the critical period catches them, so to speak, in a state of grammatical immaturity. Their language conceptual aspects are also markedly delayed. But for those aspects, there is the possibility that some important development could still occur during adolescence and early adulthood, as suggested above.

Let us see, now, whether the data on MR adolescents conform to the predictions made. Before proceeding to a review of the relevant literature, a word of caution is necessary. Most data available to date are cross-sectional ones in a longitudinal type of problem and therefore exposed to the usual reservations in this respect. Additionally, there is the possibility of a sort of cohort caveat. All the MR adolescents studied today have not or not always benefited from early specialized language intervention. Assuming at least a minimal long-term effect for this intervention, it would be inappropriate to consider that the developmental levels reached by the MR adolescents today necessarily reflect absolute norms for ultimate attainment. It is also entirely possible that future improvement in the remediation techniques could lead to better levels of functioning than those documented so far.

Lenneberg et al. (1964) reported developmental data supporting the hypothesis of a 'freeze' in language acquisition in MR subjects after 14 years. Sixty-one DS individuals aged CA 3–22 years at the beginning of the study were followed over a three-year period. Those who had attained puberty failed to make any discernible progress in acquiring language structures. This was in contrast to younger subjects for whom some growth was observed. However, judging from the unclear report of Lenneberg et al. (1964) on this point, it seems that only 4 subjects were beyond CA 14 years when tested; a too limited subsample from which to generalize.

Cromer (1974) proposed mildly MR individuals aged CA 7–16 years (most subjects in the sample being 14, 15 and 16 years old) a comprehension task with verb syntactic contrasts of the type *The bear is eager to see* vs. *The bear is easy to see*, when the two sentences have identical surface structure but different deep structures (C. Chomsky, 1969). None of the subjects, what ever their place in the age scale, was able to identify contrasting thematic roles of different verbs. Similar responses would be expected in early language development. On this basis, Cromer reasoned that this linguistic strategy had to be ascribed to the behavioural effect of the innate linguistic endowment effective only within the time boundaries of the critical period, hence its missing in MR adolescents. Cromer's argument is weak in two respects. First, the linking of the receptive strategy to innate linguistic principles is only tentative. Second, the interpretation of Cromer's data already presupposes what it aims to prove, i.e. the existence of a critical period for language acquisition.

Seitz, Goulding and Conrad (1969) claimed to have obtained results congruent with Lenneberg's interpretation. They retested on a free word-association task high-MA (mean MA 11 years 5 months; mean CA 17 years 1 month) and low-MA (mean MA 7 years 6 months; mean CA 15 years 3 months) mildly MR subjects who had been tested 30 months earlier on the same test by Keilman and Moran (1967). The higher MA group showed no significant change in its word-association characteristics from one test to the other, whereas the lower MA group did. It is hard to understand how these authors could have seen their data as relevant to Lenneberg's interpretation, as their MA groups both contained a majority of subjects with CAs over 14 years. However, a careful examination of the data presented by Seitz et al. (1969) reveals that the lower MA subjects did show some language change over time, which had to do with characteristics of the elicited word associations (e.g. use of richer networks of semantic features to mediate between words).

Rondal et al. (1981) recorded the spontaneous speech of 24 French-speaking moderately MR adolescents of mixed aetiologies aged 12–18 years (see Chapter 3, Table 3-2). Mean MLU for the 16 subjects whose ages were between 14 and 18 years was 5.52. Mean MLU for the MR subjects aged 12–14 years was 5.15, not significantly different from the older group. None of the other language measures calculated yielded a significant difference between younger and older subjects (type-token ratio; proportion of correct articles; proportion of correct verbal inflections; proportion of sentence; sentence complexity; proportion of information; or proportion of new information).

Fowler (1988) supplied conversational MLU data from a small group of adolescents with DS (aged 12;6–19 years). She split her group between lower Stanford-Binet IQ (38–48) and higher IQ (55–64) subjects. Mean MLU in words plus grammatical morphemes was 3.58 in the lower IQ group and 3.78 in the higher IQ group (with noticeable intersubject differences in the two groups). These MLU figures may be compared to the middle age DS group (7–12;6 years) also studied by Fowler (1988). Corresponding MLU data for this group were 2.56 in the lower IQ group and 4.03 in the higher one. Similar results were obtained by Fowler (1988) with a second measure labelled Index of Productive Syntax (IPS), designed by Scarborough (1985), and consisting in awarding points for the occurrence in the speech sample of 56 kinds of morphological and syntactic forms. In another study, Fowler, Gelman and Gleitman (1994) reported no further modification in MLU over the 2½ to 4 years following initial measurement in four DS adolescents (mean CA 12 years and 7 months at the beginning of the study). MLU remained in the range 3–3.50. Figure 5.1 illustrates schematically the evolution in MLU with CA in Down's syndrome. It is based on data from the following sources: Rondal (1978a, 1985b); Rondal, Lambert and Sohier (1980b, 1981); Fowler (1988, 1990); Smith, Von Tetzchner and Michalsen (1988); and Fowler, Gelman and Gleitman (1994). For additional comments on MLU development, see Section 5.5.

A word of caution is in order regarding the validity of MLU as an index

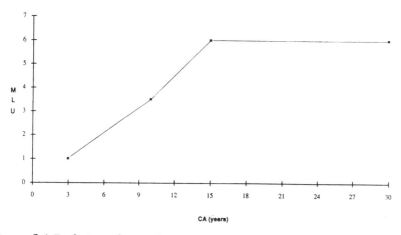

Figure 5.1 Evolution of mean length of utterance in Down's syndrome. MLU is computed in number of words plus grammatical morphemes according to the procedures outlined in Brown, 1973, and Rondal, Bachelet, and Perée, (1986)

of grammatical development. MLU is a global index of combinatorial language. It is reliable and predictively valid as a measure of morphosyntactic development only within given developmental boundaries. Putting together the relevant studies of Klee and Fitzgerald (1985), and Rondal et al. (1987), with NR children, it can be suggested that utterance length is a valid reflection of morphosyntactic complexity (estimated with reference to the LARSP analytical technique developed by Crystal, 1979, 1982, and Crystal, Fletcher and Garman, 1976, 1989, in the above two studies) up to approximatively MLU 3.00. Rondal et al. (1988) confirmed the above indication for DS subjects. They found that MLU correctly predicts complexity and diversity of bound morphemes and major syntactic structures in DS subjects between MLU 1.00 and 3.50. Scarborough et al. (1991) reached a similar conclusion in their study relating MLU to IPS in NR and language-disordered groups (Fragile-X, Down's syndrome and autistic subjects). They found a strong curvilinear association between the two measures across the MLU range from 1.00 to 4.50. However, correlations were weaker when MLU exceeded 3.00 than at earlier stages of development.

After MLU reaches 3.00 approximately, it becomes a less reliable predictor of grammatical development. The relationship between utterance length and grammatical complexity is less secure as individuals become more able to express constructions of a greater diversity. MLU remains potentially valid as an index for those aspects of grammatical development most directly tied to utterance length (such as bound morphemes, phrasal and clausal connectives). However, Fowler et al. (1994) remarked that the relatively longer utterances with correct word order produced by their DS adolescents did not necessarily imply the use of appropriate grammatical markers. MLU beyond the range 3.00–3.50 can be observed in DS. It may be more a reflection of an increased capacity to chain vocabulary items in a canonically appropriate way than of a genuine structural progress.

Regarding articulatory development, Buckley and Sacks (1987) report that over half of the adolescent girls and about 80 per cent of the adolescent boys in their survey were rated by their parents as unintelligible to strangers. Of course, it is possible that the parents' intelligibility ratings could have been based primarily on limitations in language skills (as opposed to speech). Assuming these parents were indeed rating articulation in the first place, intelligibility in DS adolescents does not seem to have changed much from the reports of Lenneberg (1967), Ryan (1975) and Rondal (1978b). Bray and Woolnough (1988) confirm that intelligibility of speech is indeed a problem in DS children and adolescents (12–16 years), even in those who have more advanced syntax.

Van Borsel (1988), in a more technical study, has supplied an analysis of the elicited speech (obtained from picture description) of five Dutch-speaking girls with DS: CAs 16 years 5 months to 19 years 9 months. The work included a phonetic analysis, a substitution analysis and a phonological process analysis. All Dutch phonemes occurred in the corpus of each subject, except the low-frequency loan-phonemes /ß/ and /Ω/. Results indicate that the speech errors of the DS adolescents are for the greater part identical to the error patterns observed in young NR children. Voiced plosives and fricatives are more frequently substituted for their voiceless cognates. The substitutions for a given phoneme concerned not only voice but manner and place of articulation as well. Also substitution by a zero element (omission) occurred frequently. However, there was a lot of variation among subjects. Percentages of substitution were highest for fricatives and liquids and lowest for glides. At present, no data are available on the misarticulations of Dutch-speaking DS children with whom Van Borsel's DS adolescents could be compared. Tentative comparisons with Anglo-Saxon studies on the speech of DS children (Dodd, 1976; Stoel-Gammon, 1980; Smith and Stoel-Gammon, 1983; Bleile and Schwarz, 1984) suggest that most phonological processes observed in children (e.g. final consonant deletion, deletion of unstressed syllables, cluster reduction, fronting of palatals, assimilation, metathesis and voicing of intervocalic voiceless obstruents) are also at work in DS adolescents. No matter how imperfect the above comparison may be, it suggests, first, that phonological development is not complete in most DS adolescents, and, second, that the speech levels reached by these older subjects do not differ markedly from those of the children, even if some slight improvement may occur with age. Corresponding data were reported by Borghi (1990). He studied 50 DS subjects between the ages of 5 and 19 years. They were given the Fisher-Logemann Test of Articulation Competence (1971). Data analysis indicates that seven phonemes are most error-prone and resistant to change. They are in descending rank order: /z/, / θ/,/ð/, /ê/, /Ê/ and /v/.

Interesting observations on several aspects of the language of French-speaking DS children, adolescents and adults can be found in Annick Comblain's doctoral work at the Laboratory for Psycholinguistics of the University of Liège. In the part of her doctoral dissertation to which we are referring, Comblain (1995) proposed a series of randomized language tasks to 11 DS children (8 girls and 3 boys), aged 6 years 10 months to 12 years 10 months, 16 DS adolescents (9 girls and 7 boys) aged 14 years 5 months to 21 years 6 months, and 15 adults (9 females and 6 males) aged 23 years 9 months to 42 years 10 months. All subjects had standard trisomy 21. The non-adults were enrolled in primary or secondary special schools for the MR. The adults were attending 'La Fermette', an occupational day centre for DS adults, located in the vicinity of Verviers, in the eastern part of Belgium. Twelve NR children (7 girls and 5 boys) with CAs between 3 years 7 months and 7 years 4 months, matched with the DS children on social class and MA (obtained through the application of the EDEI Test – Epreuves Différentielles

Table 5.1 Group means and standard deviations (between parentheses) for the measures computed by Comblain (1995) on the language of Down's syndrome (DS) children, adolescents and adults, and non-retarded (NR) children matched with DS children on mental age and social class

Categorial data	Group (n)			
	NR children (12)	DS children (11)	DS adolescents (16)	DS adults (15)
1. Chronological age (CA)	3;8	9;10	18;4	30;8
2. Mental age (MA)	—	3;7	5;9	4;5
3. Mean length of utterance (MLU)	—	2.08 (1.04)	4.75 (2.50)	4.73 (2.98)
4. TVAP	—	3;3 (0;5)	5;9 (1;11)	4;10 (1;5)
5. TVP	—	28.79 (6.62)	38.43 (11.84)	40.57 (13.23)
6. Personal pronouns	62.50 (17.32)	53.33 (13.71)	46.25 (14.55)	43.33 (24.10)
7. Articles	47.92 (13.13)	37.04 (11.44)	37.28 (12.03)	33.70 (11.20)
8. Verbal inflections	44.94 (13.50)	41.67 (8.14)	44.55 (10.12)	40.28 (7.81)
9. Coordinate clauses	65.63 (21.65)	45.83 (17.94)	70.31 (14.34)	60.83 (15.57)
10. Subordinate clauses	75.00 (19.66)	48.33 (16.42)	51.25 (26.05)	34.29 (22.43)
11. Relative clauses	89.06 (11.97)	62.08 (12.47)	80.47 (18.24)	67.86 (23.87)
12. Negative sentences	89.06 (11.06)	34.38 (21.40)	64.84 (21.99)	41.96 (34.88)
13. Passive sentences	78.91 (21.27)	64.58 (17.54)	58.59 (18.10)	51.79 (33.20)

Notes: CA, MA and TVAP ages are expressed in years and months; MAs are global scores obtained at the EDEI; categories 5–13 are expressed in per cent of correct answers; MLU is computed in number of words plus grammatical morphemes (according to Rondal, Bachelet and Perée's, 1986 procedure); TVAP: Test de Vocabulaire Actif et Passif; TVP: Test de Vocabulaire Productif; Categories 6–13 are from the BEMS (Batterie d'Evaluation Morpho-Syntaxique); Dashes indicate categorial data that were not collected.

d'Efficience Intellectuelle, Perron-Borelli and Misès, 1974) were used as controls on some of the tests.

The language measures involved: MLU obtained from free play or conversational speech, TVAP (Test de Vocabulaire Actif et Passif; Deltour and Hupkens, 1980), TVP (Test de Vocabulaire Productif; Comblain, 1993), as well as eight receptive subtests from level 1 of the BEMS (Batterie d'Evaluation Morpho-Syntaxique; Comblain, Fayasse and Rondal, 1993). The TVAP is a receptive pointing-to-picture vocabulary test containing 30 items. The TVP is an expressive test in which subjects are requested to label as many as 817 pictures (over several sessions) representing common objects or actions (taken from the *Imagier Larousse pour Enfants*, 1982) and corresponding to 20 common semantic categories (e.g. animals, fruits, body parts, tools, clothes). The subtests from the BEMS concern the comprehension of personal pronouns, definite and indefinite articles, verbal inflections, coordinate clauses, temporal, locative, causal and conditional subordinate clauses, relative clauses, negative and passive sentences. In this test, the subjects are requested either to select the picture corresponding best to the meaning of the proposed sentence, or to act out the sentence with play material, depending on the particular subtest.

The resulting data are summarized in Table 5.1.

A one-way ANOVA with either three (DS children, adolescents and adults) or four (NR children, DS children, adolescents and adults) levels to the factor was performed on each of the variables 3–13 in Table 5.1. It yielded a significant effect for all the variables except Verbal Inflections. Table 5.2 summarizes the follow-up analyses performed on the significant variables above, using the Fisher LSDP (Least Significant Difference Procedure).

Only the data concerning DS children and adolescents, and NR children, will be discussed here. The question of a possible continuation of

Table 5.2 Significant contrasts (at the $p < 0.05$ level) revealed by the follow-up analyses (using FISHER LSDP) conducted on the significant categorial variables from Table 5.1

1. NR children ‡ from DS children on articles, coordinate, subordinate and relative clauses, negative sentences.
2. NR children ‡ from DS adolescents on personal pronouns, articles, subordinate and relative clauses, negative and passive sentences.
3. NR children ‡ from DS adults on personal pronouns, articles, subordinate and relative clauses, negative and passive sentences.
4. DS children ‡ from DS adolescents on MLU, TVAP[1], coordinate and relative clauses, negative sentences.
5. DS children ‡ from DS adults on MLU, TVAP, TVP[2], coordinate clauses.
6. DS adolescents ‡ from DS adults on subordinate clauses, passive sentences.

Notes: 1: TVAP: Test de Vocabulaire Actif et Passif; 2: TVP: Test de Vocabulaire Productif; ‡ = differ from.

language development into the adult years in MR persons will be addressed in Section 5.7, where we discuss the other part of Comblain's (1995) data.

The MLU values reported by Comblain (1995) for her children and adolescents groups are globally consistent with those of Rondal et al. (1981), Fowler (1988) and Fowler et al. (1994), as reported earlier. As they stand in Table 5.1, Comblain's MLU data could easily give the impression of a marked increase in MLU in DS from childhood to adolescence. Actually, the older DS children in Comblain's study have MLUs surpassing the group mean (consistent with the mean MLU value reported by Rondal (1978b) for his older group of English-speaking DS children – mean CA 117 months, i.e. MLU 2.87; bearing in mind the caution necessary when comparing MLU data in different languages). Comblain's (1995) MLU data regarding the DS adolescents are also drawn towards a higher mean value by the inclusion in the group of one male subject with an MLU of 11.34.

The lexical measures in Comblain's (1995) data show a significant increase, from the DS children to the adolescent group, in receptive (TVAP) but not in expressive (TVP) referential ability. In absolute terms, however, the gains of the DS adolescents in MLU and referential lexicon are quite modest. The mean MLU of normally developed people in free conversation is around 12 points vs an average MLU of 4.75 for the DS adolescents in the above study. The mean receptive lexical age of the DS adolescents studied by Comblain (1995) is 5 years 9 months (in exact correspondence with the mean MA of the group). DS adolescents on average can label correctly only 39 per cent (SD 12 per cent) of the objects or actions shown on the TVP (vs 29 per cent (SD 7 per cent) for the DS children). One additional lexical indication on diversity of vocabulary of use (type-token ratio, TTR) is available in a study of MR adolescents by Rondal et al. (1981; see Chapter 3, Table 3.2). Mean TTR of the 16 subjects whose CAs were between 14 and 18 years, are close to 0.60 (only slightly and non-significantly ahead of the mean TTR of the 12–14-year group, that is 0.58). Rondal (1978b) supplied mean TTR values of 0.44 for DS children younger than CA 6 years and 0.49 between CAs 6 and 12 years in the spontaneous free-play and conversational speech of 21 English-speaking DS children. It could be, therefore, that there is a gradual increase in lexical diversity of use in older MR children and young adolescents.

As to the BEMS data, DS adolescents significantly outperform DS children only on the subtests assessing comprehension of coordinate and relative clauses, and negative sentences. However, they still perform markedly lower than NR children on the subtests evaluating comprehension of personal pronouns, definite and indefinite articles, subordinate clauses, negative and passive sentences. On the whole, their receptive scores on the subtests of the BEMS are located in the vicinity of 50 per cent correct answer (i.e. beyond chance level, as there were at least four possible answers to each sentence proposed in the tasks), except for the coordinate and the relative clauses, as well as the negative sentences, where they are higher.

There is a growing literature on *language pragmatics and linguistic communication* in MR adolescents (see Abbeduto and Rosenberg, 1987, and Rosenberg and Abbeduto, 1993, for reviews). The general impression that one derives from these studies is that the abilities regrouped under the loose label *pragmatics*, develop slowly but consistently over a long period of time in MR subjects; a period covering childhood, adolescence and early adulthood.

There are indications (e.g. Greenwald and Leonard, 1979) that young children with DS (1- to 4-year-olds) use one-word productions efficiently to *request* interesting objects placed out of reach. When matched with NR children for Piagetian level of intellectual sensorimotor development, DS children behave in the same way in the requesting tasks. This may not be true for non-verbal communicative performance (i.e. requesting, turn-taking, inviting the experimenter to play), however, as shown in a study by Mundy et al. (1988), comparing DS and non-DS MR children to MA-matched NR children.

Speech acts have received some attention in the literature on MR subjects. A speech act is the social function that a speaker intends an utterance to perform in a communicative interaction (Austin, 1962; Searle, 1969), e.g. *I promise to buy you a present*, commitment to a future course of action. Two questions are particularly relevant in this context. First, do MR people use the same type of speech acts as NR individuals, and is the development similar in the two cases? Second, do MR people express speech acts through the same linguistic means as typically developing persons?

As to the first issue, Owens and MacDonald (1982) defined a taxonomy of speech acts, which they used to analyse the language produced by 4- to 6-year-olds DS and MA-matched 2- to 3-year-olds NR children during dyadic free play with their mothers. The categories of speech acts included: question/answer, assertion, suggestion/command, naming an entity, acknowledging a maternal utterance without adding semantic content. Owens and MacDonald found few differences between children with and without DS in terms of the relative frequency with which the various speech acts were used. Similar results were reported in other studies with DS children (e.g. Coggins, Carpenter and Owings, 1983). Researchers have also examined the speech acts produced spontaneously by MR adolescents and adults. Abbeduto and Rosenberg (1980) used the following categories: assertion, commissive, expressive (i.e. a speaker indicating feelings about or evaluating an event, a proposal or a proposition), question and request. The subjects (CA 20–31 years; MA 8–13 years) were assembled in triads and recorded during mealtime conversations. Each triad produced all five categories of speech acts. Assertions and questions were the most frequently occurring speech acts (47 and 43 per cent of the initiating turns, respectively). Expressives and commissives were relatively infrequent (4 and 3 percent of the initiating turns, respectively). These data show not only that mildly MR adolescents and adults are interested in giving and receiving information, but also that they are able to talk about their future plans, feelings and opinions. Corresponding results have been reported for moderately and severely MR adolescents and adults (Zetlin and Sabsay, 1980; Owings, McManus and Scherer, 1981). There is even anecdotal evidence that subjects with profound mental retardation express a variety of speech acts in their primitive conversational interactions (Price-Williams and Sabsay, 1979).

MR individuals, however, evidence important delays in using the linguistic forms that NR people find appropriate for the expression of particular speech acts, as documented in several studies (Abbeduto, 1984; Bliss, 1985; Nuccio and Abbeduto, 1993). MR individuals may have special difficulty in the area of verbal politeness, such as appropriate polite expressions for their requests, which pragmatically may require indirect and inferred forms.

Comprehension of speech acts has been investigated in a limited number of studies (Abbeduto and Rosenberg, 1980; Zetlin and Sabsay, 1980; Abbeduto, Davies and Furman, 1988). These studies document important chronological delays in this development. However, the performance of MR children and adolescents in speech act comprehension is generally at a level appropriate for their MAs. Despite the delays, mildly and moderately MR adults eventually become skilled at understanding speech acts in familiar interactions involving minimal cognitive and linguistic demands. It is unlikely that these MR people evidence mature comprehension of speech acts in more demanding types of exchanges, but research on this point is mostly lacking. Basically, the same developmental picture emerges when a related pragmatic skill is considered, i.e. *requesting repair of conversational failures and responding to a request for repair* directed at the MR subjects themselves. Noticeable developmental delays are the rule, but by adulthood, it seems, from the limited number of studies available, many MR individuals can manage reasonably well in responding to a variety of requests for repair.

Lastly, regarding *the organization of the conversation*. Conversational turn-taking does not seem to constitute a problem for older MR children, adolescents and adults. Their turn-taking behaviour appears to be systematic and rule-governed (Abbeduto and Rosenberg, 1980; Abbeduto, 1991; Abbeduto and Rosenberg, 1992). But again, there are important delays early in this development. Jones (1977) showed that DS infants are less responsive to mothers' verbal stimulation. They take the initiative in the interaction less often than NR infants of similar ages. When they do react, DS infants tend to vocalize in continuous strings or to repeat vocalizations with a very short time lapse (less than half a second on the average), which reduces the opportunity for the partner to take a turn in the exchange. Such patterns reveal lapses of interactive turn-taking skills by DS infants. Beyond prelinguistic development, the results of several studies (e.g. Davis, Stroud and Green, 1988) suggest that the rate of turn-taking errors (e.g. undue interruption of one speaker by the other) for MR children is similar to that observed in younger NR children matched to them on measures of linguistic or cognitive development. Topic contribution and topic continuation are important pragmatic skills for which little is known at the present time in mental retardation. Certainly, MR individuals have the desire to keep a topic going and to contribute significantly to it. However, they often lack the language skills and sometimes the relevant knowledge to advance the topic (Warne and Bedrosian, cited in Bedrosian, 1988). Not surprisingly, Beveridge, Spencer and Mittler (1979) found that those MR children who were more advanced on several measures of communicative functioning were also more likely than their less advanced peers to produce utterances related to the task at hand.

Concluding this section on language and language evolution in MR adolescents, it can be suggested that *there is little progress beyond childhood in the computational aspects of language. There may be some progress in some conceptual language aspects* (e.g. receptive and productive referential lexicon, lexical diversity of use), but it appears to be limited in scope. *The area in which there may be more relative progress is pragmatics and communication.* The suggestion made earlier in this section that the critical period for first language acquisition has to be envisaged in a modular way, therefore, receives empirical support. However, one will have to consider language data from MR adults in order to ensure that this conclusion is fully warranted. So far, it would appear that MR individuals do not develop in the phonological and morphosyntactic aspects of language much beyond the levels reached towards the end of childhood. The limited MLU increase from childhood to adolescence documented in some studies does not correspond to a genuine structural progress, but probably to a better ability, in some subjects at least, to chain larger numbers of vocabulary items or expand phrases minimally in order to express more semantic information within the same utterance. The limited progress observed in MR adolescents with comparison to NR children in semantic lexical comprehension and expression may reflect additional life experience properly verbalized, and corresponding to the continued, even if limited, general conceptual development of these individuals during adolescence. In the same way, it is likely that the progress of MR adolescents in the pragmatic and communicative aspects of language is associated with continued progress in social knowledge and skills, as suggested by Rosenberg and Abbeduto (1993).

As observed by Comblain (1995), the same hierarchies of correct responses and types of errors are found in the performance of NR children, DS children, DS adolescents, and DS adults, on the various subtests of the BEMS (see Table 5.1). Van Borsel (1988) also reported that the phonological processes of his DS adolescents were similar to those of younger NR children. These observations suggest that similar mechanisms are at work in the development of the computational aspects of language in MR and NR individuals, which is consistent with the continuity-developmental perspective adopted in this book. These last observations may be in opposition to the suggestions by Lenneberg (1967) and others (e.g. Newport, 1992) that the linguistic analyses entertained by late learners differ from those of earlier learners. It may be that most of the structural learning performed by MR adolescents actually takes place during childhood, i.e., within the boundaries of the critical period for computational language development. This being the case, there would be no reason for the linguistic analyses of these subjects to differ from those of younger individuals.

5.2 Prelinguistic development

This period of development covers the major part of the first 18 months in the NR infant. The same development is extended in the moderately and severely MR child and occupies most of the first 2 or 3 years. During this period, the child learns the basic principles of human communication, first, at the non-verbal level. He or she gradually goes from a global mode of expression, involving the whole or most of the body, to more differentiated forms centering on vocal activity. The infant's vocal activity modifies itself considerably during prelinguistic development. It goes from crying and cooing to babbling, and later to the production of unconventional and then conventional words. The first year also witnesses a remarkable evolution in the mental activity of the infant. It evolves from the physiological reflexes to the beginning of structuration of the human and physical environment, the major aspects of which have been described by authors such as Piaget (1936, 1937) and Spitz (1958). Spitz analysed the infant's evolution in the first year of life, concentrating on the construction of the affective figures. Other authors, such as Schaffer and Emerson (1964) and Yarrow (1972), have described the affective bonding process between mother and infant during the first year, and the appearance around 7 or 8 months in the NR infant of the first reactions of fear in the presence of strangers. However, the infant's reconstruction of the world does not concern the affective figures only. Piaget and others, particularly Bower, have analysed in great detail the infant's early structuration of reality (e.g. Piaget, 1937; Bower, 1967): for example, the object permanence concept and the evolution of what Piaget called sensorimotor intelligence (i.e. the intellectual regulations embodied in the baby's sensorimotor activities prior to symbolic development and language; also corresponding to Vygotsky's notion of prelinguistic intelligence, Vygotsky, 1962). During this period, the infant organizes his immediate physical world into more stable entities which become targets for symbolic coding and vocal labelling. In the same way, he becomes sensitive to a number of typical relations between persons, objects and events, which supply the basis for semantic relational development.

Towards the end of the first year or the beginning of the second year, the NR child contextually understands a limited number of words and short multiword utterances. He is then close to trying to produce them. The symbolic link between significant and signified is within conceptual reach and will serve as a basis for further lexical development.

5.2.1 Sensorimotor development

Results of neurological examinations (see Cowie, 1970) show hypotonia and abnormalities in the early reflexes and automatisms of DS infants. These include the palmar and plantar grasp reflexes, the Landau reaction (ventral suspension), the Moro response and automatic stepping. Delayed dissolution of early reflexes and reactions is also commonly observed in this syndrome. Corresponding indications have been reported for other handicapped infants (cerebral palsied, chronic brain syndromes and other syndromes of mental retardation) (Foley, Cookson and Zappella, 1964; Paine et al., 1964; Zappella, 1964; Zappella, Foley and Cookson, 1964).

Motor development is usually delayed in moderate and severe MR, particularly in DS, due to congenital hypotonia. As classically noted (e.g. Paine, 1963), mental retardation is often associated with generalized hypotonia. Problems in motor development in moderate and severe MR infants may further delay early cognitive development to the extent that the latter is at least partly dependent upon moving around in a familiar physical setting, manipulating objects, and perceiving and acting on events and relationships between people and objects, objects and objects, people and people. Piaget (1936, 1937) claimed that the knowledge of young infants is in terms of the sensorimotor impressions familiar objects have on them and the motor adjustments they require. The child will not have verbal concepts until the second year of life.

5.2.2 Sound discrimination

By late foetal life, the hearing mechanism is well developed. It is believed that the foetus cannot hear sounds of normal intensity. Very likely, however, he has the capacity to perceive sounds of intensities beyond 80 or 90 decibels, particularly low-frequency sounds (also transmitted through bone vibration). Visual mechanisms are less well developed at birth than auditory ones. However, a full-term infant is capable of following visually a slowly moving object of medium size. He is sensitive to object contours and patterns within a few days of birth. Myelinization of the visual nervous fibres is not completed until several months after birth and improvement in the ability to fixate accurately and to see details continues to take place until about age 6.

As a result of prenatal and perinatal developments, NR infants display early discrimination of their mother's voice and speech, providing it is normally intonated. If the mother is requested to read sentences backwards, the infant no longer recognizes his or her mother's voice (Mehler et al., 1978). Young NR infants are also able to discriminate their maternal language (in the double sense here of the language of the cultural community first heard and the mother's language) from any other language presented. Mehler et al. (1987, 1988) presented random alternative sequences of 15-second speech samples from French and Russian to neonates (4 days old). All could reliably differentiate maternal and foreign language as indicated by modifications induced in the rates of non-nutritive sucking (operated according to the paradigm of selective habituation). Such a discriminative performance is based on an analysis of the prosodic properties of the languages. However, the babies are only able to discriminate two languages if one of the two is already familiar. These observations mean that from birth onwards the human infant is sensitive to the prosodic characteristics of what will later be recognized as sentences belonging to the community language.

Most remarkable is the capacity of the young infant to perceive syllables. Syllables play an important role in speech perception in many languages. They usually are discriminated better and with shorter response times by adult subjects than single phonemes (e.g. Savin and Bever, 1970). Young infants are capable of distinguishing syllables in alternating triplets of consonant–vowel–consonant (e.g. *pat* vs *bat*). Normal syllables shortened to 30-second stimuli can be reliably differentiated by neonates (4 days old), as opposed to 20 seconds for adults (Bertoncini et al., 1987). Treating syllables in maternal language therefore could require only minimal learning from the infant's part.

In the early 1970s, the now classic research conducted by Eimas et al. (1971) revealed that young infants perceive language sounds in a categorial way, just like adults do (i.e. language sounds are perceived in a discontinuous way with very narrow frontiers between each other – physically, of course, sounds constitute continuous series). Following on Eimas et al.'s work, researchers established that 1-month-old infants are potentially sensitive to acoustic contrasts between *all* the sounds existing in natural languages. For example, neonates are capable of discriminating language sounds on the basis of place of articulation (e.g. *p, t, k*), mode of articulation (*d, n*), oral vowels (*a, i, u*), oral and nasal vowels (*a, an*), etc. A controversy subsists between universalists and developmentalists. The universalist position concludes from numerous studies that the infant's discriminative ability is excellent at birth and only some fine-tuning is necessary. The work of Eilers et al. (1984) and others suggests, however, that some particular contrasts may only be correctly perceived after minimal linguistic experience.

Interestingly, the neonates' overall discriminative ability for language sounds gradually decreases over the first year of life, except for the phoneme sounds characteristic of their community language (or languages in multilingual situations). For example, Japanese babies are able to distinguish /r/ and /l/ sounds, whereas older Japanese children and adults no longer can, as these phonemes do not exist in the Japanese language. A number of longitudinal studies have been carried out in several languages (e.g. Werker et al., 1981; Werker and Tees, 1984) showing that decreased discriminative ability for the phonemic contrasts non-existent in maternal language, is established around 10–12 months. The gradual loss of sensitivity to unheard phonetic contrasts seems to be cognitive and/or attentional but not neurosensorial. Actually, as shown in a study by Best, McRoberts and Sithole (1988), there is no decrease in sensitivity in older infants for those sounds and contrasts that are not potential competitors for the phonemes of maternal language. Only those sounds and contrasts that share one or several dimensions with maternal phonemes are lost towards the end of the first year. The other sounds and contrasts with no equivalence or acoustic proximity in maternal language continue to be discriminated correctly in older children as well as in adults. It may be concluded that in the course of the first year, there is receptive specialization in the infant in the phonemes of maternal language(s). This specialization is established on a statistical basis. The frequency of occurrence of the phonemes in a given language increases towards the centre part of the linguistic categories preferentially used in that language. Conversely, the less a given language is practised, the lower the frequency of occurrence of the sounds close to the basic phonemic categories. This natural statistics explains why babies progressively ignore those sounds that have no distinctive value in their community language.

Mehler and Dupoux (1990) suggest that the babies' evolution in sound sensitivity over the first year is a clear example of 'learning by forgetting'. Such an explanation is reminiscent of the conception of postnatal development according to a sort of 'neural Darwinism'. In this view (e.g. Changeux, 1983; Gazzaniga, 1993), human brains comprise a large initial excess of synaptic connections and circuits. During development, the connections that are particularly useful to an organism are sustained, whereas the others are eliminated. Actually, the infants' gradual specialization in maternal speech for sound perception (and, as we shall see in what follows, for sound production as well) is as compatible with the neural constructionist perspective advocated by Purves (1988, 1994) and Purves and Lichtman (1985), for example. According to this latter conception, the brain is constructed mostly by the gradual activity-dependent accretion of circuitry, and not, or only very little, by selection of circuitry from an initial excess.

5.2.3 Babbling and infraphonological development

Indications corresponding to the evolution in sound discrimination have been reported regarding the evolution in infants' babbling over the first year. Oller and Lynch (1993) distinguish five major periods within babbling. They construe them as construction stages building upon each other towards adult speech sounds. *Stage 1* (0–2 months, approximately) witnesses reflex or quasi-reflex vocalizations with crying and other more or less vegetative sounds. Between approximately 2 and 4 months (*stage 2*), babies produce cooing sounds tied to smiles and prevocalic sounds. Oller (1990) observed a lengthening in duration of prevocalic and vocalic sounds between 3 and 5 months going from 700 to 1400 milliseconds. In *stage 3* (3–8 months), full precanonical (see below) babbling experience is going on. Researchers insist on the excellent ability of the infant to play with his or her voice, exploring its full-range spectrum and contrastive power (producing a wide variety of sounds, for example, quasi-vowels (or immature vowel-like sounds), clicks, palatalized, rounded or pharyngealized consonants, affricates, sibilants, etc., as noted years ago by Jakobson, 1941, 1968). A marked widening of the vocal spectrum is observed. Low-pitch (growls) as well as high-pitch (squeals) sounds may be produced beginning around the third month. The sounds produced by the infants also vary widely according to intensity level. *Stage 4* (5–10 months) is characterized by the production of well-formed, or so-called *canonical syllables*, of the consonant-(full) vowel (CV) type (e.g. *ba* or *da*). Oller (1990) relates the concept of canonical syllable to that of minimal rhythmic unit of natural language, and its components, the nucleus, the margin(s), and the formant transition(s). Oller and Eilers (1988) suggest that canonical syllabic babbling is first *reduplicated* (e.g. *mamama, papapapa, babababababa*) – which attests to a first clear auditory control over the vocal activity – and then *variegated* (consisting of consonants and vowels that differ). As observed by Steffens et al. (1992), however, the production of precanonical syllables and quasi-vowels, though diminishing with time, persists into the second year of life. These data provide an indication that stage models such as Oller and Lynch's (1993) are idealizations, which may be useful, but that infants do not necessarily abandon previous vocal styles when moving ahead in development. Finally, *stage 5* (9–18 months) witnesses the appearance of significant productions in the infant's babbling. It could be questioned whether this period is still babbling rather than prelexical or lexical as intended meaning begins to play a role in constraining vocal productions.

Before 6 months, approximately, infants' babbling appears to be only minimally influenced by the community language. Sounds that do not belong to maternal language are produced. Between 6 and 12 months, an influence of the linguistic environment on phonetic characteristics of the infants' babbling is most likely. Konopczynski (1986), quoting from a unpublished work by Tuaycharoen, observes that as early as 6 months Thai babies' babbling differs at the prosodic level from the babbling of babies raised in non-tonal linguistic environments. Contradictory results have been reported by Locke (1988) and Oller and Eilers (1988), finding no difference in the babbling of English and Spanish infants as well as other languages in the second half of the first year. However, a series of studies conducted by Boysson-Bardies and associates (Boysson-Bardies, Sogart and Durand, 1984; Boysson-Bardies, 1988; Boysson-Bardies and Durand, 1991; Hallé and Boysson-Bardies, 1991; Hallé, Boysson-Bardies and Durand, 1992) clearly illustrate the gradual influence of the community language on prosodic and segmental characteristics of infants' babbling in the second half of the first year.

These researchers show that phonetically naïve adults can reliably recognize prosodic features of their language (French, Algerian Arabic or Cantonese) in 15-seconds babbling samples from 8- and 10-month infants. The existence of intonational differences between the reduplicative babbling of French- and English-learning infants (5–11-months) was confirmed by Whalen, Levitt and Wang (1991). Such data corroborate the indication that infants begin to use prosodic features specific to their maternal language in the second half of the first year (Ingram, 1989). Boysson-Bardies and associates have demonstrated further that infants' babbling is differentiated according to segmental features towards the end of the first year (*circa* 10 months of age). Vowel configurations from French, Algerian Arabic and Cantonese infants, aged 10 months, were compared to speech sequences from adults of corresponding language communities for 'long-term spectrum'. Those spectra compute the spread of vocal energy for vocalic portions of speech signals lasting several minutes. The data reveal a good convergence between vowel characteristics of infant babbling and adult speech. This indication was confirmed in a direct analysis of the formant characteristics of the vowels produced in the babbling of 10-month infants exposed to French, English, Algerian Arabic and Cantonese, respectively. It seems indeed that the infants' vocalic space tends towards that of the adults towards the end of the first year. English-exposed infants and English-speaking adults have the highest formant 2 (oral)/formant 1 (pharyngeal) ratio observed, which corresponds to a prevalence in frequency of occurrence of diffuse vowels in English. Cantonese subjects produce the most compact vowels in average value. French and Algerian Arabic subjects are located in between the other two groups with formant 1 being lower in tonal value for the French subjects, which reflects the relatively high occurrence of closed rounded vowels in French (Hallé, Boysson-Bardies and Durand, 1992).

The above data regarding sound perception as well as sound production in babbling appear to corroborate the 'interactional hypothesis' in prelinguistic development. Normal infants can make most perceptual speech distinctions at birth likely because they are born with a basic capacity to perceive and produce speech. Or, as claimed by Petitto and Marentette (1991), infants are innately predisposed to discover a particular patterned input of 'phonetic and syllabic units', whatever the language modality, a predisposition to be ascribed to an amodal language capacity. These latter authors have documented babbling in the manual mode similar to babbling in the vocal mode in deaf infants exposed to sign languages from birth. Perceptual maturation is ahead of production. It may be basically complete at birth. Early sound (sign) production requires additional maturational growth. The role of language experience is not to be minimized, however. Over the course of the first year, normal infants specialize in maternal language, first, at the non-segmental level, then, at the segmental level. They do so partly at the expense of their previous 'universal' phonetic capacity.

5.2.4 Babbling and speech perception in MR infants

How do MR infants develop prelinguistically in comparison to what is known of NR infants? Data are largely missing but some indications can be proposed with particular reference to Down's syndrome. Dodd (1972) and Smith and Oller (1981) suggested that the sounds of babbling are mostly similar in types and tokens in NR and DS infants. Parameters such as number of vowel and consonant productions, number of non-speech noises, variety of consonants and vowels produced, length of vocalic and consonantal utterances, and general trends regarding the development of individual consonants and vowels, do not seem to differentiate between the two populations of infants. However, syllabic patterning may be more problematic in MR infants. In opposition to an earlier indication by Smith and Oller (1981), Lynch et al. (in press) report that reduplicated babbling is delayed and less stable in DS infants. The latter authors observe the onset of reduplicated babbling around 6 months at home and 9 months in laboratory studies in NR infants, vs 8 and 10 months, respectively, in DS infants. The discrepancies between the results of Lynch et al. (in press) and those of Smith and Oller (1981) may be due to differences in the frequency of contact between investigators and subjects. Lynch et al. sampled vocalizations more frequently.

Reduplicated babbling may be a distinct precursor to meaningful speech. In Lynch et al.'s study, the age of onset of reduplicated babbling estimated from parental report was significantly correlated with the DS infants' scores at 27 months CA on the Early Social-Communication Scales (Mundy, Seibert and Hogan, 1984). These scales have predictive value with respect to subsequent development of verbal communication (Mundy, Sigman and Kasari, 1990). It seems to be the case that DS negatively influences expressive vocal development as early as the first year of life. Possible explanatory variables for the delays of DS infants in the development of canonical syllables and reduplicated babbling are maturational delay, generalized hypotonia at birth and in the following months in many DS babies, and mild auditory deficiency in a number of DS babies. Over time, however (particularly in the first half of the second year of life), and in spite of marked individual differences, DS infants increase their production of full vowels and canonical consonant–vowel syllables, implying better coordinated articulatory movements. They decrease their production of less mature quasi-vowels and precanonical syllables (Steffens et al., 1992).

Very few systematic data have been reported on speech perception in MR babies and its evolution compared to NR babies. Eilers et al. (1985) have suggested that DS infants may be limited in perceiving place of articulation distinctions in well-formed syllables. A problem with speed of auditory processing may be involved. Indeed when syllables were slowed down through synthesis of acoustic stimuli in Eilers et al.'s research, DS infants demonstrated improved performance. More research on these aspects of prelinguistic development in MR infants is necessary. One needs to know the exact capacities of MR babies regarding early recognition of mother's voice and maternal language, sensitivity to prosodic and rhythmic aspects of adult language, to precanonical and canonical syllables and related structures of language, the early differentiation of infraphonemic contrasts, as well as the evolution of these abilities over time.

Assuming that the above-mentioned capacities belong to the species-specific predispositions for speech (or, according to Petitto and Marentette, 1991, for language no matter the modality that is being developed), they should be ascribed to MR infants as well and to the same extent as NR infants. Of course, moderately and severely MR infants being maturationally delayed, the open manifestation of the above capacities can be postponed for some time, a period for which we have no clear estimate at present.

5.2.5 Interactive babbling

As early as 3 months, prelinguistic vocalizations display particular characteristics labelled 'phrasing' in recent publications (e.g., Lynch et al., in press). Prelinguistic phrasing is defined as intermittent babbling,

approximately 3 seconds long, characterized by the rhythm and structure that later underlie speech (for example, phrase-ending syllables last
longer than other syllables, which could be interpeted as a signal prefig-
urating turn-taking organization). The DS babies (2–12 months of age)
studied by Lynch et al. (in press) display the same rhythmic organization
in prelinguistic phrases as NR infants. But they take longer to finish a
prelinguistic phrase (an average of more than 5 seconds). This extended
timeframe could explain why mothers and their DS babies are often
found to vocalize simultaneously (Jones, 1977; Buckhalt, Rutherford
and Goldberg, 1978; Berger and Cunningham, 1983).

Moderately and severely MR infants may be slower to develop prelinguistically. We need to specify better in which respects and why. Prelinguistic phrasing should be investigated carefully for it may provide an
indication of the vocal exchange patterns that contribute to the developing bond between babies and people. This bond may be necessary for
communication development.

5.2.6 Symbolic babbling

NR children are known to produce *jargon babbling* (i.e. meaningless
babbling sequences that sound like sentences because they reproduce
the intonational structures of adult speech). The onset is 12–14 months
(Petitto and Marentette, 1991). About at the same time, NR infants begin
to produce particular sounds or sequences of sounds to refer to object
entities or to suggest some course of action. Halliday (1975) supplied
examples of this stage from diary observations of his son Nigel. For
example, Nigel had two early vocalized requests for joint action of the
type expressed in adult language by *Let's*. These were the equivalent of
the adult forms *Let's go for a walk* and *Let's draw a picture*. The first was
expressed by a sound of Nigel's 'invention', a very slow vibration of the
vocal chords; the other a sound which at first was probably an imitation
of the word *draw*, and later more often as *bow-wow*, meaning originally
Let's draw a dog, but then generalized to a sense of *Let's draw a picture*.
Earlier in his vocal development, Nigel would typically comment on the
presence of a plane flying overhead with a sound which was his imitation of the noise of the plane.

The point is that the infant is developing a temporarily stable relation
between some sounds and meanings. These meanings are usually not
something that can be easily glossed in terms of the adult language. They
correspond to the infant's perception of an event or object and the
infant tries to mark these perceptions through the use of vocal sounds.
Carter (1978) confirmed Halliday's observations in a longitudinal
analysis of the communication acts of an infant between 12 and 24
months. She noted numerous examples of phonetically stable vocalizations containing elements of meaning. Golinkoff (1983) has stressed the

interactive nature of such vocalizations. She demonstrated the role played by mothers' interpretation of the infants' protowords and the true process of 'meaning negotiation' taking place between the partners in this type of interaction.

It will be remembered that this stage of development also corresponds to the establishment of cognitive object permanence (Piaget, 1936, 1937), although we acknowledge the distinct possibility that younger babies may already exhibit *perceptual* object permanence (see Bower, 1967). It then makes sense and it is possible for the infant to attempt symbolic relations between vocal sounds (and/or gestures) and permanent referents.

Few systematic observations are available on these developments in MR infants. It is likely that object permanence and sensorimotor intellectual development are delayed in these infants in proportion to their cognitive handicap. Wishart (1993; see also Wishart, in press) has analysed individual developmental profiles drawn from a series of longitudinal studies of early cognitive development in DS children. On the whole, age of initial acquisition of most object concept stages was found to lag only a few months behind control subjects. However, developmental instability was a recurrent theme. Cicchetti and Mans-Wagener (1987) also reported little delay in object permanence development in DS children. Rast and Meltzoff (1995), on the contrary, signal a marked delay. Their NR infants reached high-level object permanence (invisible displacements) at about 8–12 months, which is consistent with the usual developmental indications (Piaget, 1936; Uzgiris and Hunt, 1975), whereas their DS sample ranged from 20 to 43 months-CA for the same acquisition. Rast and Meltzoff (1995) suggest that the studies reporting little delay in object permanence for DS children actually provided training by testing the infants repeatedly. They find support for their hypothesis in the indication that positive outcomes in those studies were not maintained after termination of the regular testing schedule (Wishart, 1988).

5.2.7 Transition from babbling to speech production

It is now clear that infant vocalizations are continuous with later development of spoken language. The discontinuity hypothesis proposed by Jakobson (1941, 1968), Lenneberg, Rebelski and Nichols (1965) and Lenneberg (1967), according to which prelinguistic vocalizations have no direct relationship with further language and only illustrate the maturation of the neurophysiological apparatus for speech, no longer finds persuasive defenders. It appears, on the contrary, that for normally developing infants at least, the phonetic characteristics of babbling persist into early word production and influence early word selection (Locke, 1988; Kent and Miolo, 1995). Prelinguistic development should receive more attention from researchers for it could certainly yield additional cues as to why functional speech is markedly delayed in MR children.

5.3 Speech development

Phonology is the study of the sound system of languages. From the wide range of sounds that the human vocal tract can produce, only a small number are used distinctively in any one language (around 30–40 in French or English; more than 100 in Bochiman, the language of African Bushmen; and fewer than 20 in some Polynesian languages). The phonemes are organized into a system of contrasts. These contrasts play an important role in the explanation of phonological development.

Within phonology, two branches of study are recognized: *segmental phonology* and *non-segmental or suprasegmental phonology*. The former branch studies the way speech is analysed into discrete segments (the phonemes) along with the analysis of the phonetic features and processes which relate and differentiate these segments (Crystal, 1989). Non-segmental phonology studies those features which extend over more than one segment, such as intonation and rhythm.

The study of non-segmental phonology is less advanced than the analysis of segmental phonology. The integration of a number of relevant notions such as 'prosody', 'intonation', 'stress' (primary, secondary), 'rhythm', 'tone of voice', etc., into a coherent framework is still to come (see Halliday, 1985, and Crystal, 1989, for descriptive analyses). As a consequence, much less is known of the development of non-segmental phonology and its problems than for segmental phonology.

5.3.1 Articulatory problems in mental retardation

Articulatory problems are more prevalent among MR subjects than NR children. Prevalence varies with the psychometric level of the cognitive handicap and the specific MR syndrome. Mildly MR subjects exhibit only a slightly higher incidence of articulatory difficulties (i.e. 8 or 9 per cent) than NR subjects (approximately 5 per cent including minor articulatory difficulties; Spreen, 1965). However, between 70 and 90 per cent of the moderately and severely MR subjects have serious articulatory problems (Schlanger, 1953; Spradlin, 1963). Down's syndrome subjects are particularly prone to slowness of articulatory development and persisting difficulties. A number of problems may be responsible for the high prevalence of speech difficulties in DS people. Some of these problems apply to MR subjects with other aetiologies as well. Peripheral pathological factors associated with defective speech in DS have been long noted (e.g., Benda, 1949). They include a buccal cavity too small for the tongue and a protruding tongue (Ardran, Harker, and Kemp, 1972). It is rarely the case, however, that the tongue is markedly enlarged as some reports have suggested (for example, Oster (1953).[1]

Some DS children may have localized enlargement in the region of the lingual tonsil (resulting in narrowing of the lower pharynx and the superior laryngeal aperture). Many DS children have enlarged adenoids. Another common anatomical feature of DS persons is the displacement forwards of the mandible. Sixty per cent, according to Shapiro (1970), have a 'prognathic jaw relationship'. A large proportion of DS children show teeth deformities which are uncommon in NR children. These problems may result in defective dental occlusion and a change in the size of the oral cavity, which in turn may affect sound resonance. The palate may be short or cleft (Spitzer, Rabinowitch and Wybar, 1961). The larynx is often located high in the neck with thickening of fibrotic mucosa, vocal fold oedema, myxoedema of the pharynx, and an oedematous tongue, which is impaired in its mobility. Hypotonia of the speech muscles, involving tongue, lips, soft palate and breathing muscles, is common.

Other mechanical factors influencing speech include auditory defects. Hearing loss is more frequent in MR subjects than in NR people. This seems to be particularly true for DS individuals. These subjects have more hearing problems than other mental retardation categories at comparable mental levels (Keiser et al., 1981; Evenhuis et al., 1992). In Rigrodsky, Prunty and Glovsky's report (1961), hearing impairment was indicated to affect 60 per cent of the DS sample. The losses are mainly in the mildly to moderately impaired range (i.e., mean decibel range 25–55 bilaterally over the frequencies 500, 1000 and 2000 Hz) with the impairment being half-conductive and half sensorineural and 'mixed'. Other reports signal lower figures of hearing loss in DS subjects and prevalence of conductive losses over sensorineural and mixed ones (e.g. Clausen, 1968). Brainstem auditory evoked responses (BAEPs) in children with DS (e.g. Gigli et al., 1984; Ferri et al., 1986) confirm the existence of conductive losses in a large proportion of the subjects. Numerous DS individuals show BAEP abnormalities indicative of a brain-

---

[1] To improve tongue control, swallowing and facial appearance, increasing attention has been given in recent years to surgical modification of the tip of the tongue (see Lemperle and Radu, 1980; Rozner, 1983; Olbrisch, 1985), thereby decreasing tongue length for improved intraoral control. Some improvement in intelligibility of articulation and swallowing has been reported (e.g. Wexler et al., 1986). However, this information has come principally from parent reports, not from formal studies. Other indications (e.g. Margar-Bacal, Witzel and Munro, 1988) have been more critical regarding the possibility of improved articulation following facial plastic surgery in DS subjects, while acknowledging that it could favour physical appearance. Actually, as sound coarticulation implies the mobilization of a large number of muscles and anatomical structures, the tip of the tongue being only one of them, it is unlikely that punctual modifications could lead to marked changes in speech quality. Besides, since the articulatory problems in DS mainly result from a developmental delay, it is doubtful that interventions merely modifying a part of the peripheral mechanism could lead to markedly improved speech.

stem conduction dysfunction which seems to be positively correlated with the degree of mental retardation.

The deficits in motor coordination, timing and the generalized hypotonia characteristic of DS subjects particularly during the first years, may adversely affect the speech production system (O'Connor and Hermelin, 1963; Rosin, Swift and Bless, 1987). Things may be more complex, however. It is known that most Williams syndrome subjects also suffer from generalized hypotonia, but they are often exempt from serious articulatory problems. It is likely that no simple relationship holds between generalized hypotonia and speech development. Frith and Frith (1974) suggested that DS subjects exhibit a deficit in preprogrammed motor sequences. However, if one takes into account Liberman and Mattingly's (1989) proposal regarding the existence of a speech module, central to speech perception as well as to speech production, then a minimal repertoire of innately specified speech gestures cannot be denied to MR subjects (including those with genetic syndromes). This type of hypothesis runs contrary to a literal interpretation of Frith and Frith's (1974) suggestion.

Deficits in motor coordination and timing may be partly responsible for the higher proportion of stuttering or stuttering-like phenomena observed in moderately and severely MR subjects, particularly DS subjects. DS subjects exhibiting some kind of stuttering represent 33–50 per cent of the samples observed, depending on the particular study (Gottsleben, 1955; Zisk and Bialer, 1967; Preus, 1972; Stansfield, 1990).

Voice problems are classically described as prominent in some categories of MR subjects, particularly DS subjects. The voice quality deviations most often noted include breathiness, hoarseness and harshness. Some studies have reported a higher fundamental frequency in DS individuals (e.g. Weinberg and Zlatin, 1970). Others indicate that differences tend to vanish when proper control is exercised for factors like karyotype, verbal task, degree of closeness in matching DS and NR subjects or MR subjects of other aetiologies than DS (Montague and Hollien, 1973). As suggested by Benda (1949), there could be a relationship between specific vocal problems and anatomical–physiological features frequent in DS. For example, many DS subjects have small, blunt styloid processes as well as deviation of various other facial bones. The styloid processes and other facial bones are joints of attachment for many muscles which extend to the larynx or the hyoid bone, whose movement influences that of the larynx. These abnormalities may result in an abnormal pull on the larynx supporting the usual observation that the larynx of DS subjects tend to be located higher in the neck than is normal. These anomalies may favour deviations in voice quality.

A recent study by Pryce (1994) casts an interesting light on other possible causes of harshness and hoarseness in the voices of people with Down's syndrome. She reports that the energy level needed to activate the vocal mechanism from its 'at rest' to its voicing level (measured by a technique known as electromyographic biofeedback) is almost twice as great for DS adults (132 microvolts or thereabouts) as for control subjects (around 73 microvolts). These results may be related to the hypotonia frequent in DS subjects (although to a much lesser extent in adults than in younger children). Greater levels of energy are needed to activate a more flaccid vocal mechanism. Harshness and gruffness in DS subjects' voices could be explained at least partly by the exaggerated energy level employed by these people in activating a hypotonic vocal apparatus. Other explanatory factors are almost certainly involved, however. They include possible differences in laryngeal fundamental frequencies (having to do with the size and texture of the vocal chords in DS subjects) and a possible drying effect of the mucosal lining extending down the oral tract and covering the laryngeal areas, caused by the open mouth posture frequently associated with DS.

5.3.2 Segmental phonological development

According to Jakobson (1941, 1968), the child universally first acquires the phonemes most contrasted first. For example, the first vowel to emerge and stabilize is usually /a/, and a labial stop consonant inaugurates consonantism. This yields C–V combinations. The articulatory contrast is maximal for oppositions between vowels such as /a/ and consonants such as /p/, /b/ or /m/. In order to articulate /a/, the mouth is open. The tongue is flat in the mouth and the vocal chords must vibrate. There is no limitation in duration and a strong acoustical energy is concentrated within a relatively narrow band of frequencies ('compact' character). The articulatory-acoustical characteristics of consonantal phonemes such as /p/ are almost exactly the reverse as those of /a/. The child may therefore start phonological development with two consonants and a vowel and gradually build up his system by a general process of binary splitting. He would then distinguish /i/ and /u/ on the vowel side, and phonemes like /t/ then /k/ on the consonantal side (continuums acute–grave and compact–diffuse). Then other oral and nasal vowels would add to the phonemic repertoire, together with voiced stop consonants, nasal consonants, unvoiced and voiced continuous consonants, and laterals (such as /l/). This development begins by the end of the first year and terminates around 5 years. However, the latest consonants (continuous) may remain articulatorily unstable until 7 or 8 years in normally developing children.

There are problems with this type of formulation. First, it assumes that there is a typical, universal order of phoneme acquisition applying to all children. Second, it fails to allow for the fact that some of the phonemes belonging to a phonemic category may be acquired earlier than others. Third, it is not clear which criterion of acquisition should prevail in this context. Some investigators seem to consider that acquisition has occurred when a child produces an acceptable allophone of a consonant phoneme in initial, intervocalic and final positions, but other variables besides position affect pronounciation (e.g. consonant harmony). Fourth, dialect differences may influence phonological development (Menn and Stoel-Gammon, 1995).

Sander (1972) reanalysed studies of large groups of American-English subjects provided by Templin (1957), using single words elicited and imitated. For labial phonemes /p/, /b/, /m/, /w/, and also for /h/ and /n/, the 50 per cent mark (i.e. the ages at which 50 per cent of the children produce acceptable allophones) is reached before age 2 in Templin's test materials. Except for /b/, these phonemes reach the 90 per cent mark by age 3. The velars /k/, /g/, /ŋ/, and the alveolar stops /t/ and /d/ reach 50 per cent correct production at age 2; /b/, /k/, /g/ and /d/ reach 90 per cent by age 4, but /t/ and /ŋ/ do not so until age 6. The greatest lag between the 50 and 90 per cent marks was shown by the phoneme /s/, which reaches 50 per cent at age 3 but does not reach 90 per cent until age 8.

In spite of the fact that considerable individual differences may be found in longitudinal group studies, the order of contrast acquisition proposed by Jakobson (1941, 1968) is a good fit probabilistically. For instance, the American-English and the French vowel system (except for the nasal vowels in the latter language) are most often completed before the consonantal system is complete. In general, consonantal stops precede fricatives and affricates. Glides (or semi-vowels) /j/ and /w/ precede liquids (for example, /l/ and /r/). The order of early vowel acquisition is close to /a/, /i/, /u/, /o/ and /ʌ/, in many cases. For languages which employ more complex articulations, simply articulated sounds such as /k/ are mastered before more marked phones such as glottalized [k'].

One way in which the phonemic model of development is clearly inadequate is that it does not enable one to see how different strategies used by children can produce similar phonological results (Crystal, 1989). The suggestion was made (Stampe, 1972; Ingram, 1974, 1976) that a study of the strategies or processing rules used by children to approximate adult forms in their outputs would be illuminating. Three main classes of rules (assumed to be universal; Stampe, 1972) have been proposed. The following presentation owes much to Crystal (1989): (1) *Substitution processes*, such as *stopping*, whereby fricatives tend to be replaced by stops (e.g. say → /teɪ/); *fronting*, whereby velars and palatals are replaced by alveolars (e.g. *shoe* → /suː/); *gliding*, whereby /l/ and /r/ are replaced by /w/ or /j/ (e.g. *leg* → /jeg/); and *vocalization*, whereby syllabic consonants are replaced by vowels (e.g. *apple* → /apʊ/). (2) *Assimilatory processes*. Examples of these latter rules are *consonant* or *vowel harmony*, whereby a consonant or a vowel in one position within a word or syllable becomes more like or identical with one consonant or one vowel, respectively, from another position in the same word or syllable (e.g. *flower* → /fa:wa/). Another example of assimilatory process is *voicing*, whereby a consonant becomes voiced before a vowel and devoiced in syllable-final position (e.g., *pig* → /bik/). And (3) *syllable structure processes*, which consist in direct simplifications of the adult forms. For example, *cluster reduction*, whereby elements in adult consonant clusters are omitted or blended, so that a singleton consonant is uttered (e.g. *quick* → /kik/); *final consonant deletion*, whereby the last consonant in a CVC syllable is omitted (e.g. *bike* → /bai/); and *unstressed syllable deletion* (e.g. *banana* → /na:na/).

Ingram (1976) attempted to place phonological development in relation to Piaget's cognitive stages. He correlated the sensorimotor period (from birth to 18 or 20 months) with prelinguistic vocalizations and early phonological development (the first 50 words or so), and the preconceptual subperiod (18–20 months to 4 years) with the phonology of single morphemes (child expanding productive inventory of speech sounds and relying on phonological processes to reproduce – incorrectly – many adult words). The latter period of development ends at around 4 years when most words of single morphological structure are correctly spoken. The cognitive preoperational subperiod (4–7 years) is correlated with completion of the phonemic inventory with good production of single words and beginning of use of longer and articulatory more complex words. Corresponding to the cognitive concrete operational period (7–12 years) is morphophonemic development. At this stage, children learn more elaborate derivational structures of the language, acquiring the morphophonemic rules (that is the contextual variations in the shape of morphemes which are not due to general phonological rules). Lastly, according to Ingram, the period of formal operations corresponds to the ability to spell (spelling rules) and the metaphonological ability (see Menn and Stoel-Gammon, 1995).

Ingram (1976) is cautious, however, not to propose an overtly causal relationship between cognitive and phonological development, although he may have something of that kind in mind. Ingram probably views favourably the hypothesis according to which phonological development could be explained, at least in part, by aspects of cognitive development considered within Piaget's conceptual framework. Unfortunately, Ingram does not supply more specification regarding his point of view (including in more recent publications, e.g. Ingram, 1989). To the best of our knowledge, he is the only one to have proposed such a direct relationship between cognitive and phonological developments. So-called constructivist or functional theories in developmental phonology (e.g. Macken and Ferguson, 1983; Menn, 1983) have sometimes referred to their positions as being cognitivist, meaning that they oppose innate specifications. But the term *cognitive* or *cognitivist* used with this latter type of intension does not compare to Ingram's suggested relationship between cognitive and phonological developments.

Ingram's suggestion may seem at first glance to be highly relevant to studying phonological development in MR children, as these children are cognitively retarded by definition. As noted above, moderately and severely MR subjects usually exhibit a much higher proportion of speech problems than mildly retarded and non-retarded subjects. The former are depicted (Inhelder, 1968; Gibson, 1981) as not progressing beyond preoperational levels of development, which may appear to be a validating argument for Ingram's hypothesis. It would seem, however, that data regarding the excellent phonological abilities of a number of language-exceptional MR subjects, as analysed in Chapter 4, as well as the fact that many Williams syndrome subjects have good quality speech despite a moderate level of mental retardation, as documented in Chapter 3, are sufficient to refute any hypothesis directly tying phonological and cognitive developments.

Articulatory development is slow and difficult in many MR children (but not all) for a number of reasons including the delays and uncertainties of lexical development, but the overall progression parallels that of NR children, even if many MR children (particularly DS children) exhibit more inconsistent articulation (Dodd, 1976; Smith and Oller, 1981; Stoel-Gammon, 1980, 1981; Menn, 1983; Smith and Stoel-Gammon, 1983; Dodd and Leahy, 1989; Borghi, 1990). Vowels, semivowels and nasal and stop consonants are produced and mastered first. Fricatives /f/, /θ/, /s/, /ʒ/, /ʃ/, /v/, /ð/, /z/ and affricates /tʃ/ and /dʒ/ are more difficult to articulate. They take longer to be mastered by MR subjects and may never be achieved. The distinctive features found to be more error-prone are the fricative–affricates, combined with the features of blade/alveolar, tip/dental, blade/prepalatal, and labio/dental. In Down's syndrome, the anterior tongue appears to be particularly associated with continuing faulty articulation. Although they have been less studied, major phonological strategies seem to be similar in NR and MR children, including DS children (Stoel-Gammon, 1980; Bleile, 1982; Klink et al., 1986). Other relevant data on this point have been summarized in Section 5.1.

5.3.3 Non-segmental phonological development

The NR babies' early sensitivity to non-segmental characteristics of maternal speech is well documented (see Section 5.2). On the productive side, non-segmental features of babies' babbling come to resemble prosodic patterns of the mother tongue from as early as 6 months of age. A configuration of features is involved, using primarily pitch, rhythm and pause, which gives prosodic envelopes with recognizable intonation to the babies' productions. This culminates in jargon babbling towards the end of the first year or the beginning of the second year. Linguistic development of utterance begins as a holistic tonal pattern with a segmental and a prosodic dimension. At that time, however, it is the latter component that is the more stable.

According to Crystal (1989), early tonal development proceeds through the following major steps. Initially, the child uses only *falling* patterns. The first contrast is *falling* vs *high level*; the level tone being often accompanied by other prosodic or paralinguistic features (e.g. loudness). This is followed by a contrast between *falling and high rising tones*. The latter is used in a variety of functional contexts, such as requesting, attention-getting and offering. The next contrast is between *falling* and *high rising falling tones*. This latter tone is used in emphatic contexts (e.g. *bùs* vs *bûs*; the former label used to refer to any vehicle, the latter to a 'real' bus, for instance). Next appears a contrast between *rising* and *falling-rising tones*, the latter used especially in warning contexts (Halliday, 1975). These features appear first on isolated lexical items. Tonic contrastivity (contrastive stress) appears as linguistic productions become syntagmatically more complex, starting with two-word utterances around 20 months. As Bloom (1973) has shown, lexical items that have appeared as one-word utterances, with their own pitch and pause, at first retain their non-segmental autonomy. Gradually, the pause between them is reduced (e.g. *dáddy ... cár*). The next step is the prosodic integration of sequences of two items into a single-tone unit (e.g. *dáddy cár*). This step is of central importance in combinatorial language development, because the concatenation of two or three words under one unique utterance contour is the main means used by the younger child to express early semantic-syntactic relations (Brown, 1973).

Around 20 months in the NR child, two-word utterances are produced within single prosodic contours and tonic prominence becomes systematically distributed. In adult English, tonic prominence in one-tone-unit sentences is most often on the last lexical item (Chomsky and Halle, 1968; Crystal, 1969).

With further combinatorial development in utterance production, non-segmental patterns gradually conform to the role of prosody in the adult language. As is known, this role is particularly important in helping to delimit a variety of syntactic structures such as questions, relative clauses, coordination and direct–indirect object marking (Wode, 1980). Little research has been done on this latter development, but it is likely that it continues (both productively and receptively) until puberty and possibly later in terms of stylistic control over non-segmental phonological features of discourse (Crystal, 1989).

Systematic studies of non-segmental phonological development in MR children are almost non-existent. An interesting exception is Edwards' research (1990) with Toby, a DS child aged 4 years 7 months at the beginning of the research project. Toby had been fostered since birth and became the youngest of six children. No facts are known about his natural parents. At the time of the study, he still had persistent chest and throat infections, a minor heart defect and a history of intermittent hearing loss, although at the start of the study his hearing was thought to be within normal limits. Additionally, he was thought to have some problems with visual acuity. No IQ testing could be made of Toby when he was 4 years old. Later, at 8 years 4 months, he was considered to have a verbal IQ of 49 and a performance IQ of 51. Although the major part of Toby's language production was unintelligible, Edwards (1990) was able to segment portions of it into communicative units. She used as criteria: the pauses between stretches of vocalization, the relevant adult speech addressed to Toby and prosodic contour. These utterances contained only a few identifiable words (Edwards, 1992) but his prosodic development seemed to be in advance of his lexical. Most of the segments identified in Toby's production had clear tone units, defined as a distinctive sequence of pitches or tones within an utterance (Crystal, 1986). Examination of the child's prosody was focused on the nucleus, which is the essential feature of the tone unit: it is the syllable within the utterance which, because of the pitch change it carries, is prominent. Tone units were identified and quantified according to pitch changes in the nucleus, although it is open to debate whether Toby's utterances were linguistically contrastive enough to qualify for such terms as tone unit and nucleus. However, having completed the analysis, the data were examined in terms of proportion of utterances that had clearly defined tone units; types of units used; the function of these units between sessions and over time; and the use of prosodic contrasts. The preferential use of type of tone unit with identified lexical items was also examined to see how far this aspect of Toby's linguistic development was independent of his lexical development. Finally, Edwards made some tentative comparisons with normal speakers, although here the data are limited.

Within the literature which addresses the preverbal and early stages of language, there is a tradition which interprets the child's earliest utterances as communicative and which suggests that the child, even before first words are established, is able to use intonation to convey meanings, to label, call, request, etc. (Brown, 1973; Halliday, 1975; Menn, 1978; Dore, 1983; Crystal, 1987), although whether the adult's interpretation matches the child's intended meaning is questionable. No clear examples of consistent use of prosody to convey meaning were found in these data collected from Toby nor were any word-like utterances used with any consistent contrastive intonation patterns as reported by Menn. On the contrary, Toby's word-like utterances tended to have falling intonation, while a range of patterns were heard in his babble and, like Menn's normally developing subjects, Toby seemed to experiment with intonation patterns in his babble before using them on words.

Edwards stresses that she used a cautious approach in the analysis and interpretation as categorization was based on auditory judgements rather than acoustic analysis. Menn (1978) had found discrepancies between her auditory judgements and acoustic analysis of her data which would suggest that listeners may be unreliable and prone to over-interpretation. Furthermore, Toby, the DS subject, had poor muscular control, flaccid tonicity and repeated infections of the upper respiratory tract, which resulted in reduced vocal control, and it was therefore difficult to be confident that changes in pitch and volume were intentional and communicative rather than fortuitous. However, even with a conservative approach, three-quarters of all Toby's vocalizations carried an identifiable pitch pattern, which may account for the speech-like quality of his utterances despite the low number of identifiable lexical utterances. These vocalizations were then categorized by Edwards using a taxonomy of contrastive intonation patterns.

Between 50 and 60 per cent of the identified tones were classified as *falling*, which is in line with the 51 per cent suggested by Crystal (1969) for normal adult speech and claims that the fall is the first tone to be identified in normally developing children (Halliday, 1975; Menn, 1978; Crystal, 1989). The next largest category was that of *level tone* which may reflect poor muscular control rather than communicative contrast. Other categories such as *rise, fall–rise, rise–fall* accounted for much smaller proportions of the data, and the proportion of rising tones was somewhat smaller than would be expected in adult speech. There was some variation in these proportions over the 12 months Toby was observed, but no clear pattern of change and no strong evidence that rising tones were increasing in frequency with maturity or, indeed, with lexical proficiency.

There was some evidence in the data that Toby's intonation was clearer when he was vocalizing freely in play situations than when he was engaged in play in which his adult interlocutor constructed a conversational exchange. However, a greater definition of tone units was not found to be associated with an increase in the number of words used. Although Toby was more likely to use clear tone units when he was babbling freely and engaged in egocentric play, he was more likely to produce identifiable words when engaged in directed interaction with an adult. While the number of words used increased during the observation period, there was no consistent change in the distribution of tone units in this time. The two aspects of the linguistic system, prosodic and lexical, seemed to be developing independently.

Although no invariant relationship between Toby's use of tone units with communicative function was established, the majority of *falling tones* were found to be in 'answer' positions in the dialogue, that is they followed adults' questions. There was some association, although weaker than that for the *falling tones* and answering, between his use of *rising tones* and other communicative functions. Two functions were found to be associated with *rising tones*: routines and requests. During the play sessions Toby was observed to be using *rising tones* when handling familiar play objects. These routines resembled indicating or 'enumerating' objects, or establishing a possessive relationship between an object and his conversational partner. The use of a *rising tone* to signal a request was less marked in the data, but some examples which demonstrate this function were given.

Edwards suggests that the prosody of this DS child with severe language delay may have been slightly in advance of other linguistic skills, although in the absence of quantified normative data no firm conclusion could be reached. Toby was able to contribute to the interaction by using contrastive intonation patterns to support his emerging conversational skills, but use of contrastive intonation was not consistent and the range of functions limited when compared with reports of normally developing children. Whether these differences reflect real differences of ability or methodological differences remains to be shown.

5.4 Lexical development

Barrett and Diniz (1989) have compiled a detailed review of the studies on lexical development in MR children. Portions of this section are based on their account as well as on other reviews by Rondal (1975, 1985a) and Rosenberg and Abbeduto (1993). Recent descriptive or experimental studies of lexical development in MR subjects are relatively rare. A literature search on lexical development in mental retardation between 1988 and 1994 yielded only 40 publications, most of them training studies (Psycinfo, 1994).

Major problems regarding lexical development and functioning in MR subjects may be envisaged according to three major questions: (1) How do MR subjects learn the meanings of the words they come to know? (2) How do these subjects represent their knowledge of word meaning? (3) How do they represent the semantic relationships existing between the meanings of the words? Let us consider the information available in this order.

5.4.1 Learning words and word meaning

Lexical development is markedly delayed in moderately and severely MR children. The first recognizable words are often recorded between 24 and 30 months of age (Cunningham, 1979; Lambert and Rondal, 1980). Around 30 months-CA, the proportion of conventional words in the vocal productions of DS children is less than 5 per cent (Smith, 1977; Smith and Oller, 1981). This figure gradually increases with age. Around 4 years-CA, more numerous meaningful vocalizations are produced.

Nelson (1973) found that the average age at which normally developing children have acquired ten words is 15 months (range 13–19 months). The average age at which they have acquired 50 words is 20 months (range 14–24 months), and their average productive vocabulary size at 24 months is 186 words (range 28–436 words). Comparable data are reported in a large-scale cross-sectional study by Fenson et al. (in press). By age 2, NR children are able to produce from 50 to 600 words. They add steadily to this stock at an astonishing rate of 10 words/day, to reach a vocabulary of 14 000 words by age 6 (Templin, 1957; Carey, 1978). From there on, NR subjects average 3000 new words a year through to age 17 at least (Clark, 1995).

Overall, MR and NR children seem to present similar *patterns* of early vocabulary development. Both groups acquire social words and a few object names first, and, later, relational words and more object names (Gilham, 1979; Gopnik, 1987). The object name vocabularies acquired by young DS children have referential contents similar to those of NR children (Cunningham and Sloper, 1984). DS children comprehend object names at similar MAs (around 15 months) as NR children (Glenn and Cunningham, 1982). They have similar sized vocabularies in comprehension as MA-matched NR children between 13 and 21 months (Cardoso-Martins, Mervis and Mervis, 1985).

In their review, Barrett and Diniz (1989) claim that lexical development in MR children soon starts to fall behind that of MA-matched NR children. As development unfolds, they argue, MR children lag behind NR peers of similar MAs in expressive as well as in receptive aspects of lexical development. We disagree with such an interpretation. As alluded to in Chapter 4 (see also Rondal, 1994b), we maintain on the contrary that MA is a satisfactory predictor of at least *receptive lexical development* in MR (including DS) subjects. Chapman, Schwartz and Kay-Raining Bird (1991) have reported stepwise multiple regression analyses showing that CA and MA, collectively, accounted for 78 per cent of the variance in the vocabulary comprehension of their sample of children and adolescents with Down's syndrome. *Productive lexical use* may be further delayed and hampered, particularly in some MR (including DS) children, due to articulatory difficulties and memory limitations. This makes up for the dissociation sometimes observed between productive and receptive lexical capacity in MR subjects (Miller, 1988).

A careful review of the empirical studies summarized by Barrett and Diniz (1989) shows that many of them do in fact suggest that MA correctly predicts lexical functioning in MR subjects. Cardoso-Martins, Mervis and Mervis (1985) observed that DS children have similar sized vocabularies both in production and in comprehension as MA-matched NR children when MA is between 13 and 21 months (upper age-limit in this study). The same authors observe that DS children tend to have smaller vocabularies (both in production and in comprehension) than

NR children when the matching variable is level of sensorimotor development. However, it is known that DS children are relatively better off with sensorimotor than with more cognitively advanced aspects of development. Using level of sensorimotor development as the matching variable for comparing NR and DS children necessarily has the consequence of relating the latter to higher functioning NR children; hence the result obtained by Cardoso-Martins et al. (1985).

Other data from the studies reviewed by Barrett and Diniz (1989) support the predictive value of MA for referential aspects of lexical development and functioning in MR subjects. They are: Lyle's (1961a, b) for comprehension and production of object and action names; Bartel, Bryen and Keehn's (1973) for word comprehension; Lozar, Wepman and Hass's (1972) for vocabulary of use; Winters and Brzoska's (1976) for picture labelling with nouns; Ryan's (1975, 1977) for comprehension and production of nouns. It is correct, to note, however, that Thompson (1963) signalled impoverished spatial vocabularies in DS children (CA 5–6 years), that Rogers (1977) obtained lower scores on the Expressive Vocabulary Subscale of the Reynell Scales with DS and other MR children and adolescents of varied or uncertain aetiology (CA 4–16 years), and that Bless, Swift and Rosin (1985) reported vocabulary production and comprehension both delayed compared with non-verbal cognitive status in DS children (CA 5–8 years).

Other, at times older, studies, not appearing in Barrett and Diniz's review, also reveal much similarity in lexical development in MR and MA-matched NR subjects (see Rondal, 1975, for a review). Beier, Starkweather and Lambert (1969) reported a large commonality in basic vocabulary of use in MR and NR children at corresponding MAs. Waters (1956) observed no important difference between mildly and moderately MR subjects and NR children of corresponding MAs on the vocabulary items of the Stanford-Binet Intelligence Scale. Mein and O'Connor (1960) reported that compared to NR subjects of similar MAs, MR subjects have larger 'core' vocabularies (i.e. the set constituted by the words used by at least half the subjects in the sample studied) and smaller 'fringe' vocabularies (i.e. the remainder of the words used). MR subjects seem to make use of a vocabulary only slightly more stereotyped than NR subjects. The sample of words produced at least once by all the subjects covered 23.8 per cent of the corpus of words in the MR subjects vs 18 per cent in NR subjects. It should be noted that the larger stereotypy of vocabulary of use observed by Mein and O'Connor (1960) is a *group* measure. As will be seen below, there are indications, at the individual level, that the vocabulary used by MR subjects may be more diversified than that of MA- or MLU-matched NR children. As MA increases, the size of core vocabulary grows larger whereas the proportion of core words in the total vocabulary decreases (Wolfensberger, Mein and O'Connor, 1963). Also with increase in MA, the proportion of nouns produced by MR subjects decreases, whereas the proportions of other formal classes increase. This is the same phenomenon as observed in normally developing NR children.

In conclusion, there does not appear to exist solid empirical grounds on which to reject the indication that referential lexical development in MR subjects, particularly in its receptive aspects, proceeds in line with mental age .

What exactly covers this relation between MA and lexical development? Several aspects of lexical develoment are conceptual in nature and may be *causally* related to MA development. This is confirmed by data summarized below on process-aspects, categories and semantic-lexical networks in MR subjects. For earlier conceptual development, it does not seem that MR children develop any differently from NR children when the time dimension is not taken into account (Mervis, 1990).

Children's first object words appear to be related to the attainment of *certain levels of intellectual sensorimotor development*. The relationship between cognitive and lexical development may be quite specific on both sides. For example, Gopnik (1984) reported that words that refer to visible movements of entities (such as moving, falling down) tend to emerge during stage V object permanence, which entails performing successfully on visible object displacements. Stage VI is concerned with invisible displacements. It is only at this particular level that words referring to invisible displacements (e.g. *away, gone*) are properly understood and come to be used. Gopnik and Meltzoff (1984, 1986) found that the acquisition of words referring to success and failure tend to be related to sensorimotor stage VI means-and-ends, which involves the ability to deal with action plans in order to solve practical problems. Gopnik and Meltzoff (1987) also claim that the 'naming explosion' in NR children around 20 months is related to the better ability of the children at that time to sort objects into conceptual categories. Other explanations proposed in the literature for the naming explosion (see Woodward, Markman and Fitzsimmons, 1994) involve the realization that words are symbols and the onset of constraints on word learning (e.g. the whole object assumption, taxonomic constraint or mutual exclusivity).

No naming explosion has been reported for moderately and severely MR children, even later in development; however, see Oliver and Buckley (1994) for some indications regarding a possible acceleration of productive referential lexical development, in some DS children at least, around 30 months-CA.

It seems to be the case that early words are mapped onto already developed cognitive notions. It can happen too, however, that things work the other way around. The child's acquisition of a new word can determine the formation of a new concept (Schwartz and Terrell, 1983).

Mental retardation can also be viewed as a natural dissociation between development (conceptual, linguistic or otherwise) and life experience (associated with chronological age). Not surprisingly from this point of view, some aspects of lexical functioning may actually be more favourable in MR subjects than in necessarily younger MA- or MLU-matched NR children

Such appears to be the case of diversity in lexical use as measured with the type–token ratio index (TTR). As one would usually expect a person with a large lexical repertoire to be capable of producing speech which is more lexically diverse than somebody else with a smaller vocabulary, TTR is sometimes interpreted as supplying an indication of productive vocabulary size. MR subjects seem to use more diversified sets of vocabulary items or more diversified noun vocabularies than MA- or MLU-matched NR peers. One possible explanation (suggested in Rondal, 1978c) is that general life experience plays an important role in lexical use. This is consistent with current work on the nature of lexical knowledge and word meaning in children (see Keil, 1989). MR subjects may be more advanced in some aspects of lexical development than their MLU- or MA-matched NR peers, because they have lived longer and experienced more, even if with limited cognitive means (see Facon, 1994, for additional data along the same lines and a further discussion). It is even possible to observe MR children and adolescents exhibiting better lexical abilities (not just lexical diversity) than MA-matched NR children. Rosin, et al. (1988) and Chapman, Schwartz and Kay-Raining Bird (1991) have reported such data for DS subjects. They suggest that one potential source of disparity is the access of older children and adolescents to a wider variety of real-word and vocational activities which may create opportunities for more diverse and increased vocabulary learning and use.

In a study by Facon and Bollengier (1991), French-speaking MR subjects (MA 5 years; CAs 10 and 15 years, for two groups of MR subjects, respectively) demonstrated significantly higher scores on the Test de Vocabulaire Réceptif of Légé and Dague (1974) (the French equivalent of the PPVT) in MR subjects than MA-matched NR subjects. However, the same trend was not observed on the Raven Test of Progressive Matrices (Raven, 1981). Life experience presumably may compensate, and sometimes more than compensate, for intellectual limitations in tasks such as referential lexical activity that are particularly sensitive to environmental influence, but not to more remote ones, such as reasoning on abstract spatial material.

5.4.2 Process-oriented aspects of lexical-semantic development

There is partial evidence that similar strategies operate in word learning of MR and NR children. Chapman, Kay-Raining Bird and Schwartz (1990) reported that DS children and adolescents (CA range 5–20 years) do not differ from MA-matched NR children (CA range 2–6 years) in the ability to infer a connection between a novel word and a referent, and to comprehend the novel word, at least partially, after a single exposure in both immediate and delayed testing. Chapman et al. (1990) added that fast-mapping skills in event contexts were unrelated to expressive language deficit in their MR subjects. Mervis and associates (Mervis, 1988; Cardoso-Martins and Mervis, 1985; Cardoso-Martins, Mervis, and Mervis, 1985) have shown that although children, NR as well as MR, may differ from one another, and from adults, in the specific attributes that they use in sorting objects into different categories, the sorting principle is always that of form–function correlation (e.g. if it is spherical and it rolls, it is a ball). The basis for early word learning appears to be the same for MR and NR children. They tend to treat a new object label as referring to the object as a whole rather than to a part or an attribute of the object or an action performed by or with the object. Also the main interest of MR and NR children at the beginning of lexical development, is with objects that either move independently or can be manipulated. It would seem that MR children as well as NR children have a predisposition to segment incoming speech into significant units, as well as to use the linguistic context to help in the identification of the meanings of unfamiliar words.

5.4.3 Lexical definitions

As argued above, lexical development appears to be reasonably well in line with MA in MR subjects. However, this suggestion may not apply as well to lexical definition as an instance of metalexical ability, i.e. the verbal product of conscious awareness of the convential meanings of words. In Papania's study (1954), mildly MR children of varied aetiology (aged 9–16 years-CA) produced fewer abstract and more concrete word definitions than MA-matched NR children (see also Badt, 1958; Allen and Wallach, 1969). As CA and MA increased, the MR children produced larger proportions of abstract definitions. More recently, however, Chapman et al. (1991) have reported performance on word definition tasks in MR children and adolescents, equivalent to MA-matched NR controls.

Françoise, the language-exceptional DS subject studied by one of us (see Chapter 4), presented a lexical referential comprehension at the level of NR children aged 5–8 years. However, her word definition appeared to be markedly more limited. On the Vocabulary Subtest of the WAIS, she supplied numerous imprecise or incorrect definitions. Similar discrepant results were obtained on the Epreuves Différentielles d'Efficience Intellectuelle (Perron-Borelli and Misès, 1974), a test containing a verbal definitional task and a picture-pointing vocabulary task. In the case of Françoise, given her excellent expressive language ability, the lexical definitional limitation cannot be attributed to a difficulty in verbal expression. Another interesting demonstration that lexical use and definition may correspond to different skills is supplied by Williams syndrome subjects. As documented in Chapter 3, WS subjects may have preserved referential lexical skills. The same subjects, however, present marked difficulties with word definition.

Giving good definitions requires controlling not only word meaning but also definitional forms. Most definitional tasks assess the level of abstraction of the definition of nouns, with *concrete* or *descriptive* being the lowest level, *functional* next, and *abstract* the highest level. Definitional skills are strongly affected by opportunities to practise the required definitional forms (Snow, 1990). It is doubtful that such activities are often undertaken in the schools for MR children (particularly moderately and severely MR subjects).

5.4.4 Semantic-lexical categories and networks

An important theory concerning the mental representation of the meanings of words is the prototype theory articulated by Rosch (1977, 1978; see also Bowerman, 1978). According to this theory, when children acquire the meaning of object names, they mentally represent these meanings in the form a prototypical referential exemplar (for example, *robin* or *sparrow* for the bird category). This exemplar functions as a specification of the clearest example of the kind of objects which can be referred to by means of that word. The word is then used to refer to actual objects which share attributes with this mentally represented prototypical exemplar. Depending upon how many attributes a particular object shares with the prototypical exemplar, that object may be a more or less typical referent of the word. Thus an object which shares many attributes with the prototype would be a highly typical referent of the word, whereas an object sharing relatively few attributes with the prototype would be an atypical or peripheral referent of the word (e.g. *ducks* or *chicken* in the bird category).

Many studies conducted with NR children have established that such effects are the rule in lexical production and comprehension. For example, the phenomena of lexical underextension in children's language development are based upon the exclusion of peripheral rather than prototypical referents in a given lexical category (Kay and Anglin, 1982). Mervis (1984) assessed the comprehension of object names by DS children (CA range 17–19 months, MA range 8–14 months). She reported that these children sometimes underextend their object names by excluding the more peripheral referent category members, just like NR children of similar ages. DS children were reported occasionally to overextend their object names by including within their extensions inappropriate referents sharing either perceptual or functional attributes with the prototypical entities, again like NR children of similar ages.

Corresponding results were found by Tager-Flusberg (1985b, 1986) with a group of older retarded children of various aetiologies, matched on MA with NR children. The mean CA of the MR children was 11 years 5 months. Their mean MA was 4 years 9 months. Other studies have examined the extent to which the lexical object categories of MR subjects are similar in organization to those of NR subjects (McCauley, Sperber and Roaden, 1978; Winters and Hoats, 1986). Results from these studies using various lexical tasks confirm that, although delayed in their development relative to CA, the object categories of MR subjects are organized in a manner similar to those of NR subjects.

A well-known phenomenon in NR people, children as well as adults, is *semantic priming*, whereby category relatedness usually reduces the time needed to name a second item in a proposed pair. Sperber, Ragain and McCauley (1976) have supplied systematic observations of MR subjects consistent with the findings of research with NR subjects. They requested mildly MR adolescents (mean CA 16 years 4 months; mean MA 7 years 3 months) to name as quickly as possible pairs of pictures of objects whose names they already knew. The second item in each of the pairs was either in the same semantic category as the first item (e.g. *cat–horse*) or in a different category.

In the case of other semantic-lexical categories, such as *action names, adjectives, pronouns, demonstratives* and *connectives*, less evidence is available. Bartel, Bryen and Keehn (1973) have reported data concerning the acquisition of action names, pronouns, demonstratives and connectives. They administered the Carrow Auditory Test of Language Comprehension (CATLC; Carrow, 1973) to a sample of MR children (CA range 9–16 years; MA range 2;7–6 years). MR subjects demonstrated comprehension of *action words* such as *jump, run, catch, hit* and *give*, and *adjectives* such as *little, big, fast, slow, red, two, some, many, middle, tall, short, black, yellow, more, four, few, left, right*, at MAs close to those of NR children. However, they failed to exhibit comprehension of the adjectives *alike, different*, and the ordinal *fourth*, even at an MA of 6 years (the highest MA at which they were tested), whereas 60 per cent of the NR children of this age comprehended these particular items.

Cook (1977) reported evidence suggesting that DS children (CA range 3–6 years) understand *big* before *long*, which is the order of acquisition demonstrated by NR children, and predicted by Clark's (1974) semantic feature theory of lexical development (on the ground that the adjectives not tied to a particular physical dimension should be mastered first, and unidimensional adjectives later). It may be noted that Clark has abandoned this theory since then for a different framework, namely lexical contrast theory. In this latter framework, the building blocks of word meanings are lexical contrasts rather than semantic features (see Clark, 1993, 1995). Bartel et al. (1973) reported contrary findings to those of Cook. Their MR subjects acquired unidimensional adjectives such as *tall* and *short* at lower MA ages than the more general items *big* and *little*.

Markowitz (1976) has reported additional data on the same developmental problem which might help in overcoming the contradiction just mentioned, and that would seem to be compatible with Clark's contrast theory. He studied the comprehension of spatial adjectives in their nominal, comparative and superlative forms with a group of mildly and moderately MR adolescents (CAs between 11 and 16 years). Acquisition followed with so-called lexical age, as established on the PPVT. Three developmental stages could be distinguished. At stage 1 (mean lexical age 48 months), there was little evidence of comprehension of the adjectives proposed (*tall, short, high, low, long, big, small*). At stage 2 (mean lexical age 58 months), the positive poles of the adjectives were correctly understood (i.e. *big, tall, high, long*), whereas the 'negative' poles still determined random responses. The evolution in comprehension suggested by Markovitz does not depend on the unidimensionality of the meaning of the adjectives, but rather on their polarity. Positive terms are acquired before 'negative' or 'neutral' ones. At the third stage (mean lexical age 71 months), all nominal forms were correctly understood, as well as their comparative forms. The latter forms were understood earlier than the superlative ones.

Regarding *pronouns*, Bartel et al. (1973) reported that their MR children comprehended the forms *he, she, they, her, him* and *them* at higher MAs than NR children, while they failed to comprehend *his, her* and *their* at the highest MA at which they were evaluated. NR children demonstrated comprehension of these particular items on the CATLC at 4 years of age. On the same topic, Dooley (1976) reported that the two DS children that she studied used lexical forms such as *it, they, here, there* at an early point in their language development (i.e. MLU 1.5–1.8).

Demonstrative forms of *this, that, these* and *those* seem to be acquired at early stages of language development (CA range 3–6 years, in Coggins' (1979) expressive data), but very few observations are available on this point. For *connectives*, Bartel et al. (1973) reported that 60 per cent of their MR subjects could comprehend *and* and *or* at MAs around 4 years. Kamhi and Johnston (1982) indicated that their mildly MR children (mean CA 8 years 3 months) productively used *and* at MAs of 5 years approximately.

Concerning *prepositions*, Bartel et al. (1973) reported that their group of MR children were delayed in the comprehension of locative prepositions *on, in, up, down, by* and *between*. At the highest MA studied (6 years), they all failed to demonstrate comprehension of *under* and *in front of*, whereas NR children usually comprehend such notions by 3 or 4 years of age. The same authors signalled that MR children seem to acquire the preposition *on* before *in*. This observation is congruent with that of Cook (1977) whose subjects acquired *on*, before *in*, before *under*. This is the order exhibited by NR children, which would suggest that MR children acquire the meaning of these prepositions in a manner corresponding to that of normally developing children.

Lexical development in NR subjects also implies acquiring a knowledge of *word relatedness*, or more precisely of the relationships that exist between the meanings of different words from a semantic point of view (see below for the relationships holding between different words from a grammatical point of view). Rosch (1977, 1978) has proposed a theoretical account of lexical subordination, basic level and superordination which has been influential. One particular level of vertical categorization is the basic level. This level regroups the most general categories into a categorical hierarchy containing objects sharing common attributes. For example, *car, apple, dog*, are basic-level lexical items. Superordinate categories (e.g. *vehicles, fruits, animals*, in the above cases) are more general than basic-level categories. Subordinates categories (e.g. *Mercedes, golden, fox terrier*, in the above cases) are more specific. Rosch claims that basic-level categories are psychologically privileged. They are at the level at which things are most frequently named and are processed faster than either superordinates or subordinates items.

Basic-level items are also learned earlier than other items by NR children. There is evidence that this is also the case with MR children. Studies by Winters and Brzoska (1976), Harrison, Budoff and Greenberg (1975), Bender and Johnson (1979), Davies, Sperber and McCauley (1981) and Tager-Flusberg (1985b, 1986), conducted with moderately and mildly MR children and adolescents, show that MR subjects acquire a knowledge of superordinate and subordinate words, although this knowledge is not as advanced as their knowledge of basic-level words. The meanings of superordinate and subordinate words seem to be mentally represented by MR subjects in the same way as NR subjects at corresponding MA levels. MR subjects also appear to represent mentally the semantic relationships existing between the meanings of superordinate and subordinate words on the one hand, and superordinate and basic-level words on the other, in the same way as NR subjects.

It remains, however, that MR subjects are not as efficient in constructing semantic knowledge and in processing semantic information (particularly when more complex linguistic input is involved), as CA-matched NR peers.

5.4.5 Grammatical aspects of lexical organization

In NR children, somewhere between 6 and 8 years of age, a progressive change takes place in the nature of free word associations (Brown and Berko, 1960; Erwin, 1961; Entwistle, Forsyth and Muuss, 1964; Entwistle, 1966). Children shift from typical syntagmatic or sequential associations (e.g. *snow-white*) to paradigmatic or grammatical type of associations, that is associations between words from the same grammatical class (e.g. *snow-rain*), according to the distinction introduced by Jakobson and Halle (1956). This shift possibly represents an important milestone in the grammatical organization of the lexicon, although the reasons for its occurrence are not well understood (see Erwin, 1961, and McNeil, 1966, for theoretical suggestions).

The syntagmatic and paradigmatic word associations of mildly MR children (CAs between 10 and 15 years) have been studied by Semmel et al. (1968), using free-association tasks. MR children give fewer paradigmatic responses than CA-matched NR children. However, when equated for MA, NR and MR groups produce about the same amount of paradigmatic responses. Keilman and Moran (1967) compared two groups of mildly MR children above 10 years-CA. They reported an MA-related increase in level of paradigmatic responses. Seitz, Goulding and Conrad (1969) administered the same word-association task to Keilman and Moran's subjects some 30 months later. The younger Keilman and Moran group had moved towards the level of the older group, while the latter did not show any significant change in their word association performance. The older group had a mean CA of 15.2 years with a standard deviation of 18 months (for a mean MA of 9.6 years) at the time of the Keilman and Moran study. From these data, it can be suggested that the maximal level of paradigmatic association in mildly MR children is reached at around CA 15 years.

However, Denhière (1973, 1974) administered a task of free word associations in French, devised by Noizet and Pichevin (1966) for NR children of elementary school age, to a group of French-speaking mildly MR children and adolescents (CA range 8–18 years). He reported no significant evolution with chronological age in the proportions of syntagmatic and paradigmatic responses.

The productive oral cloze-task procedures devised by Goodstein (1970) and Semmel, Barritt and Bennett (1970) (see Chapter 2) may tap related aspects of the grammatical organization of the lexicon and sensitivity to formal class aspects of phrase constituents. Mildly MR children exhibited particular difficulties in supplying deleted adjectives and verbs. A significant positive correlation was reported by Semmel et al. (1970) between the MR subjects' performance on the productive cloze-tasks and the frequency of paradigmatic responses in a previously administered word association task (Semmel et al., 1968).

No more recent data on the syntagmatic–paradigmatic shift in mildly MR subjects are available in the literature. Similarly, no data seem to have been published on the same shift in moderately and moderately MR subjects.

In conclusion, the MR subjects' evolution in the grammatical organization of the lexicon is still not clear. It seems that even in mildly MR subjects, this organization is considerably delayed and remains incomplete. If one is willing to admit that grammatical classes supply a more appropriate classification principle than simple sequential dependencies for phrase and sentence construction (see, for example, Levelt's, 1989 *'formulator'* component in planning for speaking), then MR individuals may be poorly equipped in this respect.

5.5 Thematic semantics and morphosyntactic regulations

As indicated earlier, semantic or thematic relations or structures[2] may be the building blocks on which grammatical (or more exactly morphosyntactic) development takes place. It is likely that MR subjects (including those rare MR subjects with exceptional computational language capacities) are delayed in thematic semantic development in proportion to their cognitive deficit.

5.5.1 Semantic structural development

When they begin to combine two and three words within the same utterance (usually not before 4 years-CA), moderately and severely MR children (including DS children) appear to express the same range of relational meanings or thematic roles and relations as reported by the students of early combinatorial language in the NR child (see Brown, 1973), and pertaining to the semantic structures of the natural languages (see Fillmore's, 1967 basic propositional cases, or Chafe's (1970) componential meaning analysis). Examples of early thematic relations expressed by MR, as well as by NR, children are *notice* or *existence, denial, disappearance, recurrence, attribution, possession, location, agent, patient, instrument, source, agent-action, action-patient* and *agent-action-patient* (Dooley, 1976; Michaelis, 1976; Rondal, 1978a; Coggins, 1979; Layton and Sharifi, 1979). Kamhi and Johnston (1982) analysed the ideational complexity (i.e. the average number of idea-units in an utterance) of non-verbal MA-matched mildly MR and NR children. Mean MA and CA in the sample of children with MR were 5 years 2 months and 8 years 3 months, respectively. Mean IQ was 63. The measures used by Kamhi and Johnston had to do with the semantic relations or propositions depicted by a verb and the phrase structures with which it can occur. It was reported that the MR and the NR children do not differ in the ideational complexity of their spontaneous utterances.

---

[2] In this book, we take the expressions *semantic structure(s)*, *relational* or *structural meanings*, and *thematic relations* to be equivalent. We therefore are not adopting Pinker's (1989) or Grimshaw's (1990) distinction between primitive thematic roles (as by Fillmore and others) and the more recent semantic structure theories envisaging verbs' meanings as multidimensional structures in which various events (e.g. notions, changes) are represented in separate but connected substructures.

Fowler, Gelman and Gleitman (1994) recorded spontaneous speech samples from four DS children (CA range 10;9–13 years) matched for MLU with younger NR children. MLUs were in the range 2.75–3.25 (mean 2.98). They reported that children in both groups were explicit in expressing most of the obligatory thematic relations studied in early language development. Non-stative verbs and stative locative verbs (e.g. *sit, belong*) were expressed virtually 100 per cent of the time. Stative verbs were often implicit as they are in NR children early in thematic semantic development (Bloom, Miller and Hood, 1975). For example, DS children frequently produced utterances such as *The doll upstairs*, while placing a doll in a doll's house, implying a verb such as *belongs*. Overall, obligatory nominal arguments entering into locative relations were supplied 72 per cent of the time by children with Down's syndrome and 75 per cent of the time by the NR group. The most important tendency was to omit an obligatory nominal element involving the agent (in grammatical subject role) of agent locative utterances, as in *Put it here*. DS subjects omitted this constituent 61 per cent of the time in average value vs 25 per cent in the NR group. However, sentence subjects were most consistently supplied when functioning as patients in locative state utterances (e.g. *Tyres belong in the garage*). DS children consistently supplied the patient in object position (76 per cent in average score) vs 95 per cent in the NR group. Fowler et al. (1994) also reported the results of a longitudinal investigation of language acquisition in a young child with DS named Rebecca (IQ 57), between CA 50 and 89 months. Rebecca's encoding of major thematic relations progressed regularly. Her usage of thematic categories was consistent with that seen in NR children. The only difference was a greater reliance on stereotypic phrases and vocatives.

MR children also appear to understand correctly the same set of basic thematic meanings when they are realized in the speech of other people (Duchan and Erickson, 1976).

There is no indication that the semantic structural basis of combinatorial language, as it is put to use in early language production and reception, is markedly different in MR and NR children at corresponding levels of language development. No information is available on the organization of thematic structures in later language development of MR subjects.

5.5.2 Morphosyntactic development

Morphosyntactic development is slow and remains largely incomplete in moderately and severely MR subjects. Some progress is obvious with increased CA, at least until early adolescence (see Section 5.1). This progress is illustrated in MLU measures. Figure 5.1 shows that typical DS children reach MLU 2 around 4–5 years CA, MLU 3 around 7–8 years, and

MLU 6 around 14 or 15 years. They plateau definitively or with very little progress beyond this level (see Section 5.7). In comparison, NR children reach MLU 5 or more around 6 years.

The slowness and limitation of MLU development in moderately and severely MR children correspond to important shortcomings in morpho-syntax. Word order in those languages relying on sequential devices to express thematic relations (e.g. English, French) is usually correct, however (see Ryan, 1975; Dooley, 1976; Dale, 1977; Rondal, 1978a,b, 1985c; Chipman and Pastouriaux, 1981; Rosenberg, 1982; Rosenberg and Abbeduto, 1993; Lomonte, 1995). There is a paradox here. MR children do not seem to have particular problems with word order in simple utterances while they usually have serious difficulties with other morphosyntactic aspects of language (see below). Why should word order be spared in mental retardation? It will not suffice to say that word order is a simpler matter to master than other grammatical devices. We know that word ordering has to be learnt. It cannot be ascribed to a species-specific language background for it is not a major grammatical device in case languages. Actually, word ordering is in no way a simple matter. It is not obvious why it should be easier to process than grammatical morphology. No explanation is available regarding this paradox.

In young MR children, the production of *grammatical words* (functors) is reduced (i.e. the articles, prepositions, pronouns, modals, auxiliaries, copula and conjunctions). This gives their utterances a telegraphic character (Brown, 1973). Later in development, as attested by data collected by Fowler et al. (1994), the proportions of pronouns, prepositions, modals, WH-forms and demonstratives are similar in DS and MLU-matched NR children. The same DS children supplied overall percentages of *grammatical morphemes* which were virtually identical to those of MLU-matched NR children (i.e. around 66 per cent). There were some differences, however, regarding the patterns of acquisition for individual morphemes. DS children were more *variable* in their production, although the counts of the number of cases of full mastery (considered to be achieved at 90 per cent usage in obligatory context) across the 14 grammatical morphemes documented by Brown (1973) and de Villiers and de Villiers (1973), yielded nine cases in each group. This may not be the case for all DS children at corresponding MLU levels, however. Michaelis (1976) documented the case of Jenny, a 6-year-old DS child with an MLU of 3.47. At the time of the study, Jenny had not reached the criteria on any of the grammatical morphemes.

The longitudinal study of Rebecca by Fowler et al. (1994) supplies additional information on earlier grammatical morphological development in Down's syndrome. Over the 39 months of the study, Rebecca showed initial and relatively rapid acquisition of the plural form of the nouns, the prepositions *in* and *on* and the progressive form *ing* (this form remaining variable in her usage). These are the same first four grammatical morphemes acquired by NR children around 30 months. But Rebecca made little further progress during the rest of the observation period. At 89 months (end of the study), she had mastered only one additional grammatical marker, i.e. the contracted copula (e.g. *It's gone*), which was not always used accurately.

Rutter and Buckley (1994) claimed to have obtained more optimistic data regarding the acquisition of grammatical morphemes in DS children. They concluded that most morphemes among the 14 referred to above had been acquired at least by some of their subjects, in the same order as the one reported for NR children, and that the acquisition delay varied between 3 and 15 months-CA. The following morphemes were not mastered: non-contracted copula *be*, third person singular marking on verb, and non-contracted auxiliary *be*. However, this study was entirely based on parental reports and the investigators did not appear to employ the usual acquisition criterion in this type of work (see above). Rutter and Buckley's data therefore must be taken with caution. They probably mean that some DS children were working on some grammatical morphemes at the chronological ages reported.

Chapman, Schwartz and Kay-Raining Bird (1992) (see also Chapman, 1995) observed that older DS children and adolescents more frequently omit free and bound grammatical morphemes than MLU-matched NR controls in narrative speech samples. Similarly, Bol and Kuiken (1990) documented fewer verb agreements and less frequent use of pronouns in the language of Dutch children with DS aged 8–19 years-CA (MAs greater than 3 years and 6 months), when compared to that of NR children aged 1–4 years.

Mentally retarded individuals' persistent difficulties with grammatical morphemes have long been noted. Earlier, Mueller and Weaver (1964), Bateman and Wetherell (1965), Bilovsky and Share (1965), Lovell and Bradbury (1967), Newfield and Schlanger (1968) and Ryan (1975), using either the ITPA, a modified version of Berko's test (1958), or free speech samples, reported on the expressive problems and lack of stability of the MR subjects' performance in this aspect of language. Most often MR subjects perform on grammatical morphology at levels lower than those expected on an MA basis, but no evidence of deviance in the order of mastery of the grammatical morphemes was signalled. The more recent studies largely confirm previous data in this respect.

Fowler et al. (1994) also computed several *syntactic measures* on their cross-sectional samples of spontaneous speech from DS children, as well as from Rebecca's longitudinal corpus. The number of noun and verb phrases was similar for DS and MLU-matched NR children. However, the DS children had fewer morphemes per noun phrase. Both groups of children were making little use of complex constructions, such as passives, subject/auxiliary inversions and conjoined clauses. Multiverb utterances were rare, comprising fewer than 5 per cent of the utterances in either group of children. Rebecca's syntactic evolution was reported to parallel that of younger NR children regarding early negative and interrogative constructions. Beyond 67 months, however, she failed to make further syntactic progress. The auxiliary system underlying mature negative and interrogative sentences was almost totally lacking in her grammar. She would make persistent overuse of the term *what* in order to introduce most WH-questions. The *what* term largely replaced other WH-terms such as *when, where, how*. Correspondingly, Jenny, the 6-year-old DS child studied cross-sectionally by Michaelis (1976) was reported not to produce WH-questions.

The above studies confirm previous reports (e.g. Lenneberg, Nichols and Rosenberger, 1964; Lackner, 1968; Rondal, 1978a) on the important problems MR subjects have with *syntactic aspects of expressive language*, and their increasing delay compared with MA-matched NR controls.

There are also numerous reports pointing to the serious limitations of MR children and adolescents in the *comprehension of morphosyntactic structures* and their lagging behind MA-matched NR controls in this respect as well. Semmel and Dooley (1971), Berry (1972), Bartel, Bryen and Keehn (1973), Dewart (1979), Chipman (1979) and Barblan and Chipman (1978) (the latter two studies with French-speaking subjects) analysed the particular difficulties of mildly, moderately and severely MR subjects in the comprehension of grammatical words, gender and number agreement, double object construction in English (e.g. *She gave the lady the baby*), possessive constructions, temporal clauses and temporal relations between clauses, and passive constructions. In English, Kernan (1990) has documented the difficulty of young adults with moderate or mild mental retardation (Down's syndrome and retardation of unidentified aetiology) in processing temporal sentences. Both samples of subjects exhibited patterns of comprehension that resembled those of younger NR children (see Johnson, 1975). Sentences in which temporally related events were referred to with clause order matching the order in which the events happened, were happening or would be happening, proved easier to process by the MR subjects. This was the case for the following types of sentences 'X then Y' (e.g. *The dog jumps over the cat and then the cat jumps over the dog*), 'X before Y' (e.g. *John sat down before Mary sat down*), and 'After X, Y' (e.g. *After the cat jumped over the dog, the dog jumped over the cat*). Sentences in which the clause order did not match the order of the events (e.g. 'Before X, Y' and 'X after Y' types of sentences) yielded markedly lower proportions of correct interpretive answers.

In Section 5.1, we reported on the use of the Batterie d'Evaluation Morpho-Syntaxique (BEMS; Comblain, Fayasse and Rondal, 1993) with DS children, adolescents and adults. DS subjects were found to perform markedly lower than NR children on the subtests evaluating the comprehension of personal pronouns, definite and indefinite articles, subordinate clauses, negative and passive sentences. Corresponding data have been obtained by Fayasse, Comblain and Rondal (1995). They administered the BEMS to a group of French-speaking children, adolescents and young adults who were non-retarded or had mild or moderate mental retardation. Results of the analyses confirm the existence of remarkable similarities in the hierarchies of difficulty of the grammatical structures proposed, the types of errors observed and the developmental sequences across the groups of subjects, in spite of marked differences between the groups in absolute frequencies of errors (favouring NR and mildly MR subjects, as expected). Classifying the receptive tasks on the BEMS according to increasing order of difficulty yielded the same sequences for NR, mildly MR and moderately MR subjects. Spearman rank correlation coefficients computed on the hierarchies of grammatical difficulty revealed significant associations between the groups of subjects. Such data are supportive of the continuity hypothesis in grammatical development and functioning between NR and MR subjects, on the one hand, and between levels of mental retardation, on the other.

Voice in MR subjects' sentence processing has been little dealt with systematically. One exception is found in an unpublished study by Rondal, Cession and Vincent (1988) on the comprehension of declarative monopropositional sentences varying according to voice and semantic transitivity features (see Hopper and Thompson, 1980). A group of 17 young adults with DS (mean CA 27 years and 5 months) were individually tested for comprehension of a set of plausible and (thematic or event) reversible active and passive declarative sentences. Kinesis (i.e. degree of 'action-ness') of verbs was systematically varied. Subjects were requested to choose between two pictures. One picture correctly represented the thematic relation encoded in the sentence heard (e.g. girl pushing boy, for the sentence *The girl pushes the boy*); the other picture corresponded to a reversal of the same relation (for example, boy pushing girl, for the same sentence).

As is known, passive sentences do not differ from active ones in the thematic relations expressed but only in the overt realization of these relations. Passive sentences have their underlying logical subject realized in the surface form of an oblique object most often introduced by the preposition *by* (for example, *the boy* in the sentence *The girl was pushed by the boy*) and their underlying logical object realized in the form of the surface subject (*the girl* in the sentence above). NR children understand active as well as passive sentences earlier and better when the sentences are constructed around action verbs (e.g. *push, carry*), that is, verbs taking agent as subjects, as opposed to mental verbs (e.g. *imagine, like, see*) (Maratsos et al., 1985; Sudhalter and Braine, 1985; Rondal, Thibaut and Cession, 1990). In line with the work of Kosslyn (1980) and Paivio (1986), Rondal et al. (1990) suggested that the action verb effect could be due to a particular supporting role of the mental image to the computations involved in sentence processing, especially when the analytic task is more complex or with certain types of formal structures; the construction of a mental image being favoured in the case of concrete and action verbs (see Thibaut and Rondal, in press, for a detailed discussion). This hypothesis was corroborated in a study by Thibaut, Rondal and Kaens (1995) on the role of mental imagery in sentence comprehension. The experimental results obtained by Rondal et al. (1988) indicate that the same facilitating effect of kinesis is true of the DS adults studied as it is of NR children, except that with the former subjects the effect is limited to active sentences. DS adults with relatively higher IQs (range 40–60) correctly interpreted 83 per cent of the action-verb actives versus 73 per cent of the non-action ones. DS adults with relatively lower IQs (range 20–39) obtained 75 and 50 per cent correct interpretation, respectively. For the non-action-verb passives, the profiles of responses also diverged according to IQ level. The higher IQ group interpreted passive sentences as if they were corresponding actives in 60 per cent of the cases versus 70 per cent for the lower IQ group. The action-verb passives were interpreted at chance level in the two groups (50 and 47 per cent for the higher and the lower IQ groups, respectively).

This research shows, first, that in a large majority of cases, DS adults do not correctly understand the morphosyntactic and semantic aspects associated with the passive voice; and, secondly, that the reversible declarative active sentences are correctly understood in a good proportion of the cases, particularly when action verbs are used and at higher IQ levels. For active sentences, therefore, the same facilitating effect of semantic kinesis can be shown in DS adults as in NR children. It may be supposed that the structural complexity of the passive not only makes problems of comprehension for DS subjects, but also blocks potentially facilitating semantic actionality effects.

Using the same picture-designating technique as Rondal et al. (1988), Comblain (1989) confirmed that DS adults, as a group, interpret reversible passive sentences with action or non-action verbs at chance level or below. One aspect of Comblain's work deserves additional consideration. She presented her subjects with series of monopropositional active and passive sentences randomly mixing plausible (e.g. *The boy hits the girl*) and implausible statements (e.g. *Le vélo est détesté par le livre – The bike is hated by the book*). Treating such series of sentences, the DS adults – but not the NR adults constituting the control group – also interpreted the actives at or near chance level. This shows how relatively fragile and semantico-pragmatically dependent even the linguistic treatment of simple active declarative sentences may remain in DS individuals.

Limited information is available on the *discursive capacities* of MR subjects. Reilly, Klima and Bellugi (1991) compared cognitively matched

Williams syndrome and DS adolescents in a story-telling activity. The
subjects were introduced to a wordless picture book (*Frog, where are
you?*, Mayer, 1969) and asked to tell a story from the pictures, as they
progressed page by page through the book. In contrast with DS subjects,
the WS adolescents told coherent and complex narratives that made
extensive use of affective prosody. The WS, but not the DS, subjects
enriched the referential contents of their stories with narrative, affective
and social cognitive devices. For example, WS subjects used markedly
more features such as affective and mental verbs, emphatic and intensi-
fier forms, negative markers, causal connectors, as well as onomatopoeic
forms. Despite their cognitive impairment, subjects with WS are able not
only to deal with the structural demands of narratives, but also
consciously to manipulate affective linguistic devices for the purpose of
effective story-telling. However, consistent with the indication in
Chapter 3 regarding the difficulty of these subjects to take into account
other people's point of view and participation in the verbal interaction,
WS subjects were also reported by Reilly et al. (1991) 'to use the same
level of expressivity regardless of how many times they have told the
stories and irrespective of the audience' (p. 390), which suggests that
their narrative expressivity may turn out to be aberrant.

A study by Chapman, Kay-Raining Bird and Schwartz (1991) indirectly
confirms the particular difficulty of DS children and adolescents in on-
line story processing. In such contexts, these subjects no longer demonstrate the fast-mapping ability with novel words which they currently
exhibit in simpler event contexts. In story contexts, DS subjects
encounter additional difficulties in processing the narrative structure
and in memory for story gist generally. These difficulties interfere with
inferring the likely referent of the novel words preventing the fast-
mapping production forms observed in event contexts to occur.

More generally, however, Chapman et al. (1992) report significant
increases in the narratives of older DS adolescents (CAs between 16 and
20 years) in comparison with DS children and younger adolescents aged
5 to 16 years. Chapman (1995) suggests that these data contradict the
hypothesis of a critical period in language development of MR children
which would terminate around puberty or before. As discussed in
Section 5.1 (see also Section 5.7 below), contemporary views of the critical period hypothesis are modular and tend to restrict temporal
constraints to the computational aspects of language development. As
properly analysed by Halliday (1985), for example, the discursive dimension is not specifically concerned with the grammatical, the thematic
semantic or the information structure of language. Rather, it relates to
the network of relationships between clauses and/or paragraphs that
allow for textual cohesion. As such, and in itself, the discursive ability is
not to be ascribed to the computational aspects of language as defined
by Chomsky (1981). It can be expected that at least some MR adoles-

cents and adults can continue to progress on this aspect as well as on other cognitive aspects of the language system, given correct opportunities and stimulation.

5.5.3 Patterns of individual differences in morphosyntactic development

Individual differences in MR subjects' language development and functioning have been little studied, except in extreme cases (see Chapter 4). Two exceptions are first, the large-scale study conducted by Miller, Chapman and Mackensie (1981; see also Chapman and Nation, 1981; Miller, 1988; and Chapman, 1995) including multiple comprehension and production assessments; and, second, the study by Abbdeduto, Furman and Davis (1989) on the relation between receptive language and MA in persons with mental retardation (see also Rosenberg and Abbeduto, 1993).

Miller and associates identified frequent categories of language performance relative to cognitive status in MR children aged 7 months to 7 years-CA. Cognitive status was established by application of the Uzgiris and Hunt version of the sensorimotor scales of Piaget (Uzgiris and Hunt, 1975). Syntactic comprehension was assessed by the use of tasks requiring compliance with a set of instructions, answers to WH-questions, and the Miller–Yoder Test of Grammatical Comprehension (Miller, 1983). Lexical comprehension was assessed through the PPVT. Free-speech samples were analysed in order to evaluate syntactic production. Twenty-four per cent of the MR children fell into the first pattern, termed 'production-only delay'. In this category, only production of syntactic structures was delayed. Syntax comprehension and vocabulary were within the expected range. Seventeen per cent of the MR children were classified according to a 'delayed comprehension and production' pattern. In these cases, all language measures were delayed compared to cognitive level. Thirty-six per cent of the MR subjects exhibited a 'flat pattern', i.e. their language performance was consistent with cognitive status on all language measures. Five per cent of the NR children used as controls, but none of the MR children, exhibited more advanced linguistic skills than expected relative to cognitive level. The remaining MR children differed from the most frequently encountered three patterns only to the extent that one of the two comprehension measures was either within the expected range or was delayed. As this study indicates, MR children, considered individually, may be quite heterogeneous with respect to language levels at similar cognitive levels.

Abbeduto, Furman and Davies (1989) have supplied additional indications regarding the range of interindividual variation in language development of MR subjects. Their MR subjects were grouped at three non-verbal-MA levels: 5, 7 and 9 years, and were MA-matched with NR children. The subjects were administered a developmentally ordered standardized test of language comprehension – the Test for Reception of Grammar (TROG; Bishop, 1982). This test contains single lexical items, phrases, simple sentences and complex sentences. The MR subjects evidenced considerable interindividual variability in the relationship between TROG age and MA. Only a small number of MR individuals had TROG ages greater than their MAs. In addition, after MA 5 there was an increase in the number of MR subjects whose TROG ages were less than their MAs. Neither of these trends was characteristic of the NR children.

To be added to the above observations is the fact (stressed by Hodapp, in press-a) that the MR subjects' relative strengths and weaknesses in development are not static but may change over time. The best example here is Miller's (1992) report that changing numbers of MR children show the pattern of receptive over expressive language level, or of language below MA level. Receptive skills may exceed skills in expressive language for some MR children early on, but more and more children seem to exhibit this discrepancy and to increasingly greater degrees as they grow in age. Cole, Dale and Mills (1992) also reported changes in the cognitive-language relation for language measures (i.e. PPVT and a Test of Early Language Development (Hresko, Reid and Hammill, 1981) assessing semantic and syntactic aspects language through expressive and receptive abilities) over 1- and 2-year periods.

It could be the case, as Miller (1988) and Chapman (1995) suggest, that *overall early expressive syntactic development in MR children* mostly occurs at MAs similar or close to those of normally developing children. Later on, this aspect of language shows increasing divergence from MA-matched controls. The comprehension of syntactic structures is often advanced relative to the MR children's expressive syntax, but it begins to show delays relative to non-verbal cognition in late childhood. The delays deepen during adolescence, as documented in Section 5.1. The same evolution is not observed in more conceptual aspects of language, as demonstrated in preceding sections. Miller and Chapman's suggestions as to the changing relationship between productive and receptive syntax are interesting ones. However, their data could also, or at least partly, be a product of the cross-sectional comparisons and/or the different linguistic measures employed with children at various levels of development. Longitudinal studies are needed to assess the validity of the above suggestions.

There is no contradiction between the autonomy of grammatical development documented earlier in the book and the relationship sometimes observed between MA or IQ and morphosyntactic development. For example, Lenneberg et al. (1964) and Fowler (1988) reported that moderately and severely MR subjects with relatively higher IQs develop slightly better linguistically. Such indications solely attest, in our view, to the global influence of general level of mental efficiency on language development. This influence is mediated through the semantic component of language. It can be blocked by the existence of grammatical deficiencies (as illustrated in Rondal, Cession and Vincent's, 1988 study). The fact documented above in this chapter and earlier in this book (Chapter 4) that with further development MR subjects' morphosyntax progressively lags more and more behind MA evolution, means that general mental ability can no longer compensate for the insufficiency and/or the failure of specific grammatical mechanisms to apply.

5.5.4 Explaining individual differences

How are we to explain the individual differences between typical MR subjects in morphosyntactic development? Major explanatory variables do not reside in non-verbal cognition, as the above studies by Miller et al. and Abbeduto et al. indirectly show. Environmental variables could play a role; for example, the quality of language stimulation and the participation in well-designed language intervention programmes. However, as demonstrated in the next section, the language input to MR children may be regarded as structurally adequate for linguistic development, leaving little room for marked environmental variation. We believe that the major part of the individual variance in morphosyntactic development must be attributed to brain differences between MR subjects. In so doing, we appeal to the same explanation as for the differences documented across genetic syndromes in mental retardation (Chapter 3), and for those reported concerning exceptional cases of computational language development in MR subjects (Chapter 4). Unfortunately, the present-day state of knowledge in neurology (Crick and Jones, 1993) does not allow us to go beyond setting simple relationships between differential characteristics of brain development and morphosyntactic functioning. Some reasonable hope may be permitted with the rapid growth of new non-intrusive investigation tools – including imaging technologies (e.g. positron emission tomography). These techniques are able to take pictures of the brain in action, rendering certain activities of mind visible as they take place (see Posner and Raichle, 1994).

A number of data have been reported in the recent past on hemispheric cerebral dominance for language functions in MR subjects (particularly DS subjects) *using dichotic listening* (see Elliott, Weeks and Elliott, 1987, for a review). In such tasks, syllables, speech sounds, digits or rhymed pairs of words (e.g. *goat – coat*) are presented at exactly the same time to the ears of subjects through earphones. The neural pathways from ear to brain include both ipsilateral and contralateral routes. Consequently, the auditory stimulus is projected to both cerebral hemispheres. In the competitive dichotic presentation situation, contralateral pathways prevail allowing the investigation of lateralized perception and processing of acoustic material. In NR people, starting around 3 years of age, a right ear advantage (REA) is usually observed, which is taken to indicate a left hemispheric dominance (LHD) for speech functions. This dominance seems to be statistically more marked in males than in females (Hiscock and Decter, 1988; Kimura, 1992).

Currrent neuropsychological work as to hemispheric specialization for language functions points towards a heavy involvement of the left hemisphere in the processing of speech sounds and the assembly of phonemes into words, speech rhythms, the selection of word forms, the treatment of word morphological structures, grammatical morphology, and syntax, as well as to an important participation of the right hemisphere in semantic and pragmatic processing (Damasio and Damasio, 1992; Koenig, Wetzel and Caramazza, 1992).

Several studies with DS individuals have reported a marked tendency for a left ear/right hemisphere advantage for speech sound reception (e.g. Bowler, Cufflin and Kiernan, 1985; Elliott, Weeks and Elliott, 1987; Giencke and Lewandowski, 1989; but see Tannock, Kershner and Oliver, 1984, for contradictory results). In contrast, control groups of NR children and MR subjects of aetiologies other than DS but comparable MAs, have been shown to exhibit the usual right ear/left hemisphere superiority. According to Elliott et al. (1995), the atypical cerebral organization of functions in DS subjects is confined to speech perception. Spatial processing (evaluated in dihaptic shape-matching and visual field-dot-enumeration tasks) reveals either no lateral cerebral advantage or a left-hand advantage (RHD), depending on whether the subjects are right-handed or left-handed.

Hartley (1982) has suggested that the reverse cerebral localization for speech sounds in DS subjects is responsible for their performance dissociation between serial and parallel cognitive processing. DS individuals as a group tend to perform more poorly than other MR subjects of similar MAs on serial tasks (see Chapter 3, for a critical analysis). Conversely, DS subjects may exhibit comparable or better performance than MA-matched MR subjects of other aetiologies, on tasks of motor imitation (Rondal, Lambert and Sohier, 1981), visual pattern discrimination, and visuomotor performance (Silverstein et al., 1982).

Dual-task studies supply relevant data for analysing cerebral dominance for *speech production*. Harris and Gibson (1986) summarized in Elliott et al., (1987), and Elliott et al. (1987) had DS and NR subjects perform a rapid unimanual finger–tapping task alone and while sound shadowing high-frequency words. As expected; NR subjects outperformed those with DS in all conditions. For both groups, however, concurrent speech disrupted right-hand but not left-hand performance. This was interpreted, according to Kinsbourne and Hicks (1978), as suggesting LHD for speech production.

Synthesizing the current literature, Elliott et al. (1987) proposed that most DS individuals perceive speech with their right cerebral hemisphere but depend on their left hemisphere for speech production. The same authors speculated that the language problems of DS persons may be related to a dissociation between cerebral areas responsible for speech perception and production. Such a dissociation might cause difficulties of communication between functional systems that normally overlap. Additionally, if as currently held, the left cerebral hemisphere is primarily a sequential analyser and if the cortical mechanisms for speech reception are located within the right hemisphere in DS subjects, certain types of function in these people are remote from the neural mechanisms best equipped to handle these functions.

Elliott et al.'s hypothesis raises a number of questions. One of them is related to the specificity problem. To the extent that MR individuals of other aetiologies than DS share a number of language problems with DS subjects, it is not clear why the dissociation between cortical sites assumed to be specific to DS by Elliott et al. (1987) (a strong claim that must be tested further), should be held responsible for major aspects of the DS language problems, while the same problems would have to find other explanations in other MR syndromes.

And there is more to it. Following Hartley (1982) and Elliott et al. (1987), one can entertain the following hypothesis: the more homogeneously computational language functions are represented in the left cerebral hemisphere, the better these functions. Rondal (1995b) has supplied relevant data on this problem, which do not support the type of implication one can draw from Hartley's and Elliott et al.'s hypotheses, but instead illustrate the intricacy of the relationship between brain structures and language. Françoise, the language-exceptional person studied by Rondal (1995b), demonstrated a cerebral hemisphere dominance for speech functions that was not different from normal people. Laura, the non-DS MR adolescent studied by Curtiss (1988) and Yamada (1990),[3] presented a slight LHD. This would seem to be supportive of Hartley's and Elliott et al.'s hypothesis. However, comparable data analysed by Rondal (1995b) for a number of typical DS adults reveal a more complex picture than was previously presented. These subjects were 24 DS adults (15 males, 9 females, between 21 and 36 years). One score was computed expressing the proportion of *intrusion errors*, that is the number of times the subject reported in one ear the syllable that was actually presented to the other ear on that trial, out of the total number of speech stimuli presented. The formula computed for each ear (dichotic listening score = $\frac{30-E1}{30}100$, where 30 is the number of syllables individually presented to each ear and E1 the number of intrusion errors from the other ear) allowed to calculate an REA, and an

---

[3] Laura and Françoise are the only two language-exceptional MR subjects for whom data regarding cerebral hemispheric dominance for language functions have been reported.

LEA, or a null difference (i.e. no ear advantage). Taking a percentage difference of at least 10 points to indicate ear advantage (Hartley, 1985), it was found that among DS women, three exhibited an REA (range 30–77 per cent), four exhibited an LEA (range 16–64 per cent), and two no ear advantage. Among the DS men, six exhibited an REA (10–63 per cent) and nine an LEA (range 10–77 per cent).

Fifteen of the DS adults (8 males, 7 females) having participated in the dichotic-listening study were also administered a dual-task procedure consisting of a finger-tapping task combined with a sound-shadowing task. A relative amount of interference (RAI – compared for the right hand and the left hand with and without concurrent speech production) averaged per second (see Rondal, 1995b, for a complete report) revealed the expected interference between verbalization and right-hand finger-tapping in 6 of the 8 male subjects. Among the female subjecs, the expected interference between verbalization and right-hand finger-tapping was observed in only three of the seven cases. A number of the male and the female DS adults studied by Rondal (1995b), therefore, exhibited a noticeable interference between verbalization and right-hand movements compatible with the hypothesis of a LHD for speech production. Things seemed to be less marked with the female DS subjects than with the males. This finding is consistent with the observation of Elliott et al. (1987), according to which women, whether NR or DS, are less lateralized for speech production than males.

When comparing the language abilities of the typical DS adults studied by Rondal (1995b) and exhibiting important degrees of REA (LHD) in dichotic listening and high degrees of RAI in the dual verbalization/finger-tapping task, as well as looking into the homogeneity of LHD for speech perception and speech production among these subjects, the results do not support Hartley's and Elliot et al.'s (1987) hypotheses. Three DS females exhibited a clear REA (from 30 to 77 per cent). Six males exhibited a clear REA (from 10 to 63 per cent). Retaining those individuals for whom the REA was equal or exceeded 50 per cent, one has two female and one male DS subjects. These three subjects all had positive RAI values in the dual-task study. They may, therefore, be considered as relatively homogeneous LHD for speech perception and production. However, upon meeting them and according to the information contained in their files at the occupation centre which they attend daily, it was clear that their language abilities were unexceptional for DS persons.

It would seem that no solid prediction can be made directly linking performance on dichotic listening and dual task as indices of hemispheric dominance for speech, and the actual speech and language of DS individuals.

Rejecting degree of LHD as a major explanatory variable for the interindividual differences in computational language functions in DS in no way automatically leads to undermining the neurological explanation proposed before. It means that no single brain feature or dimension will be necessarily relevant to the difference question. Within the cerebral hemispheres (left, right, or both) particular structures are at work which permit and sustain linguistic operations. In our view, the hazards of brain development across MR syndromes and MR individuals within syndromes are mainly responsible for the differences observed in computational linguistic development and functioning among these people. At this time, however, this is only a working hypothesis. Its demonstration awaits further collaborative work between psycholinguists and neurologists.

5.6 Adult–child interaction and the development of language in the mentally retarded

5.6.1 No matter how important the species-specific and the intrinsic constraints bearing on language development or some aspects of it are, it is clear that this development does not take place in an environmental vacuum. The question has been raised since the late 1960s of the exact role played by the linguistic environment in the acquisition of a first language.

The necessity for the child to be exposed to some (at least minimal) quantity of spoken language within the time boundary of the critical period for computational language development seems established. But beyond this minimal requirement, what is the role of parents and caretakers in shaping the language organization of the developing child? Early opinions were quite negative on this point. For example, Fodor (1966) claimed (without supporting empirical data) that the linguistic environment of the child did not differ from that of the adult. Both are filled with false starts, fillers, lapses, grammatical mistakes, etc. (pp. 108, 126).

Empirical observations made in the late 1960s and 1970s (see Rondal, 1985b, for a review) proved the above opinion wrong at least with regard to the existence of systematic differences between adult-to-adult and child-directed adult speech. Indeed, maternal speech addressed to the language-learning child has been shown to be finely adapted to the developmental level of the child in various respects, i.e. prosody, articulation, lexicon, semantic structures and contents, morpho-syntax, and pragmatics. These adaptations were gauged against the speech typically exchanged between adults in corresponding tasks and situations. Fathers' speech addressed to language-learning children appeared also to be modified like mothers' speech in order to correspond to the limited linguistic capabilities of the children (Golinkoff and Ames, 1979; Rondal 1980b; Brédart-Compernol, Rondal and Perée,

1981). Most importantly, maternal speech adapts to the growing linguistic ability of the child. For example, the evolutions in mothers' and children's MLU are positively correlated from approximately 18 months on. Moerk (1975) measured this correlation between 2 and 5 years in the children. It reaches 0.69 (significant at the $p < 0.001$ level). Rondal (1978c) reported a corresponding correlation of 0.55 ($p < 0.001$) between 20 and 32 months in the children. Between 18 months and 10 years in the children, the increase in maternal MLU is almost linear. The same observation holds for children's MLU between 2.5 and 4.5 years (the upper age limit in the above studies).

The same adaptive mechanisms are at work whichever the sex of the child or the parent (e.g. Phillips, 1973; Fraser and Roberts, 1976). They are found across social classes, although some finer child language tuning may exist with middle-class parents (Snow et al., 1976). The same basic interactive mechanisms appear to exist across cultural backgrounds. They are not restricted to the Western types of child-rearing habits (Blount, 1972; Omar, 1973; Slobin, 1981).

The notion of simplicity in maternal language addressed to language-learning children has been questioned by Newport, Gleitman and Gleitman (1977). These authors remarked, for example, that the elevated frequency of occurrence of interrogatives in mothers' speech to young children (between 33 and 53 per cent with children between 12 and 32 months in the studies of Broen, 1972; Savic, 1975; Newport et al., 1977; and Rondal, 1978b) could render this type of speech structurally more complex and difficult to process. This remark may be correct in absolute terms. However, overall, it is difficult to deny that mothers' speech with language-learning children is globally simplified as to its major formal and content aspects.

On the preceding basis, Moerk (1976, 1983) and Rondal (1985b) have proposed explanatory models of the language ontogenesis in which the adult partners of the child play a determining role. It seemed that this role could be extended to older children interacting with younger ones. Shatz and Gelman (1973) have shown that older children tend to behave linguistically towards their younger siblings in a way similar to parents. Moerk (1983) did not hesitate to assimilate mothers to genuine language teachers and to define first-language acquisition as being mainly the product of long-term *explicit parental teaching*. Moerk seems to have kept to this position, witness the title of his latter book on the subject (*First Language Taught and Learned* 1992). Without going as far as Moerk, Rondal (1983, 1985b) suggested that parents could be *implicitly teaching language* to their children, in simplifying and adapting their language input to the cognitive and linguistic levels of the child, and repairing and expanding their children's utterances in appropriate ways.

There is also some evidence that maternal input may not differ very much from trained teachers (Edwards, 1991). A remarkable ability in preschool and elementary schoolteachers to calibrate the formal level of their language to the receptive language abilities of their pupils was demonstrated by Rondal, Adrao and Neves (1980). It is possible, therefore, that the implicit language teaching model could be extended to include the schoolsetting.

However, the renewed emphasis on language learnability in the late 1970s and 1980s (Culicover and Wexler, 1977; Wexler and Culicover, 1980; see also Wexler, 1994) has forced a more careful scrutiny of one aspect of adult–child verbal interactions, namely the feedback dimension and the question of negative evidence bearing on the grammaticality of children's utterances. An explicit or implicit parental language teaching mechanism obviously must encompass not only input models of the target language that are adapted to the child's level of development, but also appropriate feedbacks contingent upon the children's utterances in such a way as to make it clear for the learner which productions are grammatically acceptable and belong to the target language, and which ones do not. According to Wexler and Culicover (1980), the learner's datum at any point in time must be either a positive or a negative instance of the target language. One important question, therefore, is about the exact nature of parental feedback to language-learning children. Rondal (1985b) reported percentages of maternal verbal approval and disapproval of preceding children utterances around 15 per cent and percentages of maternal expansions of children utterances around 10 per cent. The two types of feedback decrease rapidly in frequency of occurrence beyond approximately 30 months in the children. As documented in several studies (Brown and Hanlon, 1970; Hirsh-Pasek, Treiman and Schneiderman, 1984; Demetras, Post and Snow, 1986; Rondal, 1987a; see Rondal, 1988a, in press-b, for reviews and discussions of these studies; Bohannon and Stanowicz, 1988), the problem is as follows. With the exception of punctual formal corrections of children's utterances (infrequent), parental feedbacks are much more often motivated by considerations of semantics, truth value and referential adequation than by grammatical preoccupations. As a consequence, one finds the following four situations: (1) parental approval of children's utterances that are semantically and grammatically correct; (2) disapproval of utterances that are semantically and grammatically correct; (3) approval of utterances that are semantically correct but grammatically incorrect; and (4) disapproval of utterances that are grammatically correct but semantically inappropriate. It follows that parental feedbacks may be of use in helping the child to assess the semantic correctness of his utterances but not or only little regarding the grammatical correctness of these utterances. Is this surprising? We believe that it is not. People speak to communicate and not for the purpose of indulging in grammatical exercises. They are naturally more attuned to the content than to the formal aspects of the utterances that they produce or hear. This may be a major problem for strong grammar-teaching hypotheses regarding adult models and feedbacks to language-learning children.

But could not adults or parents use indirect ways to inform children that some of their utterances are ill-formed? Brown and Hanlon (1970) asked whether one could find parental responses to children's speech that would be pragmatically differentiated, i.e. have opposite consequences depending on the formal quality of the child's utterance. The answer they gave to this question is a negative one. Brown and Hanlon (1970) found little difference in the percentages of 'sequiturs' (relevant parental responses revealing a good comprehension of the preceding child's utterance) and 'non-sequiturs' (comprehension errors, expression of lack of comprehension, clarification request, and other similar reactions) in response to children's utterances independently analysed as formally primitive or grammatically correct by the researchers.

Further attempts to identify indirect feedbacks supplying consistent grammatical information to the child similarly failed. Hirsh-Pasek et al. (1984) confirmed Brown and Hanlon's data with 40 mother–child dyads with the children aged between 2 to 5 years. They also investigated the possible existence of parental implicit grammatical feedbacks contingent upon the children's utterances. Such feedbacks could consist, for instance, in an opposition between verbatim repetition of children utterances that are grammatically well-formed, and non-repetition of grammatically ill-formed children utterances. The data gathered by Hirsh-Pasek et al. (1984) suggest that the majority of adult exact repetitions of children's utterances do indeed follow grammatical utterances significantly more often than ungrammatical ones (also Nolan Post, 1994). Actually, this is trivially guaranteed by the fact that nearly all parental speech to language-learning children is grammatical (Marcus, 1993). If the child starts with such an assumption about his parents' speech (which he probably should in the same way as for other adult modelling), there is no reason and no ground for considering that he is supplied with contrasted feedback depending on the grammaticality of his own utterances.

Additionally, there is the frequent difficulty for the child (Demetras et al., 1986), and the external observer, to identify the exact target of the adult feedback. This is the 'correspondence problem' (McKee, 1992) to which we shall return.

Demetras et al. (1986) suggested that the maternal type of response that most frequently follows correctly formed children's utterances is the 'simple pursuit' (i.e. the mother acknowledges the child's contribution and allows the interaction to continue). The most frequent maternal response following a child's ill-formed utterance is the request in clarification. The latter is also the case when the content of the child's production is not clear to the parent. Theoretically, therefore, the attentive child could have an opportunity to sort out his utterances on a grammatical basis. However, there is no empirical indication that children actually use the above differential observation for grammatical learning. Additionally, this use would considerably tax their memory.

Regarding the correspondence problem mentioned above, several elements may be defective simultaneously in any utterance produced by the young child (e.g. intonation, stress, articulation, meaning, thematic role, grammatical organization, pragmatic appropriateness, illocutionary type and strength). Implicit feedbacks, because they are implicit, are rarely clear in these respects. Therefore, their possible use by the children for purpose of grammatical learning is bound to be limited. Such learning presupposes some contribution from the child's own grammatical knowledge, which remains to be explained.

Even more damaging for the hypothesis that adult feedbacks contingent upon children's utterances could be of particular utility in grammatical learning is an analysis by Marcus (1993) framed in terms of conditional probabilities. If the adult feedbacks are motivated in the first place by semantic and referential considerations, then the child cannot rely on a single feedback to assess the grammaticality or the ill-formedness of his utterance. He must take into account a number of feedbacks bearing on the same utterance or the same structural type of utterances. This raises problems of memory limitation. If it is proposed that the child can mentally classify utterances he has produced according to structural type, there is the additional question of how and from where he would have obtained the knowledge necessary to perform such a classification. Through a complex calculus that need not to be rehearsed here (see Marcus, 1993, for the details), and based on the distribution of adult feedbacks reported by Hirsh-Pasek et al. (1984), Marcus was able to establish that the child ought to reproduce the same utterance or type of utterance 446 times and compile the relevant adult reactions, to be able to decide whether a given utterance of his is to be judged grammatical or ungrammatical with a 99 per cent chance of being correct. Using a more favourable distribution of adult feedbacks, such as the one reported by Bohannon and Stanowicz (1988), the number of utterance reproductions by the child would still be 85. In a less favourable situation (Penner, 1987), the child would have to reproduce the same utterance 679 times. It is known that children repeat their own utterances very little. Pinker (1989) analysed more than 80 000 utterances from the 'Harvard children' (Brown, 1973). He counted no repetition beyond 3 times, with the exception of one grammatical error reproduced 11 times by one of the children (Eve).

In conclusion, the following characteristics of adult feedback can be observed (Pinker, 1993). Much of these feedbacks are not about grammaticality, they are noisy (grammatical as well as ungrammatical sentences tend to be repeated); they decline after the age of 24 months in the child although grammatical development is far from complete; they are weak in the sense of demanding an unrealistic number of utterance repetitions from the child's part to supply a plausible way of eliminating grammatical errors. Additionally, there is no proof that negative evidence, even if useful, is actually used by the children, or, if used, that it is instrumental in bringing about grammatical progress. It is probably wiser to consider that acquisition mechanisms do not crucially depend on negative evidence.

However, it does not follow from the above considerations that the adult input to the language-learning child is devoid of any use in grammatical development. One should keep in mind two major observations: first, adult language addressed to children is grammatical (Marcus, 1993, estimated its grammaticality to be 99 per cent); and, second, it is simplified and adapted continuously to the child's level of language development. One may assume that these simplifications and adaptations facilitate the child's parsing and grammatical analysis of the input, and make it easier (or perhaps are a necessary condition) for the young child to have the opportunity to 'crack' the linguistic code. But it is clear that this role is only a secondary one and that *the full responsibility for grammar construction rests with the child*. No datum contradicts the suggestion of a facilitating role of the input in language development, even if it is correct to acknowledge that no experimental proof is available either. The only counterargument existing to the best of our knowledge is Bickerton's hypothetical reconstruction of the birth and early evolution of Creole languages. Bickerton (1981, 1984) suggested, in relation with his language bioprogramme hypothesis, that Creole grammars are genuine inventions on the part of the first (historical) generation having started with a Pidgin as linguistic input. If confirmed, this indication would constitute the first evidence against a particular role of the linguistic input in first-language acquisition (particularly grammar acquisition). However, Bickerton's analysis has been sharply criticized by some Creolists (e.g., Muysken,1988; Youssef, 1988).

5.6.2 Turning to MR children, it has been demonstrated that at corresponding levels of language development, they are exposed to language environments and receive language inputs that do not differ *qualitatively* in major respects from those of NR children (Buckhalt, Rutherford and Goldberg, 1978; Rondal, 1978b). Previous studies (e.g. Buium, Rynders and Turnure, 1974b) had voiced some concern that the linguistic environment of language-learning MR children could be different from that of NR children, and therefore worthy of careful consideration in any attempt to understand their language acquisition process and to reduce their delays in language development. It turns out, however, that when proper matching is made on the children's levels of language development (for example, using MLU as matching variable, as in Rondal, 1978b), no significant difference appears in the language of the mothers addressing their NR or their MR children. This confirms that the language level of the child is a factor determining parental speech and a more potent factor than whether the child is NR or MR. Rondal's (1978b) observations have been confirmed in several studies (e.g. Gutmann and Rondal, 1979; Cunningham et al.,1981; Petersen and Sherrod, 1982; Mahoney, 1988). In one of the very few studies to include fathers and mothers, Maurer and Sherrod (1987) observed no or little difference in the verbal behaviours of the fathers of DS children and those of developmentally matched NR children. In contrast, Cardoso-Martins and Mervis (1985) claimed that mothers of DS children differ from mothers of language-matched and MA-matched NR children on a number of measures including lower proportion of deictic utterances (e.g. *This is a ball*) and nouns (as opposed to pronouns). Cardoso-Martins and Mervis (1985) concluded that the mothers of DS children contribute to the delayed lexical development of their offspring by failing to provide them with a sufficient number of referent–label pairings. However, as also noted by Rosenberg and Abbeduto (1993), Cardoso-Martins and Mervis's (1985) conclusion and implication are unwarranted. They have not established a relation (even less a causal one) between maternal labelling behaviours and children's vocabulary development.

Regarding early pragmatic development, a series of studies (e.g. Leifer and Lewis, 1983; Petersen and Sherrod, 1982; Mahoney, 1988; Tannock, 1988; see Rosenberg and Abbeduto, 1993, for a detailed review) also suggest that parents of MR children supply their language-learning children with appropriate exemplars of types of question and speech act at rates corresponding to those of parents of NR children at similar levels of communicative competence and cognitive capacity. Hodapp (in press-b) reviewing the literature on parenting MR children, concludes in agreement with our stand that the available studies illustrate basic similarities in the *structural properties of input language* to MR and NR children at corresponding levels of language development. But Hodapp insists that *mothers' styles of interaction* with NR and MR children may differ. He claims that even when MR and NR children are correctly equated on MA or linguistic age, mothers of MR children are often (although not always as there appears to exist a wide variety in maternal styles of interaction) more didactic, directive and even intrusive, compared to mothers of NR children.

Possible causes for these latter behaviours are: (1) mothers of MR children may be more concerned with the teaching aspect of the interaction as a plausible way to help reducing the MR children's developmental delays; (2) MR children may actually require more intensive, intrusive interactions, for optimal development in cognition, language, and other domains. See Wishart's (1994, in press) suggestion that many DS children are characterized by a 'counterproductive, avoidant approach to learning new skills and by a failure to exercise and maintain skills once they have been finally acquired' (in press, p. 23)); (3) MR infants and children may provide less clear interactive cues and therefore be less 'readable' to mothers and other adults.

Quantitatively, no differences seem to exist either between maternal speech to MR and NR children at corresponding levels of language development. Rondal (1978a) estimated that both types of children receive the same quantity of speech addressed to them. In one rare study performed with working-class mothers and their MR children aged 18 months to 5 years-CA (some diagnosed as having DS), Davis and Oliver (1980) reported more vocal stimulation, more responsiveness and less directiveness than with the controls. Increased talkativeness in mothers of MR children was not confirmed in a subsequent investigation by Davis, Stroud and Green (1988), however. The latter authors concluded that the global amount of verbal stimulation is comparable for NR and MR children at corresponding levels of language development. At any rate, lacking specifications on minimal language exposure necessary for language development to proceed in NR and MR children (no effect of variations in frequency of parental talk has been documented so far, except in cases of extreme deprivation of language input), it is impossible to make exact sense of the above data on quantity of language input to the children.

Regarding the *adult feedback question*, although the number of specific observations is limited, it seems that the situation with MR children is not different from the one in NR children (see Rondal, 1978a, c, 1985b). Most people in the field no longer consider that spontaneous verbal imitation is a valid mechanism for explaining (natural) grammatical development (see Tager-Flusberg and Calkins, 1990). However, it could still be claimed that for those children who imitate frequently during the relatively short developmental period of time in which they imitate adult speech (i.e. between approximatively 20 and 30 months; Seitz and Stewart, 1975; Rondal, 1978b, d), verbal imitation could help maintain conversational coherence (Keenan, 1977) or serve other pragmatic purposes (Folger and Chapman, 1979). Verbal imitation could also facilitate the entry and registration of lexical items into the child's mental repertoires (Rondal, 1983). For corresponding suggestions along the same line, see Speidel and Nelson (1989). In this respect also, MR (including DS) children do not seem to differ from NR children at similar language levels. This is no surprise. Indeed, as suggested by Slobin (1968) and Slobin and Welsch (1973), children mostly imitate at their level of grammatical development. Rondal (1980d) showed that spontaneous verbal imitations are mostly similar in frequency of occurrence and in grammatical structure in DS and NR children at comparable levels of language development. The mean number of children's imitations of maternal utterances were 53.43, 20.29 and 6.14, respectively, for the DS children from language level 1 (MLU 1.00 – 1.50) to language level 3 (MLU 2.50 – 3.00). Both groups of children were equally found to imitate mainly the last part of the immediately preceding maternal utterances. Values reported for the mean length of the portion of mothers' utterances following the parts imitated by the children, in number of words plus grammatical morphemes, varied between 0.19 and 0.49, with no significant difference between child groups at each language level. A similar conclusion was reached by Sokolov (1992) in his research on the rate of linguistic imitation in NR and DS children. His group data were taken from different sources within the Child Language Data Exchange System (CHILDES, MacWhinney, 1991), including the original data from Rondal (1978a) on which the imitation analysis of Rondal (1980d) was based. Sokolov's imitation analysis was carried out independently from Rondal's analysis, however. Sokolov reported a statistically significant but tiny difference (0.017 in mean proportion with a SD of 0.10 in both groups) in verbal imitativeness (exact, expanded and so-called reduced imitations confounded) between NR and DS children matched for MLU. This difference was determined in major part by variations between groups of children at the lower MLU levels. Additionally, they may have had much to do with the exclusion in Rondal's (1978a) data of non-standard forms such as *huhuh* or *yup* which could have been imitated by the mothers of younger children and counted as instances of maternal imitation in other data, for example, Hooshyars' (1985, 1987). All in all, spontaneous verbal imitation of maternal utterances in MR children appears fairly similar or close in frequency as well as in structure to that of NR children at comparable levels of language development.

In conclusion, it seems that the MR child is placed in the same environmental situation as the NR child at corresponding developmental levels when it comes to learning the language of the cultural community. Basically, the MR child is provided with a quantitatively and qualitatively appropriate language input. He tends to receive sufficient attention regarding the semantic and referential adequacy of his utterances, but little systematic grammatical teaching or specific grammatical feedback. Just as the basic determinism of grammatical development appears to be intrinsic to the NR child, so it is for the MR child.

5.7 Language in mentally retarded adults

Life expectancy in moderately and severely MR persons has increased markedly (see Chapter 1). This is an encouraging indication for those who believe in the absolute right of all human beings to live and develop to their best potential. It makes it all the more necessary to gather comprehensive data (medical, psychological, social and otherwise) on MR adults in order to evaluate more precisely their functioning capabilities, the possible evolution of these capabilities over time, and to ensure the best possible social, emotional and vocational adjustments for MR subjects. Language has a particularly important role in these adjustments. Some people (e.g. Swetlik and Brown, 1977) claim that impaired language and communication skills constitute the major impediment to the integration of MR people in society. More studies of MR adults' language are needed in order to meet this challenge.

The cohort caveat mentioned in the preceding section regarding the language levels reached by MR adolescents applies even more in the adult context. Present-day MR adults have not usually been enrolled in early intervention programmes. It is quite possible that their ultimate levels of development are not what they could have been, had they been exposed to efficient early intervention. One should avoid considering that the present language levels of MR adults supply a correct reflection of their genuine potentialities.

This section, in its first part, summarizes the levels generally reached by MR adults in the various components of the language system.

5.7.1 Two large-scale studies of the *speech characteristics* of MR adults (Shriberg and Widder, 1990; Van Borsel, 1993) and two smaller-scale technical reports (Farmer and Brayton, 1979; Hamilton, 1993) supply a preliminary basis on which it is possible to define the phonological characteristics of adults with mental retardation. Van Borsel (1993) compiled the phonemic inventories of 20 adolescent and adult DS subjects (10 males and 10 females; CAs 15 years 4 months to 28 years 3 months; mean CA 20 years 10 months; MAs 3 years 9 months to 7 years 2 months; mean MA 5 years 8 months). He also compared the single consonant and consonant cluster inventories of these DS subjects to those of 20 NR toddlers (10 boys and 10 girls; CAs 2 years 6 months to 3 years 4 months; mean CA 3 years). Speech samples were obtained from each subject individually in a picture description task. Results clearly suggest that the speech of the DS adolescents and adults is similar in its segmental phonological dimension to that of NR children. This confirms the hypothesis of a speech development mostly delayed (but not different) in DS subjects. Both DS and NR groups showed comparable consonant error rates and made errors largely on the same phonemes, even if the DS group's phonological performance was more variable. Also, the occurrence of errors was similarly liable to phonetic context, with both groups showing more frequent errors with syllable final than syllable initial consonants, and more frequent errors with consonant clusters than consonant singletons. Additionally, in both DS and NR groups, distortions of phonemes accounted for the largest proportion of errors, followed in decreasing order by substitutions, omissions and additions. Specific analysis of error categories demonstrated that the severity of the substitutions was similar in both groups. Place of articulation, manner of articulation and voicing were involved in the substitution errors to the same degree in DS and NR subjects. Analysis of addition errors showed similar trends in occurrence of additions relative to word length and position in words. Lastly, analysis of vowel and diphthong productions showed that overall error rates did not differ between the two groups of subjects. A few differences emerged, however, with respect to the occurrence of consonantal error types. For example, NR children had significantly larger proportions of distortions than DS individuals, who tended to make more omissions, particularly of syllable final consonants. These differences, Van Borsel (1993) claims, may be ascribed to a less advanced phonological development in DS subjects.

Farmer and Brayton (1979) suggested on the basis of their investigation with 13 DS adults (mean CA 30 years 8 months) that some subjects articulating correctly on single-word responses, but exhibiting poor intelligibility in conversational speech, actually speak too rapidly for the articulators to approach their correct targets. Particularly, vowel duration is significantly reduced in these subjects.

Hamilton (1993) investigated tongue movements for speech in three English-speaking adults with DS and one NR control, using electropalatography and diadochokinetic (DDK) rate. This latter technique involves counting the number of times certain sounds can be repeated per minute. She insists on the existence of speech impairments of a dysarthric and dyspraxic nature in some DS subjects in addition to immature phonological processes. In the speech of her DS adults, Hamilton documented more palatal zone contact for alveolar sounds /t/, /d/, /n/, /l/, longer closure duration, longer consonant transition times within clusters, consistently slower DDK rates, undershoot (i.e. inadequate and incomplete tongue–palate contact) with velar articulations, difficulty with rapid tongue movements both in longer words and in the DDK tests, as well as phonological processes observed in the development of NR children that have the effect of reducing the number of phoneme contrasts used (e.g. phoneme deletion, substitution, consonant harmony, fronting, stopping of fricatives, cluster reduction). Hamilton (1993) confirms the persistence of a marked lack of intelligibility of DS adults' speech for the same reasons as in children and adolescents, i.e. mainly a continued breakdown both in the ability to move the tongue and lips in order to articulate speech sounds accurately and rapidly (dysarthria), and in the ability to select, plan and sequence the sounds needed (dyspraxia). These are in addition to purely phonological difficulties.

Another study conducted by Moran, Money and Leonard (1984) with institutionalized MR adults confirms that phonological errors (phonological processes) persist into adulthood.

Shriberg and Widder (1990) audio-recorded speech samples from 40 English-speaking 20–50-year-old non-institutionalized people with mental retardation. Technical details on this study have been supplied in Chapter 3 (Table 3.2), where it was reported that speech status failed to evidence a statistical association with gender. Shriberg and Widder's paper contains an in-depth speech and prosody analysis of the MR adults' linguistic and paralinguistic behaviours in continuous speech. They confirm that across all levels of age, aetiology and intellectual involvement, the two most common error sites are consonant clusters in all word positions (deletion, substitution and distortion of member sounds) and word-final consonant deletions. Four other common error types are weak syllable deletion, stopping, fronting and liquid simplification. Shriberg and Widder (1990) also confirm the important token-to-token articulatory variability in MR adults. Abnormal suprasegmental characteristics regarding five prosodic domains (rate, stress, loudness, pitch and quality of voice, i.e. relative harshness, hoarseness or nasality) were noted in many subjects. Shriberg and Widder suggest both a 'cognitive-capacity' and a 'sociolinguistic' constraint in order to explain the persistence of abnormal segmental and non-segmental prosodic features in the speech of MR adults. A cognitive-capacity constraint limits the speaker's ability to allocate proper resources to phonological encoding, hence the token-to-token inconsistency of articulation. Although this constraint is presented by Shriberg and Widder as a sufficient explanation, it is most likely not the only factor involved in the abnormal phonology of MR subjects (see Hamilton's and Farmer and Brayton's indications above). As to the abnormal prosodic features of the MR adults, the same authors suggest the lack of adequate models for those who had been institutionalized. This sociolinguistic limitation may well play a role in those adults who were living in institutions, but it is doubtful that it constitutes a sufficient general explanation.

As indicated in previous sections, *quantitative lexical development* in MR people is generally consistent with MA. Comblain's data (1994) reveal a mean receptive lexical age of about 5 years on the TVAP, which is approximatively the mental age reached by many DS adults (Gibson, 1981). On the expressive side, her DS adult subjects could correctly label approximately 50 per cent of the common objects and actions belonging to basic semantic categories. Rondal and Lambert (1983) analysed data on language from 22 non-institutionalized French-speaking MR adults (DS and non-DS), assembled individually with a NR interlocutor (see Chapter 3, Table 3.2, for a presentation of the study). Table 5.3 supplies a summary of the quantitative observations in that study. Only the TTR data are of immediate interest.

As indicated in Table 5.3, TTR are 0.58 and 0.57, for DS and non-DS MR adults, respectively.

As to combinatorial language and morpho-syntax, most MR adults are limited to short monopropositional utterances formally simple with reduced and unstable grammatical morphology. Conventional word order is usually appropriate. Subordinate clauses are rare: most often simple completives or subject relatives. Aspect and tense are strictly reduced. Full

Table 5.3 Group means and standard deviations (in parentheses) for the measures computed by Rondal and Lambert (1983) on the language of Down's syndrome (DS) and mentally retarded non-Down's syndrome (Non-DS MR) adults in free conversation with a non-retarded adult interlocutor

Indices	DS adults		Non-DS MR adults	
1. TTR (type–token ratio)	0.58	(0.08)	0.57	(0.05)
2. MLU (mean length of utterance)	5.98	(2.62)	6.95	(2.52)
3. Proportion of sentences	0.41	(0.31)	0.53	(0.30)
4. Sentence complexity	0.22	(0.17)	0.33	(0.24)
5. Correct marking of number and gender on noun phrase	0.56	(0.24)	0.69	(0.21)
6. Proportion of correct articles	0.38	(0.21)	0.52	(0.15)
7. Proportion of correct pronouns	0.62	(0.50)	0.88	(0.50)
8. Proportion of correct verbal inflections	0.55	(0.37)	0.78	(0.38)
9. Proportion of information	0.97	(0.04)	0.95	(0.07)
10. Proportion of new information	0.69	(0.12)	0.69	(0.11)
11. Conversational continuity	0.83	(0.08)	0.82	(0.12)

Note: For the definition of the linguistic indices, see Table 3.2 (Chapter 3).

syntactic passives are nonexistent. In the language analyses of Rondal and Lambert (1983) with a group of MR adults (see Table 5.3), only about half of the utterances produced by the MR adults were grammatical clauses. Sentence complexity (estimated through the proportion of compound verbs and subordinate clauses) remained very low. Grammatical marks of number and gender were produced on average only one time in two, or two times in three utterances. Articles were used infrequently and verbs were not regularly inflected for person. Clearly, grammatical morphology and function words continue to make problems for MR adults, even more so for DS adults (see the DS/non-DS comparison in Table 5.3). Interindividual variability is important, however (witness the relatively large standard deviations obtained on many linguistic indices in that study; see Table 5.3). So also is internal individual variability. Some structures (particularly grammatical morphemes) may be correctly produced by some MR subjects in some utterances and fail to appear in other utterances (sometimes quite close to the positive instances in the discourse). Internal individual variability has been signalled frequently in the language of MR individuals, particularly with regard to the computational aspects. It may be one of the distinct features of this language. Akin to the cognitive capacity constraint suggested by Shriberg and Widder (1990), Rondal (1985a) has suggested that the internal variability in the language of MR subjects may proceed from an inability to allocate sufficient attentional and cognitive resources to the ongoing monitoring of one's language. The more demanding the extralinguistic context, the nature of the speech act performed and the content and formal aspects of the utterance, the more likely some of the less firmly established linguistic features will be lost or cause errors. The difference between Shriberg and Widder's and Rondal's suggestion is that the latter was not intended to explain the language difficulties in themselves, but only their internal variability in MR subjects.

As indicated in Table 5.3, Rondal and Lambert (1983) observed MLU values close to 6 for DS and to 7 for non-DS MR adults. This is slightly superior to the mean MLU reported by Comblain (1994) for her DS adult group (mean MLU 4.73, SD 2.98). Comblain's mean adult MLU was drawn slightly towards upper values by the inclusion in the group of one female DS adult with an elevated MLU of 12.61. The slight difference in mean group (MLU) between Rondal and Lambert's (1983) and Comblain's (1994) data is probably best attributed to sampling variation. Figure 5.1 on page 133 illustrates schematically the plateau in the MLU evolution of DS persons beyond approximatively 15 years CA.

Regarding the *receptive morpho-syntactic abilities* of MR adults, Comblain's (1994) study contains some interesting information (summarized in Table 5.1). These data confirm the lasting weakness of DS individuals in the formal aspects of language. Comprehension of subordinate clauses (temporal, locative, causal and conditional), negative and passive sentences, is very limited when extralinguistic cues are not available. Coordinate and relative clauses may be better understood, but the average levels of comprehension do not exceed 65 per cent or thereabouts. Comprehension of grammatical morphemes also appears quite limited. The average scores on personal pronouns, definite and indefinite articles and verbal inflexions are in the region of 40 per cent only.

Lastly, Table 5.4 summarizes major information available on the *pragmatic and linguistic communication levels* of MR adults, based on recent reviews of the literature (Abbeduto and Benson, 1992; Abbeduto and Rosenberg, 1992; Rosenberg and Abbeduto, 1993). It also integrates the part of the data from Rondal and Lambert (1983) that relates to conversational continuity and informativeness in the verbal productions of MR adults (see Table 5.3; indices, 9, 10 and 11). These data are difficult to 'locate' with respect to the corresponding evolution in NR people because the differences between levels of pragmatic functioning in MR adults and mature NR people are not analysed.

In summary, it seems possible to define the language of most moderately and severely MR adults as *formally restricted but semantically and pragmatically appropriate to minimal cognitive and social demands*. The formal restrictions particularly concern the computational aspects of language (abnormal segmental and suprasegmental phonology, severely limited morpho-syntactic capacity). Despite these drastic limitations, the semantic contents of the utterances produced are correctly organized, informative and appropriate to the (simple) social context. In particular, major speech acts and conversational functions are accessible to the moderately and severely MR individuals, even if with markedly limited lexical and grammatical means.

Table 5.4 Levels of language pragmatic functioning in DS adults

Pragmatic area	Level of functioning
1. Speech acts	A. MR individuals are able to question, request, answer, assert, suggest, command, name, acknowledge, commit themselves, propose and express feelings or opinions, like NR people, but with primitive linguistic means, and not always using the indirect, softened, polite or inferred forms that normal people find appropriate. B. *Receptively*, MR individuals eventually become able at understanding speech acts in familiar interactions and settings but only associated with simple linguistic, cognitive and social demands.
2. Repairing communication failures	By adulthood, MR individuals seem to have the skills necessary for responding to a variety of requests for repair and to request repair of conversational failures.
3. Conversing and debating	MR individuals exhibit appropriate turn-taking behaviours in familiar conversational situations. They evidence conversational topic continuity with peers as well as with NR interlocutors. They can meaningfully contribute to the conversational topic. Information supplied discursively does not seem to be more redundant than customary speech between familiar NR people.

5.7.2 We shall now turn to the question whether there is still language progress in MR individuals beyond adolescence. On the basis of the data reviewed above, a tentative answer may be given immediately.

No progress is observed in the *phonological aspects of language* in the adult years. The empirical reports (Shriberg and Widder, 1990; Hamilton, 1993; Van Borsel, 1993) insist on the persistence of important speech problems. No progress in *receptive and expressive referential lexicon* is attested in Comblain's (1994) data with DS adults, nor in *diversity of lexical use* if one compares the spontaneous speech of MR adults (mean TTR around 0.57, as observed by Rondal and Lambert, 1983) and that of MR adolescents (mean TTR .60, as observed by Rondal et al., 1981; see Table 5.5 below). However, Berry et al. (1984), in a 5-year longitudinal study, reported a slight but significant increase in receptive lexical ability in 31 DS adults, as attested by their scores on the PPVT. Mean PPVT score passed from 56.9 (SD 18.4) on the first assessments when the subjects were aged 21 years on average, to 61.3 (SD 18.4) five years later. This vocabulary growth paralleled a significant increase in non-verbal mental development, as assessed by the Raven Coloured Progressive Matrices (Raven, 1965), as well as by the progress demonstrated on the Adaptive Functioning Index (an Index of Social Education, devised at the Vocational and Rehabilitation Research Institute of Calgary, Alberta, Canada) over the same period of time. There may be, therefore, some continued referential vocabulary growth in MR adults. Additional research should clarify sampling and assessment issues possibly involved in the differences between the studies mentioned.

No progress is found in *the receptive morphosyntactic aspects* of the language of MR adults when compared to MR adolescents, as shown in Comblain's (1994) BEMS data. Indeed, the DS adults in that study scored significantly lower than the DS adolescents on subordinate clauses and passive sentences (see Table 5.2). On the expressive morphosyntactic side, the mean MLU of the DS adults in Comblain's data is lower than the DS adolescents' one. A similar comparison may be made on MLU and a number of other expressive language characteristics between the French-speaking MR adult data gathered by Rondal and Lambert (1983) and those collected by Rondal et al. (1981) with MR adolescents.

The comparison between corresponding data from the group of French-speaking adults studied by Rondal and Lambert (1983) and the group of French-speaking adolescents studied by Rondal et al. (1981) reveals little systematic developmental change. Those data are consistent with the null hypothesis regarding progress in expressive morphosyntax from adolescence to adulthood in MR subjects. Comblain's (1994) data even seem to indicate a slight decline from adolescence to adulthood on some of the receptive morphosyntactic aspects. However, given the lack of independent confirmation of this effect in the other two studies concerned with the expressive morpho-syntax of MR adolescents and adults, it is probably best to attribute the differences in Comblain's data between DS adolescents and adults to sampling variation. There could be a cohort variation in the sense of the cohort caveat signalled earlier in this section, or a lack of sustained stimulation for grammar in occupational centres and the like.

Table 5.5 Group means for the measures computed by Rondal et al. (1981) on the language of MR children and adolescents in free conversation with a nonretarded adult interlocutor[1]

| Indices | MR children and adolescents (CA) groups | | |
	12–14 years n = 8	14–16 years n = 6	16–18 years n = 8
1. TTR[2]	0.58	0.61	0.60
2. MLU[3]	5.15	6.15	4.89
3. Proportion of sentences	0.47	0.50	0.46
4. Sentence complexity	0.22	0.27	0.19
5. Correct marking of number and gender on noun phrase	0.56	0.62	0.57
6. Proportion of correct articles	0.31	0.40	0.42
7. Proportion of correct pronouns	0.55	0.60	0.59
8. Proportion of correct verbal inflections	0.67	0.71	0.61

Notes: 1: See Table 3.2 (Chapter 3) for a definition of the linguistic indices as well as for technical information on the study; 2: TTR: type–token ratio; 3: MLU computed in number of words plus grammatical morphemes, according to Brown's rules (1973).

Lastly, regarding *the pragmatic aspects of language*, the literature suggests continued development from childhood into adulthood. However, the lack of specific age-related comparisons in the studies makes it impossible to establish whether there are genuine discontinuities in this development (possibly varying depending on particular pragmatic aspects) or whether it constitutes a gradual process.

Comparing the language evolution in mental retardation from childhood into adolescence on the one hand, and from adolescence into adulthood on the other, it seems that a modular conception of the critical period for computational language development finds a non-trivial support. On the whole, little progress is apparent in the phonological and morphosyntactic aspects of language of MR individuals beyond late childhood. The only changes documented concern a modest increase in MLU, reflecting a slight additional capability at listing words but no genuine structural progress, and a better comprehension of coordinate, relative and negative clauses, taking place between late childhood and middle or late adolescence. Some improvement in receptive and productive referential lexical ability and in language pragmatics seems to take place during adolescence and early adulthood. Also lexical diversity of use continues to increase slowly from childhood to late adolescence. This is compatible with the possibility of a slow continued growth in non-verbal MA in MR (including DS) people possibly until the third decade of life.

Computational language development may therefore proceed under the same maturational constraints in MR and NR individuals. The more conceptual and cognitive-social aspects of language do not seem to exhibit the same maturational time constraints, although it is certainly possible to argue that the foundations of semantic and pragmatic development must be laid during childhood.

The *implications for language intervention and remediation programming* with MR individuals are straightforward. Phonological and morphosyntactic training should be recommended at a maximal rate during childhood. Adequate potential for further development in these respects may no longer exist beyond 12–14 years. Intensive semantic, lexical and pragmatic training should also be given during childhood, but it could and should be continued during adolescence and early adulthood. For those language aspects, there continues to exist a potential for further development beyond 12–14 years. Later intervention regarding the computational aspects of the language of MR individuals will always be possible at least to some extent, given appropriate training. However, its cost-efficiency ratio will rapidly decline with the growth of MR persons in CA.

5.8 Ageing and language in mental retardation

The ageing process involves a series of changes in mental and physical functioning. These changes alter the way in which elderly people communicate, as human communication demands the synergetic participation of the speech apparatus and the language and cognitive organizations. Little research work has been done so far on the psychological, cognitive and linguistic consequences of physiological ageing in MR persons. In this section, we shall summarize information on the psycholinguistic effects of ageing in NR persons and set the major implications for language in ageing MR persons.

Additionally, in some categories of MR persons, particularly Down's syndrome individuals, there may exist an increased possibility of developing Alzheimer's disease (AZ). Pathological ageing or AZ in Down's syndrome will be dealt with in the second part of this section.

5.8.1 The normal process of linguistic ageing

A CA of 65 years is the agreed age for the commencement of older age in Western cultures, and 85 years the beginning of very old age (Maxim and Bryan, 1994). The size of the elderly population is growing in all

Western countries. In the United Kingdom, about 16 per cent of the population are over the age of 65. This figure will rise to 22 per cent by early in the next century, including the proportion of very elderly people (OECD, 1988). In Australia, it is estimated that 12 per cent of the population will be over 65 years of age by the year 2000 (Australian Bureau of Statistics, 1982). Estimates from the United States suggest that 17–20 per cent of the population will be over the age of 65 by the year 2030 (Schoenberg, 1986). Of course, it is important to distinguish chronological age and biological age (biological status). The physiological processes of ageing may occur earlier in some people and be delayed in others.

Let us consider, first, *the major age-related normal changes that affect language and communication*. We shall use Maxim and Bryan's review (1994) as a guide. One noticeable aspect of motor and psychomotor performance in older people is increased slowness. A number of anatomo-physiological modifications may affect speech production and perception. Respiratory support of speech is less efficient. Changes in laryngeal functioning contribute to changes in voice pitch in the elderly (Honjo and Isshiki, 1980). Hearing problems affect a large proportion of older people. A study of the US National Center for Health Statistics (1980) shows that approximately half the people aged 75 years and over have a hearing loss of 45dB or more. The term presbyacusis is sometimes used to refer to a deterioration of auditory functioning due to ageing (Willott, 1991). The main features of presbyacusis are: decrease in hearing sensitivity; reduced perception of fast rates of speech, speech in noise, whispered and higher pitched voices; and difficulty in communicating on the telephone.

Loss of vision in elderly people can also affect communication, either directly by determining loss of visual information, or indirectly by increasing social isolation.

Cognitive deterioration may take place particularly in what concerns selective attention; more in divided attention than in focused attention tasks, although the elderly may show difficulty in allocating attention to the target in focused attention tasks (Plude and Doussard-Roosevelt, 1989). The relationship of memory to age is a complex one; in proportion to the complexities of the organization of human memory. Three findings have appeared consistently in the specialized literature (see Malec, Ivnik and Smith, 1993, for a review). First, the ability to access remotely learned information is relatively preserved across the adult lifespan. Second, the capacity to attend and register new information does not decline with age. But, the subsequent process of learning and retention of new information becomes more limited with advancing age. Third, decline in new learning becomes prominent only in late life (beyond 80 years of age). Biological sex does not appear to have a direct effect on the maintenance of cognitive abilities with ageing. Men and women at various ages exhibit about the same capacities for new learning (Trahan and Quintana, 1990).

There is also evidence that different types of memory are diversely affected by the ageing process. There may be a mild decrease in short-term memory (STM) in older subjects, although this varies according to the complexity of the information to be recalled (Craik and Rabinowitz, 1985). A small number of studies bearing on the functioning of working memory in older persons is available (see Van der Linden, 1994a, for a review). They suggest that the WM mechanism identified by Baddeley (1986, 1990) under the name of 'central executive' could be affected by the ageing process and provide fewer attentional, planification and coordinating resources, to the particular auditory-verbal and visuo-spatial stores. However, the proper spans of these stores could also be reduced in older people as well as their processing speed (Salthouse and Babcock, 1991). There is also some evidence that the elderly have greater difficulty in WM when the input is visual rather than auditory (Cerella, Poon and Fozard, 1981).

The decline in long-term memory (LTM) capacity in older persons may be more significant. Differences between younger and older subjects in LTM relate to encoding, organizational and retrieval factors and strategies (Rankin and Collins, 1985). That is probably why such differences appear much less in recognition memory (Kausler and Hakami, 1983). Age differences also vary with the type of material to memorize (more or less structured, for example) and from person to person (depending, for example, on the intellectual efficiency of the subjects). It seems that ageing does not affect the several subsystems of LTM in the same way or to the same extent (see Tulving, 1983, 1987, for a definition of these subsystems). For instance, episodic (i.e. autobiographical) memory is more age-sensitive than memories for perceptual representation, semantic memory (the memory for meanings in language and knowledge) and procedural memory (the memory for the treatment of information and processing that we use in activities such as speaking, writing or driving). One must be cautious, however, because data are still insufficent and there have been contradictory reports (see Lovelace, 1990).

A wide range of diseases can affect the elderly in addition to the ageing process, so to speak. Outside of acute episodes such as strokes or head injuries, elderly people may present with depression, confusion states, diseases associated with particular neurological deficits, such as Parkinson's, Huntington and Alzheimer's disease (the last representing approximately 80 per cent of the dementias in older persons; Evans et al., 1989), or Pick's disease; psychoses and dementia. These pathologies may affect the ability to communicate and to use language. They will not be discussed here, with the exception of AZ.

5.8.2 What about language change in the normal elderly population?

Specific information on this question is still relatively sparse, particularly in comparison with the literature on neurogenic language disorders (e.g. aphasias), which has a long scientific history. But there is another reason for this apparent neglect. This is the premature opinion, in the 1950s and 1960s, based on psychometric testing and cross-sectional comparisons, that verbal skills do not change with age in opposition to non-language mediated tasks (see Wechsler, 1958; Cattell, 1963). There were, however, a few earlier indications that a small falling-off in language performance could take place after 60 years (Thorndike and Gallup, 1944; Feifel, 1949). Jarvik (1962), in a rare longitudinal study, found that his subjects as a group showed language changes with age, but there were important interindividual differences. Recent research has confirmed that some language change does indeed occur with older age. There is evidence that the ability of the normal elderly to *understand complex utterances* may differ from that of younger age groups. It is likely that the relationship between semantic and grammatical constraints in language comprehension may be a fruitful area for research into ageing language. Scholes (1978) showed that older people (average age 69 years) have difficulties with potentially ambiguous double-object sentences (e.g. *He showed her baby pictures*), because they may be less flexible in their ability to use different decoding strategies. Maxim (1982) compared the comprehension performance of a group of normal elderly (mean age 77 years) and a group of younger people (mean age 23 years) with sentences containing a temporal subordinate clause headed by *before* or *after*. This type of clause is mastered late by NR children (beyond CA 7 years; Clark and Clark, 1977). The younger group had an average error score of only 1 per cent versus 16 per cent (statistically significant difference) for the older people. Older people had particular difficulty understanding sentences in which the order of mention differed from the order of occurrence of the events, e.g. *He went out after having breakfast*, as opposed to *He had breakfast before going out* (which is also the major source of difficulty for young language-learning children). Cohen (1979) demonstrated differences between the young and the elderly in extracting information from spoken texts. Elderly people have more difficulty than younger subjects in answering inferential questions about texts (but not direct questions), particularly when the rate of text delivery is increased. Light, Zelinsky and Moore (1982) reported similar findings. In a related study, Light and Albertson (1990) found that although older adults can process inferences as well as younger adults, they may have difficulty with inferential information because they tend to forget certain aspects important to extracting the inference, or fail to reorganize the material properly in working memory. Light and Albertson (1990) added that the elderly have particular difficulty with inference when problem-solving and complex linguistic analysis must be carried out at the same time.

Little information is available on the language produced by older adults. Concerning sentence repair, McNamara et al. (1992) reported that normal elderly subjects self-corrected between 72 and 92 per cent of their errors on a picture description task. Yairi and Clifton (1972) found that the language of the elderly contains a significantly higher number of disfluencies than younger subjects. These disfluencies seem to be, for the most part, hesitant interjections and fillers, probably attesting to the longer time the elderly need to process utterances for production. Consistent with the indication of a possible organizational difficulty in oral language output, is Davis's observation (1979) that older adults use fewer embedded clauses than middle-aged groups. This is not observed in written language, however, where more time is available to monitor complex expression (Obler, Mildworf and Albert, 1977). Lastly, some studies have looked at *connected discourse* in the elderly. Multiple factors seem to play a role in discourse processing and may cause changes (e.g. social status, sensory impairment, speech style), but, on the whole, little difference between older and younger people has emerged. In story-telling or retelling, older people may even provide more elaborated stories than younger and less experienced story-tellers (see Adams et al., 1991).

Do elderly people evidence changes in basic language levels such as *single-word processing*? They usually are slower in fluency tasks such as producing names within one semantic category. Given additional time, however, elderly people achieve the same results as younger controls (Obler and Albert, 1981). Word-to-word priming tasks show no age effect for strength of priming in on-line processing, but rate of priming may be affected in old age (Burke and Harrold, 1990). The problem of word recall is one which the elderly themselves mention frequently, hence the augmented use of semantically indefinite words and third-person pronouns with increasing age (Sunderland et al., 1986). A decline in the ability to retrieve words from lexicon is probable in older age (Brédart, 1994). There may also be a lesser ability with age to supply 'superior' synonyms (i.e. responses appearing last in the lexical development of children) when defining lexical items (Botwinick and Storandt, 1974). However, more passive knowledge of the lexicon seems to remain stable (Botwinick, West and Storandt, 1975). Prevalent among lexical retrieval difficulties are those related to *proper nouns*. For example, Lovelace and Twohig (1990) report a marked difficulty (subjective assessment) to retrieve and orally supply a proper noun in 60 per cent of their subjects aged between 54 and 85 years. The reason for this difficulty is not well understood (see Brédart, 1994, for a discussion of tentative explanations). Proper nouns refer to individual entities and not to categories as common nouns do. This reduces the ways to activate the lexical entries for the proper nouns (priming effect) in the mental organization of the lexicon.

No phonological difficulties have been reported in normal ageing.

5.8.3 Normal ageing in MR subjects

There is no reason to expect MR subjects not to present the same ageing characteristics, psychological and otherwise, as NR people. The limited information available to date on cognitive and language ageing in MR individuals seems to confirm this indication.

Changes in sensory systems have been acknowledged as a common consequence of ageing in the MR population. Some deficits may be particularly frequent among the ageing with DS when compared to non-DS MR people. Evenhuis et al. (1992) have described hearing losses of 20dB to 90dB in the speech frequencies (*circa* 3000 Hz) in 33 out of a group of 35 Dutch DS adults aged 35–62 years. Cochlear losses were noted in 69 per cent of the cases. Hearing loss should certainly be considered as a possible contributing factor to the social and mental decline of middle-aged individuals with DS. Ocular findings from 30 DS individuals aged 21–72 years were reported by Hestens, Sand and Tostad (1991). Strabismus, cataract and visual losses were found to affect almost all subjects to various degrees.

Language studies of ageing MR persons are extremely rare. In the only systematic study that we were able to locate, Young and Kramer (1991) investigated age differences in 60 DS adults (aged 22–67 years) with no hearing impairment, reportedly. Older subjects were less likely to attend to auditory stimuli, had poorer word discrimination and were less able to understand the meaning of spoken language. Expectedly, these older subjects had more difficulty in following verbal directions.

It is possible to be more specific, at least predictively, in extrapolating from the language literature on normal ageing. Table 5.6 summarizes these predictions, pending empirical verification, of course.

Table 5.6 Additional language problems in ageing mentally retarded persons

1. Slower expressive and receptive language processing.
2. Less efficient respiratory support for speech.
3. Aggravated hearing problems; hence reduced attention to auditory stimuli, particular difficulties in perceiving whispered speech, speech in noisy conditions and in communicating on the telephone.
4. Additional difficulties in linguistic analysis and information extraction from spoken discourse. Additional problems in following verbal directions.
5. Augmented rates of dysfluencies (particularly hesitation pauses, interjections and fillers).
6. Additional difficulties in organizing spoken discourse.
7. Reduced word fluency.
8. Increased difficulty in word discrimination and in retrieving common and proper nouns.

5.8.4 Language and Alzheimer's disease

For a significant number of older DS people, there is more to ageing than physiological ageing. They develop with a higher frequency of occurrence than normal people or MR people of other aetiologies, a degenerative disease known as Alzheimer's disease (AZ). As emotional withdrawal is not infrequent among the representing symptoms of older adults with DS, the differential diagnosis of AZ must include depression (Lott, 1992).

In AZ, brain neurons develop *neurofibrillary tangles*, i.e. flame-shape alterations composed mainly of condensed cytoskeletal proteins. Another protein, β/A4 amyloid is deposited in large amounts in the form of *neuritic* (or *senile*) *plaques* and around blood vessels (*amyloid angiopathy*). The gradual accumulation of these changes plus neuronal loss (particularly in the large pyramidal cells), alteration of the motor nuclei of brainstem and reduction of neurotransmitters (particularly the choline group) render the affected parts of the brain less and less able to function properly.

There are several suspected genetic causes to AZ in non-DS people possibly involving several chromosomes, which we will not consider (see Berg, Karlinsky and Holland, 1993). In the case of DS, a possible (partial) explanation is that the amyloid percursor protein (APP) gene resides on the proximal part of the long arm of chromosome 21 (Goldgaber et al., 1987; Hyman, 1992). AZ-like pathology has been demonstrated in animals transgenic for a fragment of the APP (Kawabata, Higgins and Gordon, 1991). Neurofibrillary tangle-like structures were also reported in animals whose brains had been injected with β/A4 amyloid protein itself (Kowall et al., 1991). It is possible that overproduction of APP leads to alterations in brain morphology. Neuropathologic examination of DS individuals who died before the fifth decade shows a few neurofibrillary tangles and neuritic plaques in some areas and layers of the brain (see Hyman, 1992, for more detail). The continued accumulation of these changes leads to brain disturbance, cognitive and adaptive skills decline and emotional dysfunction, by the fifties or sixties (Hyman, 1992), or even earlier (the late thirties and forties) according to some reports (Wisniewski et al., 1985; Oliver and Holland, 1986; Thase, 1988; Rasmussen and Sobsey, 1994; Nelson et al., 1995). The brain changes involved are the same biochemically as those characterizing AZ in older non-MR individuals.

It is estimated that in non-MR people, approximately 3 per cent will develop AZ before or around 60 years. The incidence increases to about 20 per cent beyond 75 years (Evans et al., 1989). It is correct to note, however, that this figure may encompass other degenerative diseases. The same figures may be transposed (and perhaps slightly augmented) earlier in life for DS persons. Most importantly, in DS persons, there is a

15–20 year lapse between the first major brain alterations and cognitive decline. In NR people, the corresponding lapse is only approximately 7 years (Roth, 1993). The reason for this difference has not been ascertained. Wisniewski and Silverman (in press) suggest that two types of β-amyloid plaques must be distinguished: (a) those associated with fibrillization, and (b) those that do not contain fibrils. Non–fibrillar plaques are formed at earlier ages than fibrillar or neuritic plaques. Only this latter class of plaques appears to be associated with the clinical signs of AZ. In fact, non-fibrillar plaques are observed in DS people as early as 16 years, while densities of fibrillized plaques are not characteristic of cases until the forties and over. Wisniewski and Silverman (in press) posit that it is the fibrillar plaques that are associated with the disruption of normal neural functioning. If this is correct, the disparity between the clinical and neuropathological profiles of AZ among DS adults can be explained. Indeed, routine neuropathological examination does not differentiate well between fibrillar and non-fibrillar plaques. A considerable amount of ß-amyloid plaques can be present in DS adults in their thirties, but this deposit is in the non-fibrillar form. It is not until some 15 or 20 years later that significant accumulations of malign plaques are observed. This, of course, could not be the sole mechanism determining AZ dementia. Otherwise, virtually all DS individuals would end up exhibiting this dementia, which is not the case. Multiple factors must determine DS vulnerability to neuropathological age-associated changes, including AZ disease. There is, for example, increased amyloid load associated with triplication of APP on chromosome 21, unspecified ageing genes that could be on chromosome 21, and individual susceptibility to neurofibrillary pathology.

The latent period, particularly in DS, offers time for psychopharmacological and behavioural intervention with the prospect of slowing down the progress of the disease. It is possible that cognitive decline accelerates only from the time when alterations become so extensive as to overwhelm unspecified natural compensatory brain mechanisms.

Presently, there is no systematic study of *cognitive and linguistic decline in DS people with clearly diagnosed AZ*. Suggestions can be made on what to expect from the early literature on the particular language problems of NR persons with AZ.

It would seem that language is compromised in all stages in AZ, but that there is enormous variation in deficits among individuals. Despite such a large variation, general lines of major symptomatology may be traced. Language changes in AZ are most apparent at *the semantic level*, in particular the reduction of available vocabulary and the breakdown of semantical associations (Martin, 1987). Difficulty in word-finding is one of the most noticeable features of AZ. Auditory comprehension of words shows deficits as well as the comprehension of semantic complexity in sentences and paragraphs (Hart, 1988). The quality of discourse, cohesion and the whole pragmatics of language are usually found to be gravely deteriorating (see Maxim and Bryan, 1994, for a review). Most interesting is the repeated observation that the computational aspects of language (and particularly the grammatical structures) are largely spared in AZ, at least until the final collapse. They may be partly disturbed because of the breakdown in the language conceptual aspects, or as a result of a reduction in processing resource pools associated with verbally mediated tasks (see Waters, Caplan and Rochon, 1995), but not or only marginally as the primary effect of AZ pathology (Appel, Kertesz and Fishman, 1982). As mentioned in Chapter 4, Kempler, Curtiss and Jackson (1987) observed a normal range and frequency of syntactic constructions (but poor lexical use) in spontaneous speech as well as in writing with a group of 20 NR patients with AZ. These data suggest a dissociation between semantic and syntactic levels in AZ, reflecting the modular characteristics of the language organization and the fact that earlier deterioration in AZ has a predilection for certain brain sites, while leaving others untouched.

Table 5.7 briefly summarizes the probable implications of the above observations for DS individuals with AZ.

Table 5.7 Predictable language profile associated with Alzheimer's disease in Down's syndrome (DS) persons

---

Major dissociation between *language computational* (phonology and morpho-syntax) and *language conceptual, informative, and social aspects* (lexicon, semantics, pragmatics, discourse organization). The former aspects (underdeveloped in DS persons) are little touched *directly* (they may be affected indirectly as a reflexion of the cognitive-semantic breakdown), whereas the latter aspects will be found deteriorating to an extent varying from person to person.

Chapter 6
Language Remediation

We shall deal with language remediation in a reduced way as this is not the major aim of the book, limiting ourselves first, to defining and illustrating major dimensions and relevant principles to the remediation endeavour; and second, to discussing the efficiency issue with regard to current intervention programmes with MR individuals. Additional questions of interest (i.e. alternative communication, literacy training, working memory and its possible role in language development and remediation, and the use of computers in language intervention programmes) will be touched upon in a third and final section.

6.1 Dimensions and contents

In our view, language remediation with MR people, should be organized according to the set of self-embedding dimensions illustrated in Figure 6.1.

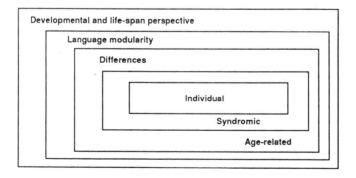

Figure 6.1 Major dimensions of language intervention with MR subjects

Remediation must be *developmental* in the sense specified in this book. Its general objective can be summarized in the following formula: *enabling the MR person to follow as quickly as possible and as completely as possible the sequences or steps characteristic of normal development.* Numerous observations suggest that language development in MR individuals proceeds in major ways like in NR individuals. This suggests that remediation programmes should follow NR development as closely as possible. We have made clear also that language in MR subjects should be envisaged according to a *life-span perspective.* Consequently, language remediation ought to be conceived according to this principle.

Language organization is basically modular. Remediation probably cannot be made in any truly effective way outside the *modularity approach.* This means defining particular intervention strategies corresponding to various language components. The specificity of the major language components is such that attempts to implement multipurpose remediation procedures are bound to generate mediocre effects.

Several levels of differences should be considered when designing language intervention. *Individual differences* have to be taken into account. The truth, unfortunately, is that as the study of these differences is little advanced in mental retardation, current programmes do not include this dimension despite lip-service being paid from time to time. Let us hope that in the not too distant future remediation programmes will be in a better position to propose individualized intervention procedures for people with MR.

It seems clear that interventions which take into account *aetiological (syndrome) characteristics* will have more chance of being effective (de Graaf, 1995). This claim was formulated by Gibson (1981; see Gibson, 1991, for additional specifications in the area of cognitive remediation and enhancement). Dykens, Hodapp and Leckman (1994) and Turk et al. (1994) insist that as patterns in development of MR individuals may be, at least partly, aetiology-specific, professionals should try as far as possible to tailor interventions to the specific aetiological groups. Intervention programmes might work better when the child's aetiology is among several important characteristics considered in designing remediation. This objective can be fully met when more data have been gathered on the various syndromes leading to mental retardation.

Last but not least, language intervention must be planned in an *age-related manner. Early intervention* is an absolute necessity (de Graaf, 1995). It carries the best hope for lasting effects given the cumulative nature of language development from prelinguistic acquisitions into later linguistic structures. It can be meaningfully carried out in close collaboration with the family of the young MR child (see, for example, the early intervention programme for DS children organized in partnership between parents and professionals by the APEM Association in Belgium; Rondal et al., 1988). *Continued intervention* during schooling should be organized in association with the schools (see Beveridge, in press). As language development is considerably spread over time in moderately and severely MR individuals, series of particular structures to be improved can be proposed in parallel with normal language acquisition at each of the school levels. Literacy training and the relationship between written and oral language development may take particular importance in school, particularly in integrated settings. Parents will often need to be advised on how to help their MR child effectively at each school level and make appropriate choices regarding curricular options (Rynders, 1994). Another topic of importance relates to the peer relations of MR children in mainstreamed groups. There, one has MR and NR children at different developmental levels interacting with each other in play and classroom activities. The work of Guralnick and associates is noted in the study of important aspects of peer-related social competence involving MR children (see Guralnick, 1992, in press; Guralnick and Paul-Brown, 1984, 1986; Guralnick and Groom, 1987; Guralnick et al., in press). The interested reader should refer to these sources for a full treatment of these questions, which is beyond the scope of the present book. Later intervention in *late adolescence and early adult years* should be recommended, particularly for the lexical and the pragmatic language aspects. It is highly advisable as a mean to enhance social-cultural and work integration with MR subjects (Rosenberg and Abbeduto, 1993; Rondal, 1995d). Lastly, language intervention with *ageing MR persons* is possible and should be encouraged adapting from current programmes with NR elderly (e.g. Maxim and Bryan, 1994). This could also supply a way of slowing down some of the language symptoms in the early stages of Alzheimer's disease in DS subjects.

Given the development emphasis in this book, the reader will not be surprised to find us stressing the necessity to model the contents of the intervention programmes after the sequences of language acquisition in NR children. Likely to be effective are the programmes closely following the developmental indications on the sequences of acquisitions in the several language components. Graduated sequences of prelinguistic, cognitive-semantic, lexical, phonological, morphosyntactic and pragmatic acquisitions can be implemented with MR children and adolescents. Such procedures have been designed by one of us (see Rondal, 1985c, 1995c, in press-a; Rondal and Perera, 1995). They are currently being experimented with in several countries. Rosenberg and Abbeduto (1993) have reviewed a number of studies aimed at improving the pragmatic aspects of language performance in MR subjects, particularly those attempting to increase the use of spoken language by MR persons when assembled with NR peers, to enhance verbal requesting behaviour, as well as to develop topic-related pragmatic skills in MR adolescents and adults (for example, how to initiate a conversation and expand on a partner's conversational topic).

Rosenberg and Abbeduto (1993) note that a number of programmes for improving social, including conversational, behaviours have been developed in recent years that depend on self-monitoring techniques. In this orientation, MR subjects (typically adults) are encouraged to monitor their own progress (for example, through audio- or videotapes) toward pre-established intervention goals (e.g. Matson and Adkins, 1980). This technique seems to have some interesting potential for bringing about improvement in pragmatic and social behaviours.

We shall not enter into the discussion of these proposals. The interested reader is referred to the sources cited for more information and for a full specification of the intervention strategies proposed.

6.2 The efficiency issue

Evaluating the effectiveness of an intervention, particularly a language intervention, is a difficult task. The goal is to enhance the subjects' learning of better linguistic structures and behaviours. Having acquired these structures, they ought to be able not only to produce or understand specific examplars involving these structures, but to exhibit generalized changes on given language aspects (Rusch and Karlan, 1983). Language training should be preceded by an adequate assessment of the language disabilities in the MR child. In this regard, language training demands extensive knowledge of the characteristics of language development and functioning in MR subjects. We are touching on the delicate question of the formation of the language professionals, pathologists or trainers. Given the complexity of the task of language intervention with MR subjects, only well-trained language professionals will stand a chance of achieving useful results.

Analyses of language intervention studies from an efficiency point of view are rare (see Snyder-McLean and McLean, 1987; Warren and Kaiser, 1988). At the end of their thorough review, Snyders-MacLean and McLean (1987) acknowledged that this type of intervention can be only moderately effective in modifying the course of these disorders. It is difficult to go beyond such a global conclusion because there are so many unsolved methodological and evaluative problems in remediation work and because few of the published intervention studies provide data regarding the maintenance and/or the generalization of treatment effects to real-word communicative contexts in which purportedly acquired skills must ultimately be used . For corresponding opinions, see Hauser-Cram (1989) and Price (1989).

Warren and Kaiser (1988) argued that proper generalization and transfer in language intervention involving MR individuals have not usually been achieved and rarely systematically explored. According to these authors, proper generalization would be manifested as an increased rate of developmental progress after the intervention; certainly a stringent criterion.

It is our opinion that remediation programmes applied to moderately and severely MR children have not met with outstanding success in teaching phonology and grammar, whereas the results in the semantic and pragmatic areas may have been more satisfactory. The latter language areas may be more accessible in general and with MR subjects in particular. Results may be easier to secure and gains easier to stabilize, within the cognitive limits of MR subjects, than with language computational aspects. Critical time periods for basic acquisitions in language conceptual aspects do not appear to exist, unlike phonology and morpho-syntax. This permits additional time and degrees of freedom for intervention. The areas of phonology and morpho-syntax are technically more complex, demanding additional knowledge on the professional's part. They are language components corresponding to specific neurological structures, and we may be touching on one of the limits of language intervention. If, as argued, computational language is largely dependent on the integrity of certain particular brain areas, and if typical moderately and severely MR subjects do not develop fully in this regard, there are bound to be definitive limitations on what can be achieved through language intervention with these subjects. More precise knowledge of the devoted brain structures coupled with marked advances in neurology could change the picture in the future. At this time, however, this is still science fiction.

Yet, one may imagine that correctly conducted remediations, carried out with sufficient frequency and intensity during the critical years, could yield better results. As Guralnick (in press) notes for early intervention programmes with MR children in general, perhaps what is most needed is an increase in the intensity of what already exists or is within reach given the actual state of knowledge. Guralnick adds, as already pointed out by Guralnick and Bricker (1987), that the formal aspects of early intervention programmes for MR children are not very demanding. At the same time, programme intensity seems to be an important remediative dimension for children with other disabilities (e.g. children with autism; see Lovaas, 1987; children at risk due to prematurity and low birthweight; see Ramey et al., 1992).

In all cases, it is clear that marked improvements in efficiency, generalization, and durability of intervention improve with increases in knowledge of the mechanisms and sequences characteristic of language development in the various entities leading to mental retardation.

6.3 Alternative and augmentative systems of communication (AASC)

AASC have three distinguishable roles in facilitating effective communication (Remington and Clarke, in press). First, they can provide a substitute for speech in individuals with little possibility of acquiring vocal fluency. Second, in children whose language is seriously delayed, they can supply a complement to the speech that these subjects have already learned or are learning. And third, in the case of individuals with profound mental retardation, they can create a 'pathway to speech', setting improved communication contexts for interpreting the sounds of speech.

A diversity of systems exists, the potential benefits of which must be evaluated in individual cases: e.g. manual sign languages such as the American or the British Sign Language (ASL, BSL), used by deaf people; simplified versions of these languages such as the Makaton system (Walker, 1978), based on BSL and widely used in the United Kingdom.

Numerous visual systems have been developed. They include Picsyms, the Makaton Visual Symbols, pictographic logographs such as the Standard Rebus Glossary (Clark, Davies and Woodcock, 1974), the Minnesota Early Language Development Sequence (MELDS; Clark, Moores and Woodcock, 1975), using a multimodality approach that combines the speech mode, rebuses and the vocabulary of ASL, presented in sequences of English syntactic patterns. Some more abstract visual symbols are also available, notably Blissymbols (Silverman, McNaughton and Kates, 1978). This system combines visual units with elementary semantic contents to make more complex semantic units. The interested reader should consult the reviews by Clark and Woodcock (1976), Vanderheiden and Harris-Vanderheiden (1976), and Vanderheiden and Lloyd (1986), for detailed descriptions of these systems and their range of applications.

Used with moderately and severely MR subjects, particularly in those cases where important associated motor impairments exist, graphic systems of communication supply interesting means for enhancing communication and promoting understanding and production of written communication (Harris-Vanderheiden et al., 1975; Sorg, 1979). Bliss symbols can be used with MR subjects at MAs as low as 2 years. Signs from ASL, BSL, or signed English have been employed to train profoundly MR subjects expressing elementary communicative intents and understanding repertoires of communicative gestures (e.g. Fristoe and Lloyd, 1977; Linville, 1977).

Signs can also be paired with words to promote lexical learning and combinatorial language development in moderately and severely MR children (Rondal and Hoffmeister, 1976). Along this line, Kotkin, Simpson and Desanto (1978) have shown that pairing words and gestures constitute an efficient learning technique for concrete referents. It can speed up the learning of lexical repertoires in MR individuals.

Remington and Clarke (in press) recommend AASC with DS children, for they may compensate for phonological and articulatory difficulties, contributing to disambiguate difficult to understand speech and allowing the opportunity to communicate in parallel through auditory and visual channels. Benefits may be particularly important for those children with important hearing losses. Vocabulary acquisition may be enhanced as well as the initial acquisition of syntax. AASC methods may aid the marking of syntactic relations (Light et al., 1989; Light, Watson, and Remington, 1990). Also non-evanescent symbols lend themselves easily to structured ways of demonstrating syntactic regulations (see, for example, Carrier and Peak, 1975).

One needs to remain cautious, however, because many important questions are still without answer in this domain, and crucial experimental work is still to be performed. In particular, it could be inappropriate to use sign language or gestures in language training with individuals in some syndromes. For example, as mentioned in Chapter 3, Fragile-X subjects with MR seem to have weaknesses in performing referential gestures, and facial and head movements, which could prevent them from benefiting from AASC training.

6.4 Literacy training

There is a growing literature on literacy training, particularly early literacy training in MR children. Notable here is the work of Buckley and associates with young DS children (Buckley, 1992; Buckley and Bird, 1993; and Buckley, Bird, and Byrne, in press). Buckley reports to have been persuaded by the progress of Sarah Duffen, as described by her father (Duffen, 1976), to the idea that children with DS could achieve functional levels of literacy and that reading might be beneficial to their overall language acquisition. Since then, she and her colleagues have been exploring this approach. They have accumulated a number of case studies of preschool DS readers who have continued to have good quality teaching. Unfortunately, it is not possible yet to give an accurate answer to the question regarding the levels of literacy skills that can be expected from DS children and moderately and severely MR children of other aetiologies.

Three strategies can be used when reading, i.e. visual, phonological or so-called context reading. Written or printed words can be stored in a visual wordstore in the brain, and then accessed and recognized directly when reading by comparison with the stored visual images. This is the direct visual route. Another route is as follows: once letter–sound correspondence rules are known, unfamiliar words can be read by sounding them out to identify their spoken forms from the store of spoken word forms that has been established in the brain as a result of lexical learning. This is the phonological route. A third route is through semantic and/or grammatical context. The unknown word can be guessed at as one that fits these contexts. Here the reader is drawing on her language and/or world knowledge to find the word rather than decoding it visually or phonologically. According to Buckley et al. (in press), DS children seem to be good visual readers. This is consistent with the reports on their relatively preserved visual and spatial abilities. They can be trained to establish a sight vocabulary from as early as 2 years-CA. Despite real difficulties that can be expected given the slowness and limitation of their language and world knowledge development, DS children seem to progress to being able to use phonological recoding for reading. They are also able to use context meaningfully. Error analyses suggest that DS children employ the same strategies as NR children when learning to read, although they progress more slowly from the logographic to the alphabetic stage.

A delicate problem regarding written language development in MR children is whether they are able to access to important degrees of *phonological awareness* like NR children once they have started learning to read and write, or whether they are confined to prephonological sensitivities. This is but another way of formulating the theoretical question whether 'genuine reading' in the case of alphabetic scripts such as English or French (for non-alphabetic written languages such as Chinese, see Huang and Hanley, 1994) is possible without (or with only minimal degrees of) phonological awareness. This question has motivated a number of publications in recent years and the debate among opposing parties is not resolved. Briefly stated (see Rondal, 1995b, for a discussion), some argue that metaphonological competence in general, or the ability to manipulate single phonemes in particular, is a prerequisite (e.g. Bradley and Bryant, 1983), or necessary sequitur (e.g. Morais et al., 1979), or both (e.g. Morais, Alegria and Content, 1987), for learning to read (see Gombert, 1990; and Goswami and Bryant, 1990, for reviews of this literature). There has been little research so far on the ability of people with moderate and severe mental retardation to analyse spoken words into their syllabic and phonemic segments. The studies that have addressed this question have met with mixed results. Cossu, Rossini and Marshall (1993) reported that adequate reading of words at a level characteristic of NR 7-year-olds could be achieved by DS children and adolescents despite a clear failure on tests of phonological awareness. These tests caused little difficulty for MA-matched NR children. Particularly interesting in this study was the fact that the DS children and adolescents were as good as the NR controls at reading non-words. What the former were not able to do was access those abilities metalinguistically. Françoise, the language-exceptional DS adult studied by Rondal (1995b), had learned to read and write to a considerable extent with limited metaphonological ability. Her case suggests that it is possible to learn to read and write, and to have considerable reading and writing practice for a long time, without being able consciously to segment words into phonemes. However, Gottardo and Rubin (1991) have documented the apparent ability of MR children and adolescents to analyse words into syllables and phonemes. Additionally, Hoogeveen et al., (1989) claimed to have established phonemic segmentation as a result of the application of operant procedures to moderately MR children. Actually, it is less than certain that the results reported in the latter study are more than specific training effects with little relevance to genuine phonological awareness. Clearly, the phonological awareness question in MR individuals awaits further research.

However, this problem should not obscure the fact that MR children may largely benefit from learning to read and write despite possibly limited phonological awareness.[1] Obviously, there are important academic implications attached to literacy training. It is needless to stress the importance of literacy training for school achievement. Additionally, written language practice may have a stabilizing effect on oral language. It could help the MR child to master some morphosyntactic aspects of his language. In one rare controlled study, Buckley (1993) reported that productive syntactic teaching which used print to support learning was more effective than speech and picture only in teaching sentence structures to DS teenagers.

6.5 Memory and language

Another interesting question concerns the relationships between short-term memory (STM) and language development in MR children. The idea that MR subjects have weakness of short-term memory is a relatively old one (e.g. O'Connor and Hermelin, 1963). MacKenzie and Hulme (1987) have supplied longitudinal data on memory span development for a group of DS children and other MR children of unknown aetiologies (MAs 5 to 7 years, CAs 11 years at the beginning of the study). Digit span was assessed using the Auditory Sequential Memory Subtest from the ITPA. The auditory-verbal short-term memory (AV-STM) span for digits increased little over a 5-year period for the DS group: from 3.1 (SD 0.57) at 11 years-CA to 3.6 (SD 0.71) at 16 years. Slightly better results were obtained with the other MR group: from 3.5 (SD 0.76) at 11 years to 4.1 (SD 1.13) at 16 years. AV-STM is late and slow to develop in moderately and severely MR subjects. Additional data from studies conducted by Maranto, Decuir and Humphrey (1984), Hulme and Mackenzie (1992) and Rondal (1995b) suggest that it remains quite limited beyond 16 years and in the adult years.

---

[1] Notwithstanding the fact that segmental systems of writing ('alphabetic' scripts) emerged only in the second millennium B.C., derived from one single ancestor: the Semitic alphabet (Sampson, 1985). From the first semasiographic systems of the Sumerians (-4500 years) to the syllabic systems of the Babylonians (-2500 years), and even later in America, the mainly logographic systems of the Aztecs and the Mayas in the fifteenth century (Queixalos, 1989), people have read for thousands of years seemingly without clear phonological awareness.

In Baddeley's model of short-term memory, named working memory (WM) (Baddeley, 1986, 1990), a controlling-attentional and resource-coordinating device (labelled 'central executive') supervises two 'slave' systems able to retain limited amounts of information at a time: the *phonological loop* responsible for the manipulation of speech-based information, and the *visuospatial sketch pad* responsible for dealing with visual images. The phonological loop comprises two subcomponents: a *phonological store* holding speech-based information, and an *articulatory control process* based on inner speech. Because the phonological loop is subject to passive loss of information over time, *rehearsal* is necessary to refresh the decaying traces of items held on the loop. Based on experimental data, it is considered that the phonological store will hold incoming information for about 2 seconds. Baddeley specifies that the capacity of the store is whatever speech material can be articulated in 2 seconds. The articulatory control process refreshes items in the store by means of subvocal rehearsal, allowing the rehearsed items to be retained in WM for longer periods of time and/or possibly to be processed in long-term memory (LTM).

Several claims have been made in the recent literature regarding the relationship between working memory or particular components of it, and aspects of oral language development. WM has been claimed to support language processing in two basic ways (Baddeley, 1990). First, it could provide temporary storage for information as language is being processed. Second, WM could support information processing in supplying a working space for the treatment operations of the material stored. More concretely, it is contemplated that WM may play an important role in the acquisition of vocabulary and the comprehension of language.

In vocabulary acquisition, WM may support phonological learning. Gathercole and Baddeley (1990, 1993) have supplied evidence demonstrating a significant correlation between non-word repetition ability (an ability known to depend on the proper functioning of the articulatory loop) and size of receptive vocabulary in NR children. A mechanism possibly accounting for this relationship is that the longer the new word is held in WM, the greater its chance of being learned. This interpretation might explain at least a part of the difficulty of MR children in learning new words. Acquiring a new word involves both (long-term) semantic construction of the underlying concept and its association to a particular phonological sequence that is a possible word in the language. It is this latter step that is presumed to depend more particularly on the articulatory loop of WM. MR subjects are not only restricted in their WM spans, they also suffer from limitations in attentional control, slow articulatory rate and from an absence or underdevelopment of rehearsal strategies and inner speech. Regarding speech rate, for example, Rondal (1995b) reported 37–79 familiar words per minute (words contained 4–5 phonemes), i.e. 1 word per second and less, in typical DS adults vs around 200 words per minute (i.e. approximately 3.3 words per second) in normal adults of corresponding ages (which is about the normal rate for continuous speech, according to Caron, 1989).

It may be hypothesized that limitations in phonological memory are responsible, in part, for the difficulties and delays in vocabulary learning of MR subjects. Presumably, limitations in phonological store and a noisier functioning of the phonological loop in these subjects render difficult and unstable the organization of temporary phonological representations of new words in WM, which then prevents or delays the construction of corresponding LTM representations. In the MR subjects, these peripheral difficulties probably add to conceptual deficits to make vocabulary development problematic.

WM has also been claimed to play a role in *language comprehension*. Language comprehension depends on a number of capacities: knowledge of vocabulary, thematic semantics, the morphosyntactic rules of the language and strategy selection, as well as the capacity to coordinate these complex phenomena. It could be that comprehension of combinatorial oral language is related to the proper functioning of the articulatory loop and the central executive of WM, although the extent of each component is not clear . Baddeley (1990) has suggested that the phonological store plays an important buffering role in retaining strings of incoming words for a period of time pending the construction of more durable representations of the structure and meaning of the sentences. It is correct to mention, however, that the current evidence for the importance of AV-STM in language comprehension is not overwhelming (see Baddeley and Wilson, 1988, for a positive point of view; and Butterworth, Shallice and Watson, 1990, for a critical position).

The above presentation, no matter how sketchy, on a topic that is still the object of heated debate in the specialized literature, is sufficient, we believe, to stress the possible role of working memory in language processing. Given that moderately and severely MR subjects have severe and lasting limitations in WM, it is clear that any language remediation with these subjects ought to have a working memory part. The WM intervention should concentrate on three major objectives: enlarging WM spans, accelerating speech rates and installing adequate rehearsal strategies.

Some reasonable hope may be permitted regarding the feasibility of such interventions with MR subjects. Preliminary research (e.g. Hulme and MacKenzie, 1992; Broadley and MacDonald, 1993; Comblain, 1994) suggests that it is possible to improve the functioning of AV-STM in MR subjects. Hulme and MacKenzie (1992) trained a group of MR adolescents to improve their recall strategies in learning lists of words. Subjects were requested to repeat overtly for themselves sequences of words to learn. Despite the fact that training lasted only 10 days, for about 10 minutes a day, the authors reported an increase in word span of 0.50 and more in some subjects. Broadley and MacDonald (1993) trained AV-STM in a group of DS children and adolescents, several times a week in 2 sessions of 20 minutes. Half the experimental group were trained to categorize the verbal material to be memorized according to appropriate semantic criteria. The other half were trained to rehearse out loud between the recall sessions. After the first 3 weeks, the training procedure were reversed for the two experimental subgroups. Following 3 more weeks of training, final tests were made. They revealed marked gains in AV-STM span in all experimental subjects, which were still operating 8 months after the training had ended (Broadley, MacDonald and Buckley, 1994). Relying on similar rehearsal techniques, Comblain (1994) obtained significant gains in AV-STM span (1 point and more) with DS children, adolescents and adults, following a 2-month period of training, which were still there mostly on a follow-up test conducted 6 months later. It is quite possible that earlier more comprehensive and more intense intervention procedures could yield more dramatic improvement in the working memory capacity of MR children.

6.6 Computer-enhanced language intervention

Another interesting issue concerns the use of *computers* in language remediation with MR subjects. Very few specific programs have been published. More generally, computers are still little used in special education. For example, in Japan, Takuma et al. (1992) report that only 10 per cent of classes for the MR are in the process of implementing programmes of computer assisted learning (concerning the teaching of fundamental skills, learning of names and shopping skills, for example). No statistics are available for other countries. A number of suggestions regarding the use of computers to improve language skills (particularly communicative acts) in school-age DS children can be found in Meyers (1988). As she recommands, computer-enhanced language interventions should always be based on the information that is known about normal development.

There are several reasons to believe that computer-enhanced intervention procedures would allow the optimization of important aspects of language remediation with MR children. First, from a general point of view, computer programmes may function as powerful *cognitive* and *linguistic scaffolds* helping children to learn language in a way not unlike the scaffolding helping in the short term in the construction of a building. The computer may provide support to the child and to the language trainer, particularly in allowing the referential display, the verbal stimulus, or both, to be repeated at will in exactly the same, appropriate way; a performance that is beyond the patience of most human educators. This advantage may be considered to be of particular significance when it comes to MR children, as it is well known that these children need a large number of repetitions to learn and to consolidate memory traces. Second, *perception of the speech signal* is often problematic in moderately and severely MR children because it is adversely affected by a high incidence of auditory deficiencies and by problems with rapid auditory processing. Human speech generally occurs at a very rapid rate and at intensities that may make problems even in cases of mild hearing loss. If the children are not in a position to process the speech signal correctly, they will not dispose of an adequate empirical basis for learning language. Computers can help MR children learn to understand and to produce the speech signal of language. Synthetised speech output can give MR children control of a slowly presented, consistent and repetitive speech signal that can be adapted to the hearing level and processing rate of each individual child. When computer software lets them generate unlimited exact repetitions of words, phrases and sentences, MR children will be in a better position to use the speech output in order to develop understanding of the linguistic material. They can improve their articulation skills by repeatedly generating the speech signal for words, phrases and sentences, imitating the signal and gradually improving their approximations to the correct articulation. Third, since the *visual skills* of MR children (particularly DS children) are often at a higher level of functioning than their auditory skills (Marcell and Armstrong, 1982), the availability of clear visual displays and cues on the computer screen accompanying the speech signal may give such children an advantage in dealing with relevant language information. Fourth, computer-enhanced language interventions can make it easier to concentrate on *specific aspects* of *language* development, one at a time, and in so doing seek better efficiency in building larger language repertoires. Fifth, *educational service distribution*: it is obvious that few correctly trained language specialists equipped with appropriate computer technologies, could serve large numbers of children. Computer-enhanced language intervention could help alleviate relevant problems in areas distant from speech and language centres, as well as in developing countries.

Rondal et al. (1995) have designed a comprehensive Computer-Enhanced Language Intervention Program (CELIP) for MR children, which is soon to undergo experimentation. CELIP is organized according to six related subprogrammes. They are concerned with: (1) sound discrimination and articulatory training; (2) receptive and expressive lexical training; (3) cognitive-semantic training; (4) receptive and productive morphosyntactic training; (5) training working memory skills (auditory-verbal and visuospatial); and (6) early reading training.

Chapter 7
Perspectives

At the conclusion of this long journey into the language organization of MR people, which perspectives and directions for future research and clinical applications should we stress? It seems that the following suggestions may apply. *First*, we need additional data on a number of aspects of language, particularly in MR adolescents, adults and elderly MR persons, in order to substantiate better the life-span approach that is generally accepted. Longitudinal studies and, whenever feasible, long-term longitudinal studies, are necessary in order to validate the present developmental indications.

Second, the questions of individual and syndrome differences in language development and functioning should receive more systematic attention. The exact range of individual variation regarding the several language components should be better specified. This represents an important number of studies to be carried out. Extreme cases of individual differences should be investigated carefully. They need to be better identified to begin with. We are convinced that there are more language-exceptional MR subjects than the dozen cases documented so far. The syndrome range of variation has to be better specified, and this adds considerably to the load of research work to consider. Only a modest start has been made in this direction. Much else lies ahead awaiting interested researchers.

Third, the dissociations between conceptual and computational language aspects in MR subjects deserves more systematic investigation, both from a theoretical and applied point of view. Theoretically, the privileged relation demonstrated between cognition and conceptual language aspects suggest explanatory paths for lexical, semantic and pragmatic development. Conversely, the lack of a close relationship between cognition and the phonological and morphosyntactic aspects of language is illustrative of a larger ontogenetic autonomy of these components. From a clinical point of view, this means that remediation programmes should be conceived along cardinal dimensions of the linguistic system. There is probably little to expect from programmes not addressing properly the specificity of the language components.

Fourth, we need to set up more systematic, better organized, time-continuous, and more intense language remediation procedures. Much work remains to be done in this respect. Let us keep in mind that remediation will always depend on progress in fundamental knowledge, for this is this type of knowledge that paves the way for efficient applications.

It is in the interest of all society that the advantaged groups thrive to aid their disadvantaged peers so that we begin to redress nature's unfair distribution of fortune. The proximity of the new century supplies us all with bountiful opportunities.

References

Abbeduto, L. (1984). Situational influences on mentally retarded and non–retarded children's production of directives. *Applied Psycholinguistics, 5*, 147–166.

Abbeduto, L. (1991). The development of linguistic communication in persons with mild to moderate mental retardation. In N. Bray (Ed.), *International Review of Research in Mental Retardation* (pp. 91–115). New York: Academic Press.

Abbeduto, L. and Benson, G. (1992). Speech act development in non–disabled children and individuals with mental retardation. In R. Chapman (Ed.), *Processes in Language Acquisition and Disorders* (pp. 257–278). Chicago: Mosby.

Abbeduto, L., Davies B. and Furman, L. (1988). The development of speech act comprehension in mentally retarded individuals and non–retarded children. *Child Development, 59*, 1460–1472.

Abbeduto, L., Davies, B., Solesby, S. and Furman, L. (1991). Identifying the referents of spoken messages: Use of context and clarification requests by children with and without mental retardation. *American Journal of Mental Retardation, 95*, 551–562.

Abbeduto, L., Furman, L. and Davies, B. (1989). Relation between the receptive language and mental age of persons with mental retardation. *American Journal on Mental Retardation, 93*, 535–543.

Abbeduto, L. and Rosenberg, S. (1980). The communicative competence of mildly retarded adults. *Applied Psycholinguistics, 1*, 405–426.

Abbeduto, L. and Rosenberg, S. (1987). Linguistic communication and mental retardation. In S. Rosenberg (Ed.), *Advances in Applied Linguistics* (Vol. 1). *Disorders of First–Language Development* (pp. 76–125). Hillsdale, NJ: Erlbaum.

Abbeduto, L. and Rosenberg, S. (1992). The development of linguistic communication in persons with mental retardation. In S. Warren and J. Reichle (Eds.), *Perspectives on Communication and Intervention* (pp. 331–359). Baltimore, MD: Brookes.

Abramsen, A., Cavallo, M. and McCluer, J. (1985). Is the sign advantage a robust phenomenon? From gesture to language in two modalities. *Merrill–Palmer Quarterly, 31*, 177–209.

Adams, C., Labouvie–Vief, G., Hobart, C. and Dorasz, M. (1991). Adult age group differences in story recall style. *Journal of Gerontology, 45*, 17–27.

Allen, R. and Wallach, E. (1969). Word recognition and definition by educable retardates. *American Journal of Mental Deficiency, 73*, 883–885.

Anderson, E. and Spain, B. (1977). *The Child with Spina Bifida*. London: Methuen.

Annis, L.F. (1978). *The Child before Birth*. Ithaca, NY: Cornell University Press.

Appel, J., Kertesz, A. and Fishman, M. (1982). A study of language functioning in Alzheimer's patients. *Brain and Language, 17*, 73–91.

Appelman, K., Allen, K. and Turner, K. (1975). The conditioning of language in a non-verbal child conducted in a special education classroom. *Journal of Speech and Hearing Disorders*, **60**, 3–12.

Ardran, G., Harker, P. and Kemp, F. (1972). Tongue size in Down's syndrome. *Journal of Mental Deficiency Research*, **16**, 160–166.

Arnold, R., Yule, W. and Martin, N. (1985). The psychological characteristics of infantile hypercalcaemia: A preliminary investigation. *Developmental Medicine and Child Neurology*, **27**, 49–59.

Ashman, A. (1982). Coding, strategic behavior and language performance of institutionalized mentally retarded young adults. *American Journal of Mental Deficiency*, **86**, 627–636.

Atkinson, J. and Braddick, O. (1989). Development of basic visual functions. In A. Slater and G. Bremmer (Eds.), *Infant Development* (pp. 7–41). Hove: Erlbaum.

Austin, J. (1962). *How to do Things with Words*. Oxford: Oxford University Press.

Australian Bureau of Statistics (1982). *Australia's Age Population* (Catalogue N°. 41090). Canberra: Commonwealth Government Printing Office.

Azoy, A. (1935). Results of the investigation of speech defects among the school children of Barcelona. *Revista de Psicologia y Pedagogia*, **3**, 265–266.

Backus, O. (1943). *Speech in Education*. New York: Longmans Green.

Baddeley, A. (1986). *Working Memory*. New York: Oxford University Press.

Baddeley, A. (1990). *Human Memory: Theory and Practice*. Hove: Erlbaum.

Baddeley, A. and Wilson, B. (1988). Comprehension and working memory: A single case neuropsychological study. *Journal of Memory and Language*, **27**, 479–498.

Badt, M. (1958). Levels of abstraction in vocabulary definitions of mentally retarded school children. *American Journal of Mental Deficiency*, **63**, 241–246.

Baer, D. and Guess, D. (1971). Receptive training of adjectival inflections in mental retardates. *Journal of Applied Behavior Analysis*, **4**, 129–139.

Baer, D., Peterson, R. and Sherman, J. (1967). The development of imitation by reinforcing behavioral similarity to a model. *Journal of Experimental Analysis of Behavior*, **10**, 405–416.

Baird, P. and Sadovnick, A. (1988). Life expectancy in Down's syndrome adults. *Lancet*, 1354–1356.

Baltes, P. and Schaie, K. (Eds.) (1973). *Life–span Developmental Psychology: Personality and Socialization*. New York: Academic Press.

Bandura, A. (1976). *Social Learning Theory*. Englewood Cliffs, NJ: Prentice–Hall.

Barblan, L. and Chipman, H.H. (1978). Temporal relationships in language: A comparison between normal and language retarded children. In G. Drachman (Ed.), *Salzburger Beitrage zur Linguistik* (pp. 46–65). Salzburg: Neugenbauer.

Barrett, M. and Diniz, F. (1989). Lexical development in mentally handicapped children. In M. Beveridge, G. Conti–Ramsden and Y. Leudar (Eds.), *Language and Communication in Mentally Handicapped People* (pp. 3–32). London: Chapman and Hall.

Bartel, N. (1970). The development of morphology in retarded children. *Education and Training of the Mentally Retarded*, **4**, 164–168.

Bartel, N., Bryen, S. and Keehn, S. (1973). Language comprehension in the moderately retarded child. *Exceptional Children*, **39**, 375–382.

Basser, L. (1962). Hemiplegia of early onset and the faculty of speech with special reference to the effects of hemispherectomy. *Brain*, **85**, 427–460.

Bateman, B. and Wetherell, J. (1965). Psycholinguistic aspects of mental retardation. *Mental Retardation*, **3**, 8–13.

Bates, E., Benigni, L., Bretherton, I., Camaioni, I. and Volterra, V. (1979). *The Emergence of Symbols : Cognition and Communication in Infancy*. New York: Academic Press.

Bates, E., Bretherton, I. and Snyder, L. (1988). *From First Word to Grammar. Individual Differences and Dissociable Mechanisms*. Cambridge: Cambridge University Press.

Bates, E. and MacWhinney, B. (1987). Competition, variation and language learning. In B. MacWhinney (Ed.), *Mechanisms of Language Acquisition* (pp. 157–193). Hillsdale, NJ: Erlbaum.

Baumeister, A. (1967). Problems in comparative studies of mental retardates and normals. *American Journal of Mental Deficiency*, 71, 869–875.

Baumeister, A. and Williams, J. (1967). Relationship of physical stigmata to intellectual functioning in mongolism. *American Journal of Mental Deficiency*, 71, 586–592.

Bayles, K. (1982). Language function in senile dementia. *Brain and Language*, 16, 265–280.

Bayley, N. (1969). *Bayley Scales of Mental and Motor Development*. New York: Psychological Corporation.

Becker, L., Mito, T., Takashima, S. and Onodera, K. (1991). Growth and development of the brain in Down's syndrome. In C. Epstein (Ed.), *The Morphogenesis of Down's Syndrome* (pp. 133–152). New York: Wiley–Liss.

Bedrosian, J. (1988). Adults who are mildly to moderately mentally retarded: Communicative performance, assessment and intervention. In S. Calculator and J. Bedrosian (Eds.), *Communication Assessment and Intervention for Adults with Mental Retardation* (pp. 265–307). Boston, MA: College–Hill Press.

Beech, H. and Fransella, F. (1968). *Research and Experiment in Stuttering*. London: Pergamon.

Beech, J. and Harding, L. (1992). *Assessment in Speech and Language Therapy*. London: Routledge.

Beery, K. and Buktenica, N. (1967). *Developmental Test of Visual–Motor Integration*. Cleveland, OH: Modern Curriculum Press.

Beier, E., Starkweather, J. and Lambert, M. (1969). Vocabulary usage of mentally retarded children. *American Journal of Mental Deficiency*, 73, 927–934.

Beilin, H. and Sack, H. (1975). The passive: Linguistic and psychological theory. In H. Beilin (Ed.), *Studies in the Cognitive Basis of Language Development* (pp. 116–138). New York: Academic Press.

Bell, J., Pearn, J. and Firman, D. (1989). Childhood deaths in Down's syndrome curves and causes of death from a total population study in Queensland, Australia, 1976 to 1985. *Journal of Medical Genetics*, 26, 764–768.

Bellugi, U., Bihrle, A., Jernigan, T., Trauner, D. and Doherty, S. (1990). Neuropsychological, neurological and neuroanatomical profile of Williams syndrome. *American Journal of Medical Genetics Supplement*, 6, 115–125.

Bellugi, U., Bihrle, A., Neville, H., Doherty, S. and Jernigan, T. (1992). Language, cognition and brain organization in a neurodevelopmental disorder. In M. Gunnar and C. Nelson (Eds.), *Developmental Behavioral Neuroscience. The Minnesota Symposia on Child Psychology* (pp. 201–232). Hillsdale, NJ: Erlbaum.

Bellugi, U., Marks, S., Bihrle, A. and Sabo, H. (1988). Dissociation between language and cognitive functions in Williams syndrome. In D. Bishop and K. Mogford (Eds.), *Language Development in Exceptional Circumstances* (pp. 177–189). London: Churchill Livingstone.

Bellugi, U., Marks, S., Neville, H. and Jernigan, T. (1987, May). *Brain Organization Underlying Unusual Language and Cognitive Functions* (abstract).

Communication to the meeting of the Western Psychological Association. Long Beach, CA.

Bellugi, U., Sabo, H. and Vaid, J. (1988). Spatial deficits in children with Williams syndrome. In J. Stiles–Davis, M. Kritchevsky and U. Bellugi (Eds.), *Spatial Cognition: Brain Bases and Development* (pp. 273–298). Hillsdale, NJ: Erlbaum.

Bellugi, U., Wang, P. and Jernigan, J. (1993). Williams syndrome: An unusual neuropsychological profile. In S. Borman and J. Grafman (Eds.), *Atypical Cognitive Deficits in Developmental Disorders: Implication for Brain Function* (pp. 23–56). Hillsdale, NJ: Erlbaum.

Benda, C. (1949). *Mongolism and Cretinism*. New York: Grune and Stratton.

Bender, N. and Johnson, N. (1979). Hierarchical semantic organization in educable mentally retarded children. *Journal of Experimental Child Psychology*, 27, 277–285.

Benett, C. (1938). An inquiry into the genesis of poor reading. *Teachers College Education*, N°. 755.

Bennett, F., La Veck, B. and Sells, C. (1978). The Williams elfin facies syndrome: The psychological profile as an aid in syndrome identification. *Pediatrics*, 61, 303–305.

Bennett, F., Sells, C. and Brandt, C. (1979). Influences on measured intelligence in Down's syndrome. *American Journal of Disabilities in Childhood*, 133, 700–703.

Benson, D. (1994). *The Neurology of Thinking*. New York: Oxford University Press.

Benton, A. (1965). *Sentence Memory Test*. Iowa City, IA: Author (address not supplied; quoted in MacDonald and Roy, 1988).

Benton, A., Hamsher, K., Varney, N. and Spreen, O. (1983). *Test of Facial Recognition*, Form SL. New York: Oxford University Press.

Benton, A., Hannary, J. and Varney, N. (1975). Visual perception of line direction in patients with unilateral brain disease. *Neurology*, 25, 907–910.

Berg, J., Karlinsky, H. and Holland, A. (Eds.) (1993). *Alzheime'sr Disease, Down 'sSyndrome and their Relationship*. New York: Oxford University Press.

Berger, J. and Cunningham, C. (1983). The development of early vocal behaviours and interactions in Down's syndrome and non–handicapped infant–mother. *Developmental Psychology*, 19, 322–331.

Berko, J. (1958). The child's learning of English morphology. *Word*, 14, 150–177.

Berko–Gleason, J. (1979). Sex differences in the language of children and parents. In O. Garnica and M. King (Eds.), *Language, Children and Society* (pp. 48–72). Oxford: Pergamon Press.

Berndt, R. and Caramazza, A. (1980). A redefinition of the syndrome of Broca's aphasia. *Applied Psycholinguistics*, 1, 225–278.

Bernstein, B. (1975). *Langage et classes sociales*. Paris: Editions de Minuit.

Berry, H., Brunner, R., Hunt, M. and White, P. (1988). Application of valine, isoleucine and leucine (VIL) to treatment of phenylketonuria. In W. Fraser (Ed.), *Key Issues in Mental Retardation Research* (pp. 85–93). London: Routledge.

Berry, P. (1972). Comprehension of possessive and present continuous sentences by non–retarded, mildly retarded and severely retarded children. *American Journal of Mental Deficiency*, 76, 540–544.

Berry, P. Groenweg, G., Gibson, D. and Brown, R. (1984). Mental development of adults with Down's syndrome. *American Journal of Mental Deficiency*, 89, 252–256.

Bertoncini, J., Bijeljac–Babic, R., Blumstein, S. and Mehler, J. (1987). Discrimination of very short CVs in neonates. *Journal of the Acoustical Society of America*, 82, 1–37.

Best, C., McRoberts, G. and Sithole, N. (1988). Examination of perceptual reorganization for non–native speech contrasts: Zulu click discrimination by English–speaking adults and infants. *Journal of Experimental Psychology: Human Perception and Performance*, **14**, 345–360.

Beuren, A., Apitz, J. and Harmjanz, D. (1962). Supravalvular aortic stenosis in association with mental retardation and a certain facial appearance. *Circulation*, **26**, 1235.

Beveridge, M. (in press). School integration for Down's syndrome children: Policies, problems and processes. In J.A. Rondal, J. Perera, L. Nadel and A. Comblain (Eds.), Down's syndrome: *Psychological, Psychobiological and Socio-Educational Perspectives*. London: Whurr.

Beveridge, M., Spencer, J. and Mittler, P. (1979). Self–blame and communication failure in retarded adolescents. *Journal of Child Psychology and Psychiatry*, **20**, 129–138.

Bickerton, D. (1981). *Roots of Language*. Ann Arbor, MI: Karoma.

Bickerton, D. (1984). The language bioprogram hypothesis. *Behavioral and Brain Sciences*, 7, 173–188.

Bihrle, A., Bellugi, U., Delis, D. and Marks, S. (1989). Seeing either the forest or the trees: Dissociation in visuospatial processing. *Brain and Cognition*, **11**, 37–49.

Bijou, S. and Baer, D. (1961). *Child Development I. A Systematic and Empirical Theory*. New York: Appleton–Century–Crofts.

Bijou, S. and Baer, D. (1965). *Child Development II. Universal Stage of Infancy*. New York: Appleton–Century–Crofts.

Bilovsky, D. and Share, J. (1965). The ITPA and Down's syndrome: An exploratory study. *American Journal of Mental Deficiency*, **70**, 78–83.

Binet, A. (1911). *Les Idées modernes sur les enfants*. Paris: Flammarion.

Binet, A. and Simon, T. (1907, 1934). *Les Enfants anormaux. Guide pour l'admission des enfants anormaux dans les classes de perfectionnement*. Paris: 1907 (republished by Colin, Paris).

Birch, J. and Matthews, J. (1951). The learning of mental defectives: Its measurement and characteristics. *American Journal of Mental Deficiency*, **55**, 384–393.

Bishop, D. (1982). *Test for Reception of Grammar*. Unpublished manuscript, University of Manchester, Manchester, UK.

Bishop, D. (1983). Linguistic impairment after left hemidecortication for infantile hemiplegia? A reappraisal. *Quarterly Journal of Experimental Psychology*, **35**, 199–207.

Bishop, D. (1988a). Can the right hemisphere mediate language as well as the left? A critical review of recent research. *Cognitive Neuropsychology*, **5**, 353–367.

Bishop, D. (1988b, 1993). Language development after focal brain damage. In D. Bishop and K. Mogford (Eds.), *Language Development in Exceptional Circumstances* (pp. 203–219). London: Churchill Livingstone (republished by Erlbaum, Hillsdale, NJ).

Blanchard, I. (1964). Speech pattern and etiology in mental retardation. *American Journal of Mental Deficiency*, **68**, 612–617.

Blank, M., Gessner, M. and Esposito, A. (1978). Language without communication: A case study. *Journal of Child Language*, 6, 329–352.

Bleile, K. (1982). Consonant ordering in Down's syndrome phonology. *Journal of Communication Disorders*, **15**, 275–285.

Bleile, K. and Schwarz, I. (1984). Three perspectives on the speech of children with Down's syndrome. *Journal of Communication Disorders*, **17**, 87–94.

Bless, D., Swift, E. and Rosin, M. (1985). *Communication Profiles of Children with Down's Syndrome*. Unpublished manuscript. Cited in Barrett and Diniz (1989).

Bliss, L. (1985). The development of persuasive strategies by mentally retarded children. *Applied Research in Mental Retardation*, 6, 437–447.

Bloom, L. (1973). *One Word at a Time*. The Hague,: Mouton.

Bloom, L. and Lahey, M. (1978). *Language Development and Language Disorders*. New York: Wiley.

Bloom, L. Miller, P. and Hood, L. (1975). Variation as aspect of competence in language development. In A. Pick (Ed.), *Minnesota Symposium on Child Language* (pp. 3–55). Minneapolis, MN: University of Minnesota Press.

Blount, B. (1972). Parental speech and language acquisition: Some Luo and Samoan examples. *Anthropological Linguistics*, 14, 119–130.

Boehm, A. (1971). *The Boehm Test of Basic Concept*. New York: Psychological Corporation.

Bohannon, J. and Stanowicz, L. (1988). The issue of negative evidence: Adult responses to children's language errors. *Developmental Psychology*, 24, 684–689.

Bol, G. and Kuiken, F. (1990). Grammatical analysis of developmental language disorders: A study of the morphosyntax of children with specific language disorders, with hearing impairment and with Down's syndrome. *Clinical Linguistics and Phonetics*, 4, 77–86.

Borer, H. and Wexler, K. (1987). The maturation of syntax. In T. Roeper and E. Williams (Eds.), *Parameter Setting* (pp. 123–172). Boston: Reidel.

Borghgraef, M., Fryns, J. P., Dielkens, A., Pyck, K. and Van den Berghe, H. (1987). Fragile X syndrome: A study of the psychological profile in 23 prepubertal patients. *Clinical Genetics*, 32, 179–186.

Borghi, R. (1990). Consonant phoneme and distinctive feature error patterns in speech. In D. Van Dyke, D. Lang, F. Heide, S. Van Duyne and M. Soucek (Eds.), *Clinical Perspectives in the Management of Down's syndrome* (pp. 147–152). New York: Springer.

Botwinick, J. and Storandt, M. (1974). Vocabulary ability in later life. *The Journal of Genetic Psychology*, 125, 303–308.

Botwinick, J., West, R. and Storandt, M. (1975). Qualitative vocabulary responses and age. *Journal of Gerontology*, 30, 574–577.

Bower, T. (1967). The development of object–permanence: Some studies of existence constancy. *Perception and Psychophysics*, 2, 411–418.

Bowerman, M. (1978). The acquisition of word meaning: An investigation into some correct conflicts. In C. Snow and N. Waterson (Eds.), *The Development of Communication* (pp. 263–287). New York: Wiley.

Bowler, D., Cufflin, J. and Kiernan, C. (1985). Dichotic listening of verbal and non–verbal material by Down's syndrome children and children of normal intelligence. *Cortex*, 21, 637–644.

Boysson–Bardies, B. de (1988). Du babillage au langage: Variabilité interindividuelle et influence de l'environnement linguistique. *Rééducation Orthophonique*, 26, 111–119.

Boysson–Bardies, B. de and Durand, C. (1991). Tendances générales et influence de la langue maternelle dans le babillage et les premiers mots. *L'Année Psychologique*, 91, 139–157.

Boysson–Bardies, B. de, Sogart, L. and Durand, C. (1984). Discernible differences in the babbling of infants according to target language. *Journal of Child Language*, 11, 1–15.

Bradbury, B. and Lunzer, E. (1972). The learning of grammatical inflections in normal and subnormal children. *Journal of Child Psychology and Psychiatry*, 13, 239–248.

Bradley, L. and Bryant, P. (1983). Categorising sounds and learning to read: A causal connection. *Nature*, **301**, 419–421.

Bray, M. and Woolnough, L. (1988). The language of children with Down's syndrome aged 12 to 16 years. *Child Language Teaching and Therapy*, **4**, 311–321.

Brédart, S. (1994). Accès aux noms propres et vieillissement. In M. Van der Linden et M. Hupet (Eds.), *Le Vieillissement cognitif* (pp. 177–200). Paris: Presses Universitaires de France.

Brédart–Compernol, C., Rondal, J.A. and Perée, F. (1981). More about maternal and paternal speech to language–learning children in various dyadic and tryadic situational contexts. *International Journal of Psycholinguistics*, **24**, 149–168.

Bresson, F. (1991). Phylogeny and ontogeny of languages. In G. Piérault le Bonniec and M. Dolotsky (Eds.), *Language Bases and Discourse Bases* (pp. 11–29). Amsterdam: Benjamins.

Brimer, M. and Dunn, L. (1966). *English Picture Vocabulary Test* (2nd edn.). London: National Foundation for Educational Research.

Broadley, I. and MacDonald, J. (1993). Teaching short term memory skills to children with Down's syndrome. *Down's Syndrome*, **1**, 56–62.

Broadley, I., MacDonald, J. and Buckley, S. (1994). Are children with Down's syndrome able to maintain skills learned from a short–term memory training programme? *Down's Syndrome*, **2**, 116–122.

Broen, P. (1972). The verbal environment of the language–learning child. *American Speech and Hearing Association Monographs*, **17** (whole issue).

Bronckart, J. P. (1973). The regulating role of speech. A cognitive approach. *Human Development*, **6**, 417–439.

Bronckart, J. P. (1976). *Genèse et organisation des formes verbales*. Brussels: Mardaga.

Bronfenbrenner, U. (1979). *The Ecology of Human Development: Experiments by Nature And Design*. Cambridge, MA: Harvard University Press.

Brookshire, R. (1967). Speech pathology and the experimental analysis of behavior. *Journal of Speech and Hearing Disorders*, **28**, 215–227.

Brown, L. and Rice, J. (1967). Psycholinguistic differentiation of low IQ children. *Mental Retardation*, **5**, 16–20.

Brown, R. (1973). *A First Language*. Cambridge, MA: Harvard University Press.

Brown, R. and Berko, J. (1960). Word association and the acquisition of grammar. *Child Development*, **31**, 1–14.

Brown, R. and Hanlon, C. (1970). Derivational complexity and order of acquisition. In J. Hayes (Ed.), *Cognition and the Development of Language* (pp. 37–63). New York: Wiley.

Brown, W., Jenkins, E., Cohen, I., Fish, G., Wolf–Schein, E., Gross, A., Waterhouse, L., Fein, D., Mason–Brothers, A., Ritvo, E., Ruttenberg, B., Bentley, W. and Castells, S. (1986). Fragile X and autism: A multi–center study. *American Journal of Medical Genetics*, **23**, 341–352.

Brownell, W. and Smith, D. (1973). Communication patterns, sex and length of verbalization in speech of four year old children. *Speech Monographs*, **40**, 310–316.

Brownfield, E. and Keehn, J. (1966). Operant eyelid conditioning in trisomy 18. *Journal of Abnormal Psychology*, **71**, 413–415.

Bruner, J. (1964). The course of cognitive growth. *American Psychologist*, **19**, 1–15.

Bruner, J. (1976, August). *On Prelinguistic Prerequisites of Speech*. Paper presented at the NATO Conference on Language Development, Stirling, Scotland.

Buckhalt, J., Rutherford, R. and Goldberg, I. (1978). Verbal and non–verbal interaction of mothers with their Down's syndrome and non–retarded infants. *American Journal of Mental Deficiency*, **82**, 337–343.

Buckley, S. (1992). The development of the child with Down's syndrome: Implications for effective education. In P. Rogers and M. Coleman (Eds.), *Medical Care in Down's Syndrome. A Preventive Medicine Approach* (pp. 29–67). New York: Dekker.

Buckley, S. (1993). Developing the speech and language skills of teenagers with Down's syndrome. *Down's Syndrome*, 1, 63–71.

Buckley, S. and Bird, G. (1993). Teaching children with Down's syndrome to read. *Down's Syndrome*, 1, 34–39.

Buckley, S., Bird, G. and Byrne, A. (in press). The practical and theoretical significance of teaching literacy skills to children with Down's syndrome. In J. A. Rondal, J. Perera, L. Nadel and A. Comblain (Eds.), *Down's Syndrome: Psychological, Psychobiological and Socio–educational Perspectives*. London: Whurr.

Buckley, S. and Sacks, B. (1987). *The Adolescent with Down's Syndrome – Life for the Teenager and for the Family*. Portsmouth, UK: Portsmouth Down's Syndrome Trust.

Buium, N., Rynders, J. and Turnure, J. (1974a). *A Semantic Relation Concepts Based Theory of Language Acquisition as Applied to Down's Syndrome Children*. Unpublished research report N°. 62, University of Minnesota, Research, Development and Demonstration Center in Education of Handicapped Children, Minneapolis.

Buium, N., Rynders, J. and Turnure, J. (1974b). Early maternal linguistic environment of normal and Down's syndrome language–learning children. *American Journal of Mental Deficiency*, 79, 52–58.

Burke, D. and Harrold, R. (1990). Automatic and effortful semantic processes in old age: Experimental and naturalistic approaches. In D. Burke and L. Light (Eds.), *Language, Memory and Ageing* (pp. 142–174). Cambridge: Cambridge University Press.

Burr, D. and Rohr, A. (1978). Patterns of psycholinguistic development in the severely retarded: A hypothesis. *Social Biology*, 25, 15–22.

Butterworth, B., Shallice, T. and Watson, F. (1990). Short–term retention without short–term memory. In G. Vallar and T. Shallice (Eds.), *Neuropsychological Impairments of Short–term Memory* (pp. 187–213). Cambridge: Cambridge University Press.

Cabanas, R. (1954). Some findings in speech and voice therapy among mentally deficient children. *Folia Phoniatrica*, 6, 34–37.

Caccamo, J. and Yater, A. (1972). The ITPA and negro children with Down's syndrome. *Exceptional Children*, 38, 642–643.

Caramazza, A. (1986). On drawing inferences about the structure of normal cognitive systems from the analysis of patterns of impaired performance: The case for single–patient studies. *Brain and Cognition*, 5, 41–66.

Caramazza, A., Gordon, J., Zurif, E. and DeLuca D. (1976). Right hemispheric damage and verbal problem–solving behavior. *Brain and Language*, 3, 41–49.

Cardoso–Martins, C. and Mervis, C. B. (1985). Maternal speech to prelinguistic children with Down's syndrome. *American Journal of Mental Deficiency*, 89, 451–458.

Cardoso–Martins, C., Mervis, C.B. and Mervis, C.A. (1985). Early vocabulary acquisition by children with Down's syndrome. *American Journal of Mental Deficiency*, 90, 177–184.

Carey, S. (1978). The child as a word learner. In M. Halle, J. Bresnan and G. Miller (Ed.), *Linguistic Theory and Psychological Reality* (pp. 264–293). Cambridge, MA: MIT Press.

Carlin, M. (1988a). Longitudinal data shows improved prognosis in Cri–du–chat syndrome. *American Journal of Human Genetics*, **41**, A50.

Carlin, M. (1988b). The improved prognosis in Cri–du–chat (5p–) syndrome. In W. Fraser (Ed.), *Key Issues in Mental Retardation Research* (pp. 64–73). London: Routledge.

Caron, J. (1989). *Précis de psycholinguistique*. Paris: Presses Universitaires de France.

Carr, D. (1964). The concept formation and psycholinguistic abilities of normal and retarded children of comparable mental age. *Dissertation Abstracts*, **25**, 997.

Carr, J. (1970). Mental and motor development in young mongol children. *Journal of Mental Deficiency Research*, **14**, 205–220.

Carr, J. (1994). Long term outcome for people with Down's syndrome. *Journal of Child Psychology and Psychiatry*, **35**, 425–439.

Carrier, J. (1970). A program of articulation therapy administered by mothers. *Journal of Speech and Hearing Disorders*, **35**, 344–353.

Carrier, J. and Peak, T. (1975). *Non–speech Language Initiation Program*. Lawrence, KS: H. and H. Enterprises.

Carrow, E. (1973). *Test for Auditory Comprehension of Language*. Austin, TX: Urban Research Group.

Carter, A. (1978). From sensori–motor vocalizations to words: A case study of the evolution of attention–directing communication in the second year. In A. Lock (Ed.), *Gesture and Symbol: The Emergence of Language* (pp. 126–148). New York: Academic.

Carter, C. (1958). A life–table for mongols with the causes of death. *Journal of Mental Deficiency Research*, **2**, 64–74.

Cattell, R. (1963). The theory of fluid and crystallized intelligence: A critical experiment. *Journal of Educational Psychology*, **54**, 1–22.

Centerwall, S. and Centerwall, W. (1960). A study of children with mongolism reared in the home compared to those reared away from home. *Pediatrics*, **25**, 678–685.

Cerella, J., Poon, L. and Fozard, J. (1981). Mental rotation and age reconsidered. *Journal of Gerontology*, **36**, 620–624.

Cession, A., Kilen, A., Denhière, G. and Rondal, J. A. (1987). Maman ... Une histoire! Etude de l'influence du milieu social et de l'âge des enfants sur la mémorisation de récits standards et de récits produits par la mère. *Enfance*, **40**, 341–358.

Chafe, W. (1970). *Meaning and the Structure of Language*. Chicago: The University of Chicago Press.

Changeux, J. P. (1983). *L'Homme neuronal*. Paris: Jacob.

Chapman, R. (1995). Language development in children and adolescents with Down's syndrome. In P. Fletcher and B. McWhinney (Eds.), *The Handbook of Child Language* (pp. 641–663). Oxford: Blackwell.

Chapman, R., Kay–Raining Bird, E. and Schwartz, S. (1990). Fast mapping of words in event contexts by children with Down's syndrome. *Journal of Speech and Hearing Disorders*, **55**, 761–770.

Chapman, R., Kay–Raining Bird, E. and Schwartz, S. (1991, November). *Fast Mapping in Stories: Deficits in Down's Syndrome*. Paper presented at the Annual Meeting of the American Speech–Language–Hearing Association, Atlanta, GA.

Chapman, R. and Nation, J. (1981). Patterns of learning performance in educable mentally retarded children. *Journal of Communication Disorders*, **14**, 245–254.

Chapman, R., Schwartz, S. and Kay–Raining Bird, E. (1991). Language skills of children and adolescents with Down's syndrome: I. Comprehension. *Journal of Speech and Hearing Research*, **34**, 1106–1120.

Chapman, R., Schwartz, S. and Kay–Raining Bird, E. (1992, August). *Language Production of Children and Adolescents with Down's Syndrome*. Paper presented at the 9th World Congress of the International Association for the Scientific Study of Mental Deficiency, Gold Coast, Australia.

Charcot, J. B. (1893). *Oeuvres complètes. Leçons sur les localisations dans les maladies du cerveau et de la moelle épinière* (Vol. 4). Paris: Alcan.

Cherry, L. and Lewis, M. (1975). Mothers and two–year–olds: A study of sex–differentiated aspects of verbal interaction. *Developmental Psychology*, **51**, 278–282.

Chi, J., Dooling, E. and Gilles, F. (1977). Left–right asymmetries of the temporal speech areas of the human foetus. *Archives of Neurology*, **34**, 346–348.

Chipman, H. (1979, August). *Understanding Language Retardation: A Developmental Perspective*. Communication presented at the 5th Conference of the International Association for the Scientific Study of Mental Deficiency (I.A.S.S.M.D.), Jerusalem.

Chipman, H. and Pastouriaux, F. (1981). La construction de phrases simples chez le jeune enfant normal et arriéré mental. In J. A. Rondal, J. L. Lambert and H. Chipman (Eds.), *Psycholinguistique et handicap mental* (pp. 68–88). Brussels: Mardaga.

Chomsky, C. (1969). *The Acquisition of Syntax in Children from 5 to 10*. Cambridge, MA: MIT Press.

Chomsky, N. (1957a). *Syntactic Structures*. The Hague: Mouton.

Chomsky, N. (1957b). Review of B.F. Skinner's 'Verbal Behavior'. *Language*, **35**, 26–58.

Chomsky, N. (1965). *Aspects of the Theory of Syntax*. Cambridge, MA: MIT Press.

Chomsky, N. (1966). *Cartesian Linguistics*. New York: Harper and Row.

Chomsky, N. (1979). *Language and Responsibility* (based on conversations with Mitsou Ronat). New York: Pantheon Books.

Chomsky, N. (1980). *Rules and Representations*. New York: Columbia University Press.

Chomsky, N. (1981). *Lectures on Government and Binding*. Dordrecht: Foris.

Chomsky, N. (1982). *Some Concepts and Consequences of the Theory of Government and Binding*. Cambridge, MA: MIT Press.

Chomsky, N. (1984). *Modular Approaches to the Study of Mind*. San Diego, CA: San Diego State University Press.

Chomsky, N. (1994). Interview with J. A. Rondal: Pieces of minds in psycholinguistics. *International Journal of Psychology*, **29**, 147–163.

Chomsky, N. and Halle, M. (1968). *The Sound Pattern of English*. New York: Harper and Row.

Chundley, A. (1984). Behavioral phenotype: The fragile X and X–linked mental retardation. *American Journal of Medical Genetics*, **17**, 45–50.

Cicchetti, D. and Beeghly, M. (1990) An organizational approach to the study of Down's syndrome: Contributions to an integrative theory of development. In D. Cicchetti and M. Beeghly (Eds.), *Children with Down's Syndrome: A Developmental Perspective* (pp. 29–62). New York: Cambridge University Press.

Cicchetti, D. and Mans–Wagener, L. (1987). Sequences, stages and structures in the organization of cognitive development in infants with Down's syndrome. In I. Uzgiris and J. Hunt (Eds.). *Infant Performance and Experience: New Findings with the Ordinal Scales* (pp. 281–310). Urbana, IL: University of Illinois Press.

Cicchetti, D. and Pogge–Hesse, P. (1982). Possible contributions of the study of organically retarded persons to developmental theory. In E. Zigler and D. Balla (Ed.), Mental retardation: *The Developmental–Difference Controversy* (pp. 277–318). Hillsdale, NJ: Erlbaum.

Cicchetti, D and Sroufe, A. (1978). An organization view of affect: Illustration from the study of Down's syndrome infants. In M. Lewis and L. Rosenblum (Eds.), *The Development of Affects* (pp. 309–350). New York: Plenum.

Clahsen, H. (1989). The grammatical characterization of developmental dysphasia. *Linguistics*, **27**, 897–920.

Clahsen, H., Rothweiler, M. and Woest, A. (1992). Regular and irregular inflection in the acquisition of German noun plurals. *Cognition*, **45**, 225–255.

Clark, C., Davies, C. and Woodcock, R. (1974). *Standard Rebus Glossary*. Circle Pines, MN: American Guidance Service.

Clark, C., Moores, D. and Woodcock, R. (1975). *The Minnesota Early Language Development Sequence*. Unpublished manuscript, University of Minnesota, Minneapolis.

Clark, C. and Woodcock, R. (1976). *Graphics systems of communication*. In L. Lloyd (Ed.), *Communication Assessment and Intervention Strategies* (pp. 549–605). Baltimore, MD: University Park Press.

Clark, E. (1974). Non–linguistic strategies and the acquisition of word meaning. *Cognition*, **2**, 161–182.

Clark, E. (1993). *The Lexicon in Acquisition*. New York: Cambridge University Press.

Clark, E. (1995). Later lexical development and word formation. In P. Fletcher and B. MacWhinney (Eds.), *The Handbook of Child Language* (pp. 393–412). Oxford: Blackwell.

Clark, E. and Clark, H. H. (1977). *Psychology and Language: An Introduction to Psycholinguistics*. New York: Harcourt Brace Jovanovich.

Clark, H. and Sherman, J. (1975). Teaching generative use of sentence answers to three forms of questions. *Journal of Applied Behavior Analysis*, **8**, 321–330.

Clarke, A. M., Clarke, A. D. B. and Berg, J. (1985). *Mental Deficiency: The Changing Outlook*. London: Methuen.

Clarke, C., Edwards, J. and Smallpiece, J. (1961). Trisomy/normal mosaicism in an intelligent child with some mongoloid characters. *Lancet*, 1028–1030.

Clarke–Stewart, K. (1973). Interactions between mothers and their young children: Characteristics and consequences. *Monographs of the Society for Research in Child Development*, **38**, N°. 153.

Clausen, J. (1966). *Ability Structure and Subgroups in Mental Retardation*. Washington, D.C.: Spartan.

Clausen, J. (1968). Behavioral characteristics of Down's syndrome subjects. *American Journal of Mental Deficiency*, **73**, 118–126.

Coggins, T. (1979). Relational meaning encoded in two–word utterance of stage 1 Down's syndrome children. *Journal of Speech and hearing Research*, **22**, 166–178.

Coggins, T., Carpenter, R. and Owings, N. (1983). Examining early intentional communication in Down's syndrome and non–retarded children. *British Journal of Disorders of Communication*, **18**, 99–107.

Cohen, B., Normand, M., Peled, I., Blonder, Y., Tumarkin, M., Elitzur, A. and Hadar, R. (1988). Maternal hyperphenylalaninemia in Israel. In W. Fraser (Ed.), *Key Issues in Mental Retardation Research* (pp. 74–83). London: Routledge.

Cohen, G. (1979). Language comprehension in old age. *Cognitive Psychology*, **11**, 412–429.

Cohen, I., Vietze, P., Sudhalter, V., Jenkins, E. and Brown, W. (1991). Effects of age and communication level on eye contact in fragile X males and non–fragile X autistic males. *American Journal of Medical Genetics*, **38**, 498–502.

Cohen, S. and Beckwith, L. (1976). Maternal language in infancy. *Developmental Psychology*, **12**, 371–372.

Cole, K., Dale, P. and Mills, P. (1992). Stability of the intelligence quotient–language quotient relation: Is discrepancy modeling based on a myth? *American Journal on Mental Retardation*, 97, 131–143.

Collacot, R., Duckett, D., Mathews, D. and Warrington, J. (1990). Down's syndrome and fragile–X syndrome in a single patient. *Journal of Mental Deficiency Research*, 34, 61–86.

Comblain, A. (1989). *Compréhension de la voix passive chez l'adulte trisomique 21*. Unpublished master's thesis, University of Liège, Belgium.

Comblain, A. (1993). *Test de Vocabulaire Productif*. Unpublished experimental version, University of Liège, Belgium.

Comblain, A. (1994). Working memory in Down's syndrome: Training rehearsal strategy. *Down's Syndrome*, 2, 123–126.

Comblain, A. (1995). *Mémoire de travail et langage dans le syndrome de Down*. Doctoral dissertation, University of Liège, Belgium.

Comblain, A., Fayasse, M. and Rondal, J. A. (1993). *Batterie d'Evaluation Morpho–syntaxique (BEMS)*. Unpublished experimental version, University of Liège, Belgium.

Concise Oxford Dictionary of Current English (1964, 5th ed.).

Conrad, R. (1964). Acoustic confusion in immediate memory. *British Journal of Psychology*, 55, 75–84.

Cook, N. (1977, August). *Semantic Development in Children with Down's Syndrome*. Communication presented at the 85th Annual Convention of the American Psychological Association, San Francisco, CA.

Copeland, R. and Schiefelbusch, R. (1961). *Surveys of Training and Service Facilities for Retarded Children*. Unpublished manuscript, The University of Kansas, Lawrence.

Cornil, F. (1970). *La Régulation verbale du comportement chez les enfants handicapés mentaux*. Unpublished master's thesis, University of Liège, Belgium.

Corrigan, R. (1978). Language development as related to Stage 6 object permanence development. *Journal of Child Language*, 5, 173–189.

Cossu, G., Rossini, F. and Marshall, J. (1993). When reading is required but phonological awareness is not: A study of literacy in Down's syndrome. *Cognition*, 46, 129–138.

Courchesne, E., Yeung–Courchesne, R., Press, G., Hesselink, J. and Jernigan, T. (1988). Hypophasia of cerebellar vermal lobules VI and VII in autism. *New England Journal of Medicine*, 318, 1349–1354.

Cowie, V. (1970). *A Study of the Early Development of Mongols*. London: Pergamon.

Craik, F. and Rabinowitz, J. (1985). The effects of presentation rate and encoding task on age–related memory deficits. *Journal of Gerontology*, 40, 309–315.

Crews, D. (1994). Animal sexuality. *Scientific American*, January, 96–103.

Crick, F. and Jones, E. (1993). Backwardness of human neuroanatomy. *Nature*, 361, 109–110.

Crisco, J., Dobbs, J. and Mulhern, R. (1988). Cognitive processing of children with Williams syndrome. *Developmental Medicine and Child Neurology*, 30, 650–656.

Crome, L. and Stern, J. (1967). *The Pathology of Mental Retardation*. London: Churchill.

Cromer, R. (1974). Are subnormals linguistic adults? In N. O'Connor (Ed.), *Language Cognitive Deficits and Retardation* (pp. 169–187). London: Butterworths.

Cromer, R. (1988). Differentiating language and cognition. In R. Schiefelbusch and L. Lloyd (Eds.), *Languages Perspectives: Acquisition, Retardation and Intervention* (pp. 128–156). Austin, Texas: Pro–Ed.

Cromer, R. (1991). *Language and Thought in Normal and Handicapped Children*. London: Blackwell.

Crystal, D. (1969). *Prosodic Systems and Intonation in English*. Cambridge: Cambridge University Press.

Crystal, D. (1979). *Working with LARSP*. New York: Elsevier.

Crystal, D. (1982). *Profiling Linguistic Disability*. London: Arnold.

Crystal, D. (1986). Prosodic development. In P. Fletcher and M. Garman (Eds.), *Language Acquisition* (pp. 76–94). Cambridge: Cambridge University Press.

Crystal, D. (1987). *The Cambridge Encyclopedia of Language*. Cambridge: Cambridge University Press.

Crystal, D. (1989). *Clinical Linguistics*. London: Whurr.

Crystal, D., Fletcher, P. and Garman, M. (1976, 1989). *The Grammatical Analysis of Language Disability*. London: Arnold (revised edition, Whurr, London).

Cuckle, H., Wald, N. and Lindenbaum, R. (1984). Maternal serum alpha–fetoprotein measurement: A screening test for Down's syndrome. *Lancet*, 28 April.

Culicover, P. and Wexler, K. (1977). Some syntactic implications of a theory of language learnability. In P. Culicover, T. Wason and A. Akmajian (Eds.), *Formal syntax* (pp. 105–157). New York: Academic.

Cummins, J. and Das, J.P. (1978). Simultaneous and successive synthesis and linguistic processes. *International Journal of Psychology*, **13**, 129–142.

Cunningham, C. (1979). *Aspects of Early Development in Down's Syndrome Infants*. Unpublished doctoral dissertation, University of Manchester, UK.

Cunningham, C., Reuler, E., Blackwell, J. and Deck, J. (1981). Behavioral and linguistic development in the interactions of normal and retarded children with their mothers. *Child Development*, **51**, 62–70.

Cunningham, C. and Sloper P. (1984). The relationship between maternal ratings of first word vocabulary and Reynell language scores. *British Journal of Educational Psychology*, **54**, 160–167.

Curtiss, S. (1977). *Genie: A Psycholinguistic Study of a Modern–day 'Wild Child'*. New York: Academic Press.

Curtiss, S. (1981). Dissociation between language and cognition. *Journal of Autism and Developmental Disorders*, **11**, 15–30.

Curtiss, S. (1982). Developmental dissociations of language and cognition. In L. Obler and L. Menn (Eds.), *Exceptional Language and Linguistics* (pp. 285–312). New York: Academic.

Curtiss, S. (1988). The special talent of grammar acquisition. In L. Obler and D. Fein (Eds.), *The Exceptional Brain* (pp. 364–386). New York: Guilford.

Curtiss, S. (1989). Abnormal language acquisition and the modularity of language. In F. Newmeyer (Ed.), *Linguistics: The Cambridge Survey* (Vol. 2, pp. 96–116). New York: Cambridge University Press.

Curtiss, S., Fromkin, V. and Yamada, J. (1979). How independent is language? On the question of formal parallels between grammar and action. *UCLA Working Papers in Cognitive Linguistics*, **1**, 131–157.

Curtiss, S., Kempler, D. and Yamada, J. (1981). The relationship between language and cognition in development. *UCLA Working Papers in Cognitive Linguistics*, **3**, 1–59.

Curtiss, S. and Yamada, J. (1981). Selectively intact grammatical development in a retarded child. *UCLA Working Papers in Cognitive Linguistics*, **3**, 82–124.

Curtiss, S. and Yamada, J. (1992). *The Curtiss–Yamada Comprehensive Language Evaluation (CYCLE)*. Unpublished manuscript, University of California, Los Angeles.

Dale, P. (1977, August). *Syntactic Development in Down's Syndrome Children*. Communication presented at the 85th Annual Convention of the American Psychological Association, San Francisco, CA.

Damasio, H. and Damasio, A. (1989). *Lesion Analysis in Neuropsychology*. London: Oxford University Press.

Damasio, A. and Damasio, H. (1992). Brain and Language. *Scientific American*, September, 89–95.

Dameron, L. (1963). Development of intelligence of infants with mongolism. *Child Development*, **34**, 733–738.

Davies, D., Sperber, R. and McCauley, C. (1981). Intelligence–related differences in semantic processing speed. *Journal of Experimental Child Psychology*, **31**, 387–402.

Davis, E. (1937). *The Development of Linguistic Skills in Twins, Singletons with Siblings and Only Children from Age Five to Ten Years*. Minneapolis, MN: University of Minnesota Press.

Davis, H. and Oliver, B. (1980). A comparison of aspects of the maternal speech environment of retarded and non–retarded children. *Child: Care, Health and Development*, **5**, 135–145.

Davis, H., Stroud, A. and Green, L. (1988). Maternal language environment of children with mental retardation. *American Journal on Mental Retardation*, **93**, 144–153.

Davis, O. (1967). Teachers' behavior toward boys and girls during first grade reading instruction. *American Educational Research Journal*, **4**, 261–270.

Davis, S. (1979). *An Investigation into the Language of the Elderly*. Unpublished master's thesis, University of London.

Day, P. and Ulatowska, H. (1979). Perceptual, cognitive and linguistic development after early hemispherectomy: Two case studies. *Brain and Language*, **7**, 17–33.

Deblauw, A., Dubbler, C., Van Roosmalen, G. and Snow, C. (1979). Sex and social class differences in early mother–child interaction. In O. Garnica and M. King (Eds.), *Language, Children and Society* (pp. 53–64). New York: Pergamon.

Deltour, J.J. (1982). *Test des Relations Topologiques*. Issy–les–Moulineaux, France: Editions Scientifiques et Psychologiques.

Deltour, J.J. and Hupkens, D. (1980). *Test de Vocabulaire Actif et Passif*. Issy–les–Moulineaux, France: Editions Scientifiques et Psychologiques.

Demetras, M., Post, K. and Snow, C. (1986). Feedback to first language learners: The role of repetitions and clarification questions. *Journal of Child Language*, **13**, 275–292.

Denhière, G. (1973). *Organisation paradigmatique et organisation syntagmatique du discours: Etude génétique avec des enfants débiles mentaux de 8 à 18 ans*. Unpublished manuscript, University of Paris VI, Vincennes.

Denhière, G. (1974). Apprentissages intentionnels à allure libre: Etude comparative d'enfants normaux et débiles mentaux. *Enfance*, **4**, 149–174.

Dennis, M. (1980a). Capacity and strategy for syntactic comprehension after left or right hemidecortication. *Brain and Language*, **10**, 287–317.

Dennis, M. (1980b). Strokes in childhood 1: Communicative intent, expression and comprehension after left hemisphere arteriopathy in a right–handed nine–year–old. In R. Rieber (Ed.), *Language Development and Aphasia in Children* (pp. 45–67). New York: Academic.

Dennis, M. and Kohn, B. (1975). Comprehension of syntax in infantile hemiphegia after cerebral hemidecortication: Left hemisphere superiority. *Brain and Language*, **2**, 472–482.

Dennis, M. and Whitaker, H. (1976). Language acquisition following hemidecortication: Linguistic superiority of the left over the right hemisphere. *Brain and Language*, 3, 404–433.

De Renzi, E. and Vignolo, L. (1962). The Token Test: A sensitive test to detect receptive disturbances in aphasics. *Brain*, **85**, 665–678.

Despert, L. (1968). *Schizophrenia in Children*. New York: Brunner.

Dever, R. (1972). A comparison of the test results of a revised version of Berko's test of morphology with the free speech of mentally retarded children. *Journal of Speech and Hearing Research*, **15**, 169–178.

Devinsky, O., Sato, S., Conwit, R. and Schapiro, M. (1990). Relation of EEG alpha background to cognitive function, brain atrophy and cerebral metabolism in Down's syndrome. *Archives of Neurology*, **47**, 58–62.

Devries, L. and Dubowitz, L. (1985). Cystic leukomalacia in preterm infant: Site of lesion in relation to prognosis. *Lancet*, **2**, 1075–1076.

Dewart, H. (1979). Language comprehension processes of mentally retarded children. *American Journal of Mental Deficiency*, **84**, 117–183.

Dewart, M. (1972). Social class and children understanding of deep structures in sentences. *British Journal of Educational Psychology*, **42**, 198–203.

Dodd, B. (1972). Comparison of babbling patterns in normal and Down's syndrome infants. *Journal of Mental deficiency*, **16**, 35–40.

Dodd, B. (1976). A comparison of the phonological systems of mental age matched normal, severely subnormal and Down's syndrome children. *British Journal of Communicative Disorders*, **11**, 27–42.

Dodd, B. and Leahy, J. (1989). Phonological disorders and mental handicap. In M. Beveridge, G. Conti–Ramsden and Y. Leudar (Eds.), *Language and Communication in Mentally Handicapped People* (pp. 33–56). London: Chapman and Hall.

Dolk, H., De Wals, P., Gillerot, Y., Lechat, M., Aymé, S., Beckers, R., Bianchi, F., Borlée, I., Calabor, A., Calzolari, E., Cuschieri, A., Galanti, C., Goujard, J., Hansen–Koening, D., Harris, F., Kargut, G., Lillis, D., Lungarotti, M., Lye, F., Marchi, M., Nervin, N., Radie, A., Stool, C., Stone, D., Svel, I., Ten Kate, L. and Zori, R. (1990). The prevalence at birth of Down's syndrome in 19 regions of Europe 1980–86. In W. Fraser (Ed.), *Key Issues in Mental Retardation Research* (pp. 3–11). London: Routledge.

Dooley, J. (1976). *Language Acquisition and Down's Syndrome: A Study of Early Semantic and Syntax*. Unpublished doctoral dissertation, Harvard University, Cambridge, MA.

Dore, J. (1983). Feeling, form and intention in the baby's transition to language. In R. Golinkoff (Ed.), *The Transition from Prelinguistic to Linguistic Communication* (pp. 115–131). Hillsdale, NJ: Erlbaum.

Dowing, J., Ollila, L. and Oliver, P. (1977). Concepts of language in children from differing socio–economic backgrounds. *Journal of Educational Research*, **70**, 277–281.

Down, L. (1866). Observations on an ethnic classification of idiots. *London Hospital Clinical Lectures and Reports*, **3**, 259–262.

Down, L. (1887). *On Some of the Mental Affections of Childhood and Youth*. London: Churchill.

DSM–III–R (*Manuel diagnostique et statistique des troubles mentaux, collectif*) (1989). Paris: Masson.

Duchan, J.F. and Erickson, J.G. (1976). Normal and non–retarded children's understanding of semantic relations in different verbals contexts. *Journal of Speech and Hearing Research*, **19**, 767–776.

Duffen, L. (1976). Teaching reading to teach language. *Remedial Education*, **11**, 139–142.

Dunn, L. and Dunn, L. (1965). *Peabody Picture Vocabulary Test*. Circles Pines, MN: American Guidance Service.

Dykens, E. (1995). Measuring behavioral phenotypes: Provocations from the 'new genetics'. *American Journal on Mental Retardation*, **99**, 522–532.

Dykens, E., Hodapp, R. and Leckman, J. (1994). *Behavior and Development in Fragile X Syndrome*. London: Sage Publications.

Dykens, E. and Leckman, J. (1990). Developmental issues in fragile X syndrome. In R. Hodapp, J. Burack and E. Zigler (Eds.), *Issues in the Developmental Approach to Mental Retardation* (pp. 226–245). New York: Cambridge University Press.

Dykstra, R. and Tunney, R. (1969). Sex differences in reading readiness. *Reading and Realism*, **13**, 623–628.

Edwards, D. (1973). Sensori–motor intelligence and semantic relations in early child grammar. *Cognition*, **2**, 395–424.

Edwards, S. (1990). *Conversational Interaction between Adults and Young Severely Mentally Handicapped Children*. Unpublished doctoral dissertation, Reading University, Reading.

Edwards, S. (1991). Comparing how mothers and teachers talk to children: Is it different and does it matter? *Child Language Teaching and Therapy*, **7**, 298–309.

Edwards, S. (1992). The single–word lexicon of a severely mentally handicapped child. *Clinical Linguistics and Phonetics*, **6**, 87–100.

Eels, K., Davis, A., Havighurst, R., Herrick, V. and Tyler, R. (1951). *Intelligence and Cultural Differences*. Chicago: University of Chicago Press.

Eilers, R., Bull, D., Oller, D. and Lewis, D. (1985). The discrimination of rapid spectral speech cues by Down's syndrome and normally developing infants. In S. Harel and N. Anastasiow (Eds.), *The At–risk Infant. Psycho/Social/Medical Aspects* (pp. 115–132). Baltimore, MD: Brookes.

Eilers, R., Oller, D., Bull, D. and Gavin, W. (1984). Linguistic experience and infant perception. *Journal of Child Language*, **11**, 467–475.

Eimas, P., Siqueland, E., Jusczyk, P. and Vigorito, J. (1971). Speech perception in infants. *Science*, **171**, 303–306.

Einfeld, S. (1993). Fragile–X syndrome. *Current Opinion in Psychiatry*, **6**, 655–658.

Eisele, J. (1991). Selective deficits in language comprehension following early left and right hemisphere damage. In I. Pavao Martins, A. Castro–Caldas, H. Van Dongen and A. Van Hout (Eds.), *Acquired Aphasia in Children* (pp. 225–238). Boston, MA: Kluwer.

Elliott, D., Pollock, B., Chua, R. and Weeks, D. (1995). Cerebral specialization for spatial processing in adults with Down's syndrome. *American Journal on Mental Retardation*, **99**, 605–615.

Elliott, D., Weeks, D. and Elliott, C. (1987). Cerebral specialization in individuals with Down's syndrome. *American Journal on Mental Retardation*, **92**, 263–271.

Elliott, D., Edwards, J., Weeks, D., Lindley, S. and Carnahan, H. (1987). Cerebral specialization in young adults with Down's syndrome. *American Journal on Mental Retardation*, **91**, 480–485.

Ellis, N. (1963). The stimulus trace and behavioral inadequacy. In N. Ellis (Ed.), *Handbook of Mental Deficiency* (pp. 134–158). New York: McGraw–Hill.

Ellis, N., Barnett, C. and Pryer, M. (1960). Operant behavior in mental defectives: Exploratory studies. *Journal of Experimental Analysis of Behavior*, **3**, 63–69.

Ellis, N. and Cavalier, A. (1982). Research perspectives in mental retardation. In E. Zigler and D. Balla (Eds.), Mental retardation: *The Developmental–Difference Controversy* (pp. 121–159). Hillsdale, NJ: Erlbaum.

Engler, M. (1949). *Mongolism*. Baltimore, MD: Williams and Wilkins.

Entus, A. (1977). Hemispheric asymmetry in processing of dichotically presented speech and non-speech stimuli. In S. Segalowitz and F. Gruber (Eds.), *Language Development and Neurological Theory* (pp. 63–73). New York: Academic.

Entwistle, D. (1966). *Children's Word Associations*. Baltimore, MD: Johns Hopkins University Press.

Entwistle, D., Forsyth, D. and Muuss, R. (1964). The syntagmatic–paradigmatic shift in children's word associations. *Journal of Verbal Learning and Verbal Behavior*, 3, 19–29.

Epstein, C. (1986). Trisomy 21 and the nervous system: From causes to cure. In C. Epstein (Ed.), *The Neurobiology of Down's Syndrome* (pp. 1–15). New York: Raven Press.

Epstein, C. (1987). The consequence of altered gene dosage in trisomy 21. In S. Pueschel, C. Tingey, J. Rynders, A. Crocker and D. Crutcher (Eds.), *New Perspectives on Down's Syndrome* (pp. 69–80). Baltimore, MD: Brookes.

Erwin, S. (1961). Change with age in the verbal determinant of word associations. *American Journal of Psychology*, 74, 361–372.

Esperet, E. (1987). Aspects sociaux de la psychologie du langage. In J.A. Rondal and J.P. Thibaut (Eds.), *Problèmes de psycholinguistique* (pp. 327–389). Brussels: Mardaga.

Esperet, E. (1990). L'acquisition différentielle du langage. In M. Reuchlin, J. Lautrey, C. Marendaz and T. Ohlmann (Eds.), *Cognition. L'individuel et l'universel* (pp. 217–252). Paris: Presses Universitaires de France.

Esquirol, J. (1838). *Des maladies mentales considérées sous les rapports médical, hygiénique, et medico–legal* (2 Vols). Paris: Baillière.

Evans, D. (1977). The development of language abilities in mongols: A correlational study. *Journal of Mental Deficiency Research*, 21, 103–117.

Evans, D., Funkenstein, H., Albert, M., Schezz, P., Cook, N., Chown, M., Hebert, L. Hennekens, C. and Taylor, J. (1989). Prevalence of Alzheimer's disease in a community population of older persons. *Journal of the American Medical Association*, 262, 2551–2556.

Evans, D. and Hampson, M. (1968). The language of mongols. *British Journal of Disorders of Communication*, 3, 171–181.

Evenhuis, H., Van Zanten, G., Brocaar, M. and Roerdinkholder, W. (1992). Hearing loss in middle–age in persons with Down's syndrome. *American Journal on Mental Retardation*, 97, 47–56.

Facon, B. (1994). *Deficience mentale: Influence de la dissociation entre intelligence et expérience*. Unpublished doctoral dissertation, Université Charles De Gaulle, Roubaix, France.

Facon, B. and Bollengier, J. (1991). *Contribution à l'étude des effets de la dissociation entre efficience et expérience sur le profil psychologique des retardés–mentaux*. Unpublished master's thesis, Université Charles De Gaulle, Roubaix, France.

Fantz, R., Fagan, J. and Miranda, S. (1975). Early visual selectivity. In L. Cohen and P. Salapatek (Eds.), *Infant Perception from Sensation to Cognition* (Vol. 1: *Basic Visual Processes*) (pp. 249–346). New York: Academic Press.

Farber, B. (1968). *Mental Retardation. Its Social Context and Social Consequences*. Boston, MA: Houghton Mifflin.

Farmer, A. and Brayton, E. (1979). Speech characteristics of fluent and dysfluent Down's syndrome adults. *Folia Phoniatrica*, 31, 284–290.

Fay, W. and Schuler, A. (1980). *Emerging Language in Autistic Children*. London: Arnold.

Fayasse, M., Comblain, A. and Rondal, J. A. (1995). *Compréhension et production des classes formelles et des structures phrasiques chez les enfants et adolescents retardés mentaux*. Manuscript submitted for publication.

Feifel, H. (1949). Qualitative differences in the vocabulary responses of normals and abnormals. *Genetic Psychology Monographs*, **39**, 151–204.

Feldman, H. (1994). Language development after early unilateral brain injury: A replication study. In H. Tager–Flusberg (Ed.), *Constraints on Language Acquisition. Studies of Atypical Children* (pp. 75–90). Hillsdale, NJ: Erlbaum.

Feldman, H., Evans, J., Brown, R. and Wareham, N. (1992). Early language and communicative abilities of children with periventricular leukomalacia. *American Journal on Mental Retardation*, **97**, 222–234.

Fenson, L. Dale, P., Reznick, J., Bates, E. and Thal, D. (in press). Variability in early communicative development. *Monograph of the Society for Research in Child Development*.

Ferreiro, E. (1971). *Les Relations temporelles dans le langage de l'enfant*. Genève: Droz.

Ferri, R., Bergonzi, P., Colognola, P., Musumeci, S., Sanfillipo, S., Tomassetti, P., Viglianesi, A. and Gigli, G. (1986). Brainstem auditory evoked potentials (BAEP) in subjects with mental retardation and different kariotypes. In V. Gallai (Ed.), *Maturation of CNS and Evoked Potentials* (pp. 369–392). Amsterdam: Excerpts Medica.

Ferrier, L, Bashir, A., Meryash, D., Johnston, J. and Wolff, P. (1991). Conversational skills of individuals with fragile–X syndrome: A comparison with autism and Down's syndrome. *Developmental Medicine and Child Neurology*, **33**, 766–788.

Fillmore, C. (1967). The case for case. In E. Bach and R. Harms (Eds.), *Universals in Linguistic Theory* (pp. 1–88). New York: Holt, Rinehart and Winston.

Finer, D. and Roeper, T. (1989). From cognition to thematic roles. In R. Matthews and W. Demopoulos (Eds.), *Learnability and Linguistic Theory* (pp. 177–210). Boston: Kluwer.

Finley, S., Finley, W., Phillips, C. and Rosecrans, C. (1965). Exceptional intelligence in a mongoloid child of a family with a 13–15/partial 21 (D/partial G) translocation. *New England Journal of Medicine*, **272**, 1089–1092.

Fisch, G. (1992). Is autism associated with the Fragile–X syndrome? *American Journal of Medical Genetics*, **43**, 47–55.

Fisch, G., Shapiro, L. Simensen, R., Schwartz, C., Fryns, J. P., Borghgraef, M., Curfs, L. Howard–Peebles, P., Arinami, T. and Mavron, A. (1992). Longitudinal changes in IQ among fragile X males: Clinical evidence of more than one mutation. *American Journal of Medical Genetics*, **43**, 28–34.

Fisher, H. and Logemann, J. (1971). *The Fisher–Logemann Test of Articulation Competence*. Boston, MA: Houghton Mifflin.

Fisher, M. and Zeaman, D. (1970). Growth and decline in retardate intelligence. In N. Ellis (Ed.), *International Review of Research in Mental Retardation* (Vol. 4, pp. 151–191). New York: Academic.

Fishler, K. (1975). Mental development in mosaic Down's syndrome as compared with trisomy 21. In R. Koch and F. de la Cruz (Eds.), *Down's Syndrome* (pp. 157–179). New York: Brunner/Mazel.

Fishler, K. and Koch, R. (1991). Mental development in Down's syndrome mosaicism. *American Journal on Mental Retardation*, **96**, 345–351.

Fishler, K., Share, J. and Koch, R. (1964). Adaptation of Gesell Developmental Scales for evaluation of development in children with Down's syndrome (mongolism). *American Journal of Mental Deficiency*, **68**, 642–646.

Flavell, J. (1963). *The Developmental Psychology of Jean Piaget*. New York: Van Nostrand.

Flavell, J. (1977). *Cognitive Development*. Englewood Cliffs, NJ: Prentice–Hall.

Florez, J., Del Arco, C., Gonzalez, A., Pascual, J. and Pazos, A. (1990). Autoradiographic studies of neurotransmitter receptors in the brain of new born infants with Down's syndrome. *American Journal of Medical Genetics Supplement*, **7**, 301–305.

Foale, M. and Patterson, J. (1954). The hearing of mental defectives. *American Journal of Mental Deficiency*, **59**, 254–258.

Fodor, J. (1966). How to learn to talk: Some simple ways. In F. Smith and G. Miller (Eds.), *The Genesis of Language* (pp. 105–128). Cambridge, MA: MIT Press.

Fodor, J. (1983). *The Modularity of Mind*. Cambridge, MA: MIT Press.

Foley, J., Cookson, M. and Zappella, M. (1964). The placing and supporting reactions in cerebral palsy. *Journal of Mental Deficiency Research*, **8**, 17–24.

Folger, J.P. and Chapman, R. (1979). A pragmatic analysis of spontaneous imitation. *Journal of Child Language*, **5**, 25–38.

Forsman, H. and Akesson, H. (1965). Mortality in patients with Down's syndrome. *Journal of Mental Deficiency Research*, **11**, 106–107

Foucault, M. (1961). *Histoire de la folie à l'âge classique*. Paris: Union Générale d'Editions.

Fowler, A. (1988). Determinants of rate of language growth in children with Down's Syndrome. In L. Nadel (Ed.), *The Psychobiology of Down's Syndrome* (pp. 217–245). Cambridge, MA: MIT Press.

Fowler, A. (1990). Language abilities in children with Down's syndrome: Evidence for a specific syntactic delay. In D. Cicchetti and Beeghly (Eds.), *Children with Down Syndrome. A Developmental Perspective* (pp. 302–328). New York: Cambridge University Press.

Fowler, A., Gelman, R. and Gleitman, L. (1994). The course of language learning in children with Down's syndrome. In H. Tager–Flusberg (Ed.), *Constraints on Language Acquisition. Studies of Atypical Children* (pp. 91–140). Hillsdale, NJ: Erlbaum.

Fraser, C., Bellugi, U. and Brown, R. (1963). Control of grammar in imitation, comprehension and production. *Journal of Verbal Learning and Verbal Behavior*, **2**, 121–135.

Fraser, C. and Roberts, N. (1976). Mothers' speech to children of four different ages. *Journal of Psycholinguistic Research*, **4**, 9–16.

Fraser, F. and Sadovnick, A. (1976). Correlations of IQ in subjects with Down's syndrome and their parents and sibs. *Journal of Mental Deficency Research*, **20**, 179–182.

Fraser, M. and Mitchell, A. (1976). Kalmuc idiocy. *Journal of Mental Science*, **22**, 169–179.

Freeman, G. and Lukens, J. (1962). A speech and language program for educable mentally handicapped children. *Journal of Speech and Hearing Disorders*, **27**, 285–287.

Frisk, V. and Whyte, H. (1994). The long–term consequences of periventricular brain damage on language and verbal memory. *Developmental Neuropsychology*, **10**, 313–333.

Fristoe, M. and Lloyd, L. (1977). Manual communication for the retarded and others with severe communication impairment: A resource list. *Mental Retardation*, **15**, 18–21.

Frith, U. and Frith, C. (1974). Specific motor disabilities in Down's syndrome. *Journal of Child Psychology and Psychiatry*, **15**, 293–301.

Frome–Loeb, D. and Leonard, L. (1988). Specific language impairment and parameter theory. *Clinical Linguistics and Phonetics*, 2, 317–327.

Fryns, J. P., Jacobs, J., Kleczkowska, A. and Van den Berghe, H. (1984). The psychological profile of the fragile X syndrome. *Clinical Genetics*, 25, 131–134.

Fuchs–Schachter, F., Shore, E., Hodapp, R., Chafflin, S. and Bundy, C. (1978). Do girls talk earlier? Mean length of utterance in toddlers. *Developmental Psychology*, 14, 388–392.

Furth, H. (1969). *Piaget and Knowledge*. Englewood Cliffs, NJ: Prentice–Hall.

Galaburda, A. (1984). Anatomical asymmetries. In N. Geschwind and A. Galaburda (Eds.), *Cerebral dominance. The Biological Foundations* (pp. 11–25). Cambridge, MA: Harvard University Press.

Galaburda, A., Sherman, G., Rosen, E., Aboitiz, F. and Geschwind, N. (1985). Developmental dyslexia: Four consecutive patients with cortical anomalies. *Annals of Neurology*, 18, 222–233.

Galaburda, A., Wang, P., Bellugi, U. and Rossen, M. (1994). Cytoarchitectonic anomalies in a genetically based disorder: Williams syndrome. *Cognitive Neuroscience and Neuropsychology*, 5, 753–757.

Garai, J. and Scheinfeld, D. (1968). Sex differences in mental and behavioral aids. *Genetic Psychology Monographs*, 77, 169–299.

Garcia, E. (1974). The training and generalization of a conversational speech form in non–verbal retardates. *Journal of Applied Behavior Analysis*, 7, 137–149.

Garcia, E. and Batista–Wallace, M. (1977). Parental training of the plural morpheme in normal toddlers. *Journal of Applied Behavior Analysis*, 10, 505.

Garcia, E. and DeHaven, E. (1974). Use of operant techniques in the establishment and generalization of language: A review and analysis. *American Journal of Mental Deficiency*, 79, 169–178.

Garcia, E., Guess, D. and Byrnes, J. (1973). Development of syntax in a retarded girl using procedures of imitation, reinforcement and modelling. *Journal of Applied Behavior Analysis*, 6, 299–311.

Gardiner, M. and Walter, D. (1977). Evidence of hemispheric specialization from infant EEG. In S. Harnad (Ed.), *Lateralization in the Nervous System* (pp. 148–163). New York: Academic Press.

Garfield, J. (Ed.). (1987). *Modularity in Knowledge Representation and Natural–language Understanding*. Cambridge, MA: MIT Press.

Gasser, J. (1995). *Aux origines du cerveau moderne. Localisations, langage et mémoire dans l'oeuvre de Charcot*. Paris: Fayard.

Gathercole, S. and Baddeley, A. (1990). The role of phonological memory in vocabulary acquisition: A study of young children learning new names. *British Journal of Psychology*, 81, 439–454.

Gathercole, S. and Baddeley, A. (1993). *Working Memory and Language*. Hove: Erlbaum.

Gazzaniga, M. (1993). *Nature's mind: The Biological Roots of Thinking, Emotions, Sexuality, Language and Intelligence*. New York: Basic Books.

Gens, G. (1951). The speech pathologist looks at the mentally deficient child. *Training School Bulletin*, 48, 19–27.

Geschwind, N. and Galaburda, A. (1985). Cerebral lateralization. *Archives of Neurology*, 42, 428–459.

Gesell, A. and Amatruda, C. (1941). *Developmental Diagnosis*. New York: Hoeber.

Ghazinddin, M., Tsai, L. and Ghazinddin, N. (1992). Autism in Down's syndrome: Presentation and diagnosis. *Journal of Intellectual Disability Research*, 36, 449–456.

Gibson, D. (1967). Intelligence in the mongoloid and his parent. *American Journal of Mental Deficiency*, **71**, 1014–1016.

Gibson, D. (1973). Karyotype variation and behavior in Down's syndrome: Methodological review. *American Journal of Mental Deficiency*, **78**, 128–133.

Gibson, D. (1981). *Down's syndrome: The Psychology of Mongolism*. Cambridge: Cambridge University Press.

Gibson, D. (1991). Down's syndrome and cognitive enhancement: Not like the others. In K. Marfo (Ed.), *Early Intervention in Transition: Current Perspectives on Programs for Handicapped Children* (pp. 61–90). New York: Praeger.

Gibson, D. and Frank, H. (1961). Dimensions of mongolism. I. Age limits for cardinal mongol stigmata. *American Journal of Mental Deficiency*, **66**, 30–34.

Gibson, D. and Pozsonyi, J. (1965). Morphological and behavioral consequences of chromosome subtype in mongolism. *American Journal of Mental Deficiency*, **69**, 801–804.

Gibson, D., Pozsonyi, J. and Zarfas, D. (1964). Dimensions of mongolism. II. The interaction of clinical indices. *American Journal of Mental Deficiency*, **68**, 503–510.

Giencke, S. and Lewandowski, L. (1989). Anomalous dominance in Down's syndrome young adults. *Cortex*, **25**, 93–102.

Gigli, G., Ferri, R., Musumeci, S., Tomassetti, P. and Bergonzi, P. (1984). Brain–stem auditory evoked responses in children with Down's syndrome. In J. Berg (Ed.), *Perspectives and Progress in Mental Retardation* (Vol. 2, pp. 277–286). London: International Association for the Scientific Study of Mental Deficiency (IASSMD).

Gilham, B. (1979). *The First Words Language Programme: A Basic Language Programme for Mentally Handicapped Children*. London: Allen and Unwin.

Girardeau, F. (1962). The effect of secondary reinforcement on the operant behavior of mental defectives. *American Journal of Mental Deficiency*, **67**, 441–449.

Glanville, B., Best, C. and Levenson, R. (1977). A cardiac measure of cerebral asymmetries in infant auditory perception. *Developmental Psychology*, **13**, 54–59.

Gleitman, L. (1983). Biological dispositions to learn language. In W. Demopoulos and A. Marras (Eds.), *Language Learning and Concept Acquisition* (pp. 114–129). Norwood, NJ: Ablex.

Glenn, S. and Cunningham, C. (1982). Recognition for the familiar words of nursery rhymes by handicapped and non–handicapped infants. *Journal of Child Psychology and Psychiatry*, **23**, 319–327.

Glovsky, L. (1966). Audiological assessment of a mongoloid population. *Training School Bulletin*, **63**, 27–36.

Glovsky, L. (1970). A comparison of two groups of mentally retarded children on the ITPA. *Training School Bulletin*, **67**, 4–14.

Goertzen, S. (1957). Speech and the mentally retarded child. *American Journal of Mental Deficiency*, **62**, 244–253.

Golden, M. and Birns, B. (1976). Social class and infant intelligence. In M. Lewis (Ed.), *Origins of Intelligence* (pp. 46–68). New York: Wiley.

Golden W. and Pashayan, H. (1976). The effect of parental education on the eventual mental development of non–institutionalized children with Down's syndrome. *Journal of Pediatrics*, **89**, 603–605.

Goldgaber, D., Lerman, M., McBride, O., Saffiotti, U. and Gajdusek, D. (1987). Characterization and chromosomal localization of a cDNA encoding brain amyloid of Alzheimer's disease. *Science*, **235**, 877–880.

Goldman–Eisler, F. (1968). *Psycholinguistics: Experiments in Spontaneous Speech* (pp. 46–68). New York: Academic Press.

Goldman–Eisler, F. (1972). Pauses, clauses, sentences. *Language and Speech*, **15**, 103–113.

Goldstein, K. (1943). Concerning rigidity. *Character and Personality*, **11**, 209–226.

Golinkoff, R. (1983). The preverbal negotiation of failed messages: Insights into the transition period. In R. Golinkoff (Ed.), *The Transition from Prelinguistic to Linguistic Communication* (pp. 42–63). Hillsdale, NJ: Erlbaum.

Golinkoff, R. and Ames, G. (1979). A comparison of father's and mother's speech with their young children. *Child Development*, **50**, 28–32.

Gombert, J. (1990). *Le Développement métalinguistique*. Paris: Presses Universitaires de France.

Goodglass, H. and Kaplan, E. (1972). *Assessment of Aphasia and Related Disorders*. Philadelphia: Lea and Febiger.

Goodstein, H. (1970). The performance of mentally handicapped and average IQ children on two modified cloze–tasks for oral language. *American Journal of Mental Deficiency*, **75**, 290–297.

Goodwin, B. and Huether, C. (1987). Revised estimates and projections of Down's syndrome births in the United States and the effects of prenatal diagnosis utilization, 1970–2002. *Prenatal Diagnosis*, **7**, 261–271.

Gopnik, A. (1984). The acquisition of 'gone' and the development of the object concept. *Journal of Child Language*, **11**, 273–292.

Gopnik, A. (1987, July). *Language before Stage 6*. Paper presented at the Fourth International Congress for the Study of Child Language (IASSCL), Lund, Sweden.

Gopnik, A. (1990a). Feature blindness: A case study. *Language Acquisition*, **1**, 139–164.

Gopnik, A. (1990b). Dysphasia in an extended family. *Nature*, **344**, 715.

Gopnik, A. and Meltzoff, A. (1984). Semantic and cognitive development in 15– to 21–month–old children. *Journal of Child Language*, **11**, 495–513.

Gopnik, A. and Meltzoff, A. (1986). Relations between semantic and cognitive development in the one–word stage: The specificity hypothesis. *Child Development*, **57**, 1040–1053.

Gopnik, A. and Meltzoff, A. (1987). The development of categorization in the second year and its relation to other cognitive and linguistic development. *Child Development*, **58**, 523–531.

Gordon, W. and Panagos, J. (1976). Developmental transformational capacity of children with Down's syndrome. *Perceptual and Motor Skills*, **43**, 967–973.

Goswami, U. and Bryant, P. (1990). *Phonological Skills and Learning to Read*. Hillsdale, NJ: Erlbaum.

Gottardo, A. and Rubin, H. (1991). Language analysis skills of children with mental retardation. *Mental Retardation*, **29**, 269–274.

Gottsleben, R. (1955). The incidence of stuttering in a group of mongoloids. *Training School Bulletin*, **51**, 209–218.

Goulet, L. and Baltes, P. (Eds.). (1970). *Life–span Developmental Psychology: Research and Theory*. New York: Academic Press.

Graaf, E. de (1995). Early intervention for children with Down's syndrome. In A. Vermeer and W. Davis (Eds.), *Physical and Motor Development in Mental Retardation* (pp. 120–143). Basel: Karger.

Graham, J. and Graham, L. (1971). Language behavior of the mentally retarded: Syntactics characteristics. *American Journal of Mental Deficiency*, **75**, 623–629.

Graham, N. (1968). Short–term memory and syntactic structure in educationally subnormal children. *Language and Speech*, **11**, 209–219.

Graham, N. and Gulliford, R. (1968). A psychological approach to the language deficiencies of educationally subnormal children. *Educational Review*, **20**, 136–145.

Greenwald, C. and Leonard, L. (1979). Communicative and sensorimotor development of Down's syndrome children. *American Journal of Mental Deficiency*, **84**, 296–303.

Grimshaw, J. (1990). *Argument Structure*. Cambridge, MA: MIT Press.

Grodzinsky, Y. (1984). The syntactic characterization of agrammatism. *Cognition*, **16**, 99–120.

Grodzinsky, Y. (1986). Language deficits and the theory of syntax. *Brain and Language*, **27**, 135–159.

Grodzinsky, Y. (1990). *Theoretical Perspectives on Language Deficits*. Cambridge, MA: MIT Press.

Grossman, H., (Ed.) (1983). *Classification in Mental Retardation*. Washington, DC: American Association on Mental Deficiency.

Guess, D. (1969). A functional analysis of receptive language and productive speech: Acquisition of the plural morpheme. *Journal of Applied Behavior Analysis*, **2**, 55–64.

Guess, D. and Baer, D. (1973a). Some experimental analysis of linguistic development in institutionalized retarded children. In B. Lahey (Ed.), *The Modification of Language Behavior* (pp. 3–60). Springfield, IL: Thomas.

Guess, D. and Baer, D. (1973b). An analysis of individual differences in generalization between receptive and productive language in retarded children. *Journal of Applied Behavior Analysis*, **6**, 311–329.

Guess, D., Rutherford, G., Smith, J. and Ensminger, E. (1970). Utilization of sub-professional persons in teaching language skills to mentally retarded children: An interim report. *Mental Retardation*, **82**, 17–23.

Guess, D., Sailor, W., Rutherford, G. and Baer, D. (1968). An experimental analysis of linguistic development: The productive use of the plural morpheme. *Journal of Applied Behavior Analysis*, **1**, 297–306.

Guess, D., Smith, D. and Ensminger, E. (1971). The role of non–professional persons in teaching language skills to mentally retarded children. *Exceptional Children*, **37**, 447–453.

Gulliford, R., Smith, B. and Philipps, C. (1971). *Neo–natal Jaundice Research: Language Assessment*. Unpublished manuscript, Birmingham University.

Gunnar, M. and Donahue, M. (1980). Sex differences in social responsiveness between six months and twelve months. *Child Development*, **51**, 262–265.

Guralnick, M. (1992). A hierarchical model for understanding children's peer–related social competence. In S. Odom, S. McConnell and M. McEvoy (Eds.), *Social Competence of Young Children with Disabilities: Issues and Strategies for Intervention* (pp. 37–64). Baltimore, MD: Brookes.

Guralnick, M. (1996). Future directions in early intervention for children with Down'ssyndrome. In J.A. Rondal, J. Perera, L. Nadel and A. Comblain (Eds.), *Down Syndrome: Psychological, Psychobiological and Socio–educational Perspectives*. London: Whurr.

Guralnick, M. and Bricker, D. (1987). The effectiveness of early intervention for children with cognitive and general developmental delays. In M. Guralnick and F. Bennett (Eds.), *The Effectiveness of Early Intervention for At–risk and Handicapped Children* (pp. 115–173). New York: Academic.

Guralnick, M., Connor, R., Hammoud, M., Gottman, J. and Kinnish, K. (in press). The peer relations of preschool children with communication disorders. *Child Development*.

Guralnick, M. and Groom, J. (1987). The peer relations of mildly delayed and non-handicapped preschool children in mainstream playgroups. *Child Development*, **58**, 1556–1572.

Guralnick, M. and Paul–Brown, D. (1984). Communicative adjustments during behavior–request episodes among children at different developmental levels. *Child Development*, **55**, 911–919.

Guralnick, M. and Paul–Brown, D. (1986). Communicative interactions of mildly delayed and normally developing preschool children: Effects of listener's developmental level. *Journal of Speech and Hearing Research*, **29**, 2–10.

Gustavson, K., Blomquist, H. and Holgren, G. (1986). Prevalence of the fragile X syndrome in mentally retarded children in a Swedish country. *American Journal of Medical Genetics*, **23**, 581–587.

Guthrie, R., Whitney, S. and Stuckey, R. (1963). *PKU Screening Program*. Unpublished Progress report N°. 4, State University of New York, Buffalo.

Gutmann, A. and Rondal, J. A. (1979). Verbal operants in mothers' speech to non–retarded and Down's syndrome children matched for linguistic level. *American Journal of Mental Deficiency*, **83**, 446–452.

Hadenius, A., Hagberg, B., Hyttnas–Bensch, K. and Sjogren, I. (1962). The natural prognosis of infantile hydrocephalus. *Acta Pediatrica*, **51**, 47–118.

Hagerman, R. (1992). Annotation: Fragile–X syndrome: Advances and controversy. *Journal of Child Psychology and Psychiatry*, **33**, 1127–1139.

Hagerman, R., Kemper, M. and Hudson, M. (1985). Learning disabilities and attentional problems in boys with the fragile X syndrome. *American Journal of Diseases of Children*, **139**, 674–678.

Haggerty, A. (1959). The effects of long–term hospitalisation and institutionalisation upon the language development of children. *Journal of Genetic Psychology*, **94**, 205–209.

Hall, B. and Smith, D. (1972). Prader–Willi syndrome. *Journal of Pediatrics*, **81**, 286–292.

Hallé, K. and Boysson–Bardies, B. de (1991). Beginnings of prosodic organization: Intonation and duration pattern of disyllables produced by Japanese and French infants. *Language and Speech*, **34**, 299–318.

Hallé, K., Boysson–Bardies, B. de and Durand, C. (1992). Babillages et premiers mots. *Glossa*, **29**, 4–15.

Halliday, M. (1975). *Learning How to Mean. Explorations in the Development of Language*. London: Arnold.

Halliday, M. (1985). *An Introduction to Functional Grammar*. London: Arnold.

Halverson, C. and Waldrop, M. (1970). Maternal behavior toward own and other preschool children: The problem of 'ownness'. *Child Development*, **41**, 839–845.

Hamerton, J., Giannelli, F. and Polani, P. (1965). Cytogenetics of Down's syndrome (mongolism) I. Data on consecutive series of patients referred for genetic counselling and diagnosis. *Cytogenetics*, **4**, 171–185.

Hamilton, C. (1993). Investigation of the articulatory patterns of young adults with Down's syndrome using electropalatography. *Down's Syndrome*, **1**, 15–28.

Hampson, E. (1990a). Variations in sex–related cognitive abilities across the menstrual cycle. *Brain Cognition*, **14**, 26–43.

Hampson, E. (1990b). Estrogen–related variations in human spatial and articulatory–motor skills. *Psychoneuroendocrinology*, **15**, 97–111.

Hampson, E. and Kimura, D. (1992). Sex differences and hormonal influences on cognitive functions in humans. In J. Becker, S. Breedlove and D. Crews (Eds.), *Behavioral Endocrinology* (pp. 357–398). Cambridge, MA: MIT Press.

Hanson, D., Jackson, A. and Hagerman, R. (1986). Speech disturbances (cluttering) in mildly impaired males with Martin–Bell/Fragile–X syndrome. In J. Opitz, J. Reynolds and L. Spano (Eds.), *X–linked Mental Retardation* (pp. 128–142). New York: Liss.

Harris, D. (1963). *Children's Drawings as Measures of Intellectual Maturity*. New York: Harcourt, Brace and World.

Harris, J. (1983). What does mean length of utterance mean? Evidence from a comparative study of normal and Down's syndrome children. *British Journal of Disorders of Communication*, **18**, 153–169.

Harrison, S. (1959). Integration of development language activities with an educational program for mentally retarded children. *American Journal of Mental Deficiency*, **63**, 967–970.

Harrison, R., Budoff, M. and Greenberg, G. (1975). Differences between EMR and non–retarded children in fluency and quality of verbal associations. *American Journal of Mental Deficiency*, **79**, 583–591.

Harris–Vanderheiden, D., Brown, D., Mackenzie, P., Reinen, S. and Scheibel, C. (1975). Symbol communication for the mentally handicapped: An application of Bliss symbols as an alternative communication mode for non–vocal mentally retarded children with motoric impairment. *Mental Retardation*, **13**, 34–37.

Hart, B. (1988). Language and dementia: a review. *Psychological Medicine*, **18**, 99–112.

Hartley, X. (1982). Receptive language processing of Down's syndrome children. *Journal of Mental Deficiency Research*, **26**, 263–269.

Hartley, X. (1985). Receptive language processing and ear advantage in Down's syndrome children. *Journal of Mental Deficiency Research*, **29**, 197–205.

Hauser–Cram, P. (1989). The efficiency of early intervention. *Ab Initio*, **1**, 1–2.

Haviland, R. (1972). A stimulus to language development: The institutional environment. *Mental Retardation*, **10**, 19–21.

Hecaen, H. and Albert, M. (1978). *Human Neuropsychology*. New York: Wiley.

Hecaen, H. and Anglelergues, R. (1965). *Pathologie du langage*. Paris: Larousse.

Herbst, D. and Miller, J. (1980). Non–specific X–linked mental retardation II: The frequency in British Columbia. *American Journal of Medical Genetics*, **7**, 461–470.

Hermelin, B. and O'Connor, N. (1960). Like and cross–modality responses in normal and subnormal children. *Quarterly Journal of Experimental Psychology*, **12**, 48–53.

Hestens, A., Sand, T. and Tostad, K. (1991). Ocular findings in Down's syndrome. *Journal of Mental Deficiency Reserch*, **35**, 194–203.

Hill, P. and McCune–Nicholich, L. (1981). Pretend play and patterns of cognition in Down's syndrome children. *Child Development*, **52**, 1168–1175.

Hillgard, S. and Pichon, T. (1987). Electrophysiology of cognition. In F. Plum (Ed.), *Handbook of Physiology: Vol. 1. The Nervous System and Higher Functions of the Brain* (pp. 519–584). Baltimore, MD: American Physiological Society.

Hinton, V., Dobkin, C., Halperin, J., Jenkins, E., Brown, W., Ding, X., Cohen, I., Rousseau, F. and Miezejeski, C. (1992). Mode of inheritance influences behavioural expression and molecular control of cognitive deficits in female carriers of Fragile X syndrome. *American Journal of Medical Genetics*, **43**, 87–95.

Hirsh–Pasek, K., Treiman, R. and Schneiderman, M. (1984). Brown and Hanlon revisited: Mothers' sensitivity to ungrammatical forms. *Journal of Child Language*, **11**, 81–88.

Hiscock, M. and Decter, M. (1988). Dichotic listening in children. In K. Hughdahl (Ed.), *Handbook of Dichotic Listening: Theory, Methods and Research* (pp. 431–473). New York: Wiley.

Hodapp, R. (in press–a). Cross–domain relations in Down's syndrome. In J. A. Rondal, J. Perera, L. Nadel and A. Comblain (Eds.), *Down's Syndrome: Psychological, Psychobiological and Socio–educational Perspectives*. London: Whurr.

Hodapp, R. (in press–b). Parenting children with Down's syndrome and other type of mental retardation. In M. Bornstein (Ed.), *Handbook of Parenting: Vol. 1. How Children Influence Parents* (pp. 233–253). Hillsdale, NJ: Erlbaum.

Hodapp, R., Burack, J. and Zigler, E. (1990). The developmental perspective in the field of mental retardation. In R. Hodapp, J. Burack and E. Zigler (Eds.), *Issues in the Developmental Approach to Mental Retardation* (pp. 3–261). New York: Cambridge University Press.

Hodapp, R., Leckman, J., Dykens, E., Sparrow, S., Zelinsky, D. and Ort, S. (1992). K–ABC profiles in children with Fragile X syndrome, Down's syndrome and non-specific mental retardation. *American Journal on Mental Retardation*, **97**, 39–46.

Hodapp, R. and Zigler, E. (1990). Applying the developmental perspective to individuals with Down's syndrome. In D. Cicchetti and M. Beeghly (Eds.), *Children with Down's syndrome. A Developmental Perspective* (pp. 1–28). New York: Cambridge University Press.

Hodapp, R. and Zigler, E. (1995). Past, present and future issues in the developmental approach to mental retardation and developmental disabilities. In D. Cicchetti and D. Cohen (Eds.), *Developmental Psychopathology: Vol. 2. Risk, Disorder and Adaptation* (pp. 299–331). New York: Wiley.

Hogg, J. (1975). Behaviour modification on mental handicap. *Royal Society of Health Journal*, December issue (n.p.).

Hollien, H. and Copeland, R. (1965). Speaking fundamental frequency of mongoloid girls. *Journal of Speech and Hearing Disorders*, **30**, 344–349.

Hollis, J. and Sherman, J. (1967). *Operant Control of Vocalizations in Profoundly Retarded Children with Normal Hearing and Moderate Bilateral Loss.* Working paper N°. 167, Parsons Research Center, Parsons, KS.

Honjo, I. and Isshiki, N. (1980). Laryngoscopic and voice characteristics of aged persons. *Archives of Otolaryngology*, **106**, 149–152.

Hoogeveen, F., Birkhoff, A., Smeets, P., Lancioni, G. and Boelens, H. (1989). Establishing phonemic segmentation in moderately retarded children. *Remedial and Special Education*, **10**, 47–53.

Hooshyar, N. (1985). Language interaction between mothers and their non–handicapped children. *International Journal of Rehabilitation Research*, **4**, 475–477.

Hooshyar, N. (1987). The relationship between maternal language parameters and the child's language constancy and developmental condition. *International Journal of Rehabilitation Research*, **10**, 321–324.

Hopper, P. and Thompson, S. (1980). Transitivity in grammar and discourse. *Language*, **56**, 251–299.

Horel, J. (1994). Local and global perception examined by reversible suppression of temporal cortex with cold. *Behavioral Brain Research*, **65**, 157–164.

Hresko, W., Reid, D. and Hammill, D. (1981). *Test of Early Language Development.* Austin, TX: Pro–Ed.

Huang, H. and Hanley, J. (1994). Phonological awareness and visual skills in learning to read Chinese and English. *Cognition*, **54**, 73–98.

Hulme, C. and MacKenzie, S. (1992). *Working Memory and Severe Learning Difficulties.* Hove: Erlbaum.

Hurford, J. (1991). The evolution of the critical period for language acquisition. *Cognition*, **40**, 159–201.

Hurst, J., Baraitser, M., Anger, E., Graham, F. and Norell, S. (1990). An extended family with a dominantly inherited speech disorder. *Developmental Medicine and Child Neurology*, **32**, 352–355.

Huston–Stein, A. and Baltes, P. (1976). Theory and method in life–span developmental psychology: Implications for child development. In H. Reese (Ed.), *Advances in Child Development and Behavior* (Vol. 11, pp. 169–188). New York: Academic Press.

Huttenlocher, J. (1975). Synaptic and dendritic development and mental deficits. In N. Buchwald and M. Brazier (Eds.), *Brain Mechanisms in Mental Retardation* (pp. 123–140). New York: Academic.

Hyman, B. (1992). Down's syndrome and Alzheimer disease. In L. Nadel and C. Epstein (Eds.), *Down's syndrome and Alzheimer disease. Progress in Biological Research* (Vol. 379, pp. 123–142). New York: Wiley–Liss.

Imagier Larousse pour Enfants (1982). Paris: Larousse.

Ingram, D. (1974). Phonological rules in young children. *Journal of Child Language*, **1**, 49–64.

Ingram, D. (1976). *Phonological Disability in Children*. London: Arnold.

Ingram, D. (1989). *First Language Acquisition. Method, Description and Explanation*. New York: Cambridge University Press.

Inhelder, B. (1944). *Le Diagnostic du raisonnement chez les débiles mentaux*. Neuchâtel: Delachaux et Niestlé.

Inhelder, B. (1968). *The Diagnosis of Reasoning in the Mentally Retarded*. New York: Day.

Irigaray, L. (1973). *Le Langage des déments*. The Hague: Mouton.

Itard, J. (1801, 1964). *Mémoire sur les premiers développements de Victor de l'Aveyron*. Paris. (Reprinted in L. Malson, *Les Enfants sauvages, mythe et réalité*, Paris, Union Générale d'Editions.)

Itard, J. (1807). *Rapport sur les nouveaux développements de Victor de l'Aveyron*. Unpublished manuscript, Paris.

Ivanov–Smolensky, A. (1951). Les interactions du premier et du second système de signalisation dans quelques conditions physiologiques et pathologiques. *La Raison*, **2**, 54–67.

Jacobs, P., Baikie, A., Court–Brown, W. and Strong, J. (1959). The somatic chromosomes in mongolism. *Lancet*, **1**, 710–711.

Jacobson, J. and Mulick, J. (1993, Summer). Behavior modification and technologies. Walkin' the walk: APA takes a step forward in professional practice. *Psychology in Mental Retardation and Developmental Disabilities, Division 33 of American Psychological Association*, **19**, (1), 4–8.

Jakobson, R. (1941, 1968). *Kindersprache, Aphasie, und Allgemeine Lautgesetze*. Uppsala: Almqvist and Wiksell (English trans: *Child Language, Aphasia and Phonological Universals*, The Hague, Mouton).

Jakobson, R., Fant, C. and Halle, M. (1963). *Preliminaries to Speech Analysis: The Distinctive Features and their Correlates*. Cambridge, MA: MIT Press.

Jakobson, R. and Halle, M. (1956). *Fundamentals of Language*. The Hague: Mouton.

Jarvik, K. (1962). Biological differences in intellectual functioning. *Vita Humana*, **5**, 195–203.

Jellinger, J. (1972). Neuropsychological features in unclassified mental retardation. In J. Cavanaugh (Ed.), *The Brain in Unclassified Mental Retardation* (pp. 293–306). Baltimore, MD: Williams and Wilkins.

Jenkins, E., Duncan, C., Wright, C., Giordano, F., Wilbur, L. Wisniewski, K., Sklower, S., French, J., Jones, C. and Brown, W. (1983). Atypical Down's syndrome and partial trisomy 21. *Clinical Genetics*, **24**, 97–102.

Jenkins, J. (1965). Mediation theory and grammatical behavior. In S. Rosenberg (Ed.), *New Directions in Psycholinguistics* (pp. 48–72). New York: Macmillan.

Jenkins, J. and Palermo, D. (1964). Mediation processes and the acquisition of linguistic structure. In U. Bellugi and R. Brown (Eds.), *The Acquisition of Language. Monographs of the Society for Research in Child Development*, **29**, 141–169.

Jernigan, T. (1992, June). *Cerebral Morphological Distinctions between Williams and Down's Syndromes.* Paper presented at the Symposium 'Two genetic syndromes of contrasting cognitive profiles: A neuropsychological and neurobiological dissection' of the American Psychological Society, San Diego, CA.

Jernigan, T., Bellugi, U., Sowell, E., Doherty, S. and Hesselink, J. (1993). Cerebral morphologic distinctions between Williams and Down's syndromes. *Archives of Neurology*, **50**, 186–191.

Johnson, H. (1975). The meaning of before and after for preschool children. *Journal of Experimental Child Psychology*, **19**, 88–99.

Johnson, J. and Newport, E. (1991). Critical period effects on universal properties of language: The status of subjacency in the acquisition of a second language. *Cognition*, **39**, 215–258.

Johnson, P. and Farrel, M. (1954). Auditory impairments among resident school children at the Walter E. Fernald State School. *American Journal of Mental Deficiency*, **58**, 640–643.

Johnson, R. and Abelson, R. (1969). Intellectual, behavioral and physical characteristics associated with trisomy, translocation and mosaic types of Down's syndrome. *American Journal of Mental Deficiency*, **73**, 852–855.

Johnson, W. and Darley, F. and Spriesterbach, D. (1963). *Diagnostic Methods in Speech Pathology.* New York: Harcourt, Brace and World.

Johnston, J. (1988). Specific language disorders in the child. In N. Lass, L. McReynolds, J. Northern and D. Yoder (Eds.), *Handbook of Speech Pathology and Audiology* (pp. 268–298). Philadelphia: Decker.

Jones, H. (1963). *An Investigation to Determine the Validity of Voice Quality as a Criterion of Mongolism.* Unpublished master's thesis, Louisiana State University, Baton Rouge, LA.

Jones, K. (1990). Williams syndrome: An historical perspective of its evolution, natural history and etiology. *American Journal of Medical Genetics Supplement*, **6**, 89–96.

Jones, K. and Smith, D. (1975). The Williams elfin facies syndrome: A new perspective. *Journal of Pediatrics*, **86**, 718–723.

Jones, O. (1977). Mother–child communication with prelinguistic Down's syndrome and normal infants. In H. Schaffer (Ed.), *Studies in Mother–Infant Interaction* (pp. 126–149). New York: Academic.

Jones, S. and Moss, H. (1971). Age, state and maternal behavior associated with infant vocalizations. *Child Development*, **42**, 1039–1051.

Kahn, J. (1975). Relationship of Piaget's sensorimotor period to language acquisition of profoundly retarded children. *American Journal of Mental Deficiency*, **79**, 640–643.

Kamhi, A. and Johnston, J. (1982). Toward an understanding of retarded children's linguistic deficiencies. *Journal of Speech and Hearing Research*, **25**, 435–445.

Kanner, L. (1943). Autistic disturbances of affective contact. *Nervous Child*, **2**, 217–250.

Kanner, L. (1960). Itard, Seguin, Howe. Three pioneers in the education of retarded children. *American Journal of Mental Deficiency*, **65**, 2–10.

Kanner, L. (1964). *A History of the Care and Study of the Mentally Retarded.* Springfield, IL: Thomas.

Karlin, I. and Strazzulla, M. (1952). Speech and language problems of mentally deficient children. *Journal of Speech Disorders*, **17**, 286–294.

Karmiloff–Smith, A. (1979). *A Functional Approach to Child Language*. Cambridge: Cambridge University Press.

Kaufman, A. and Kaufman, N. (1983). *Kaufman Assessment Battery for Children*. Cercle Pines, MN: American Guidance Service.

Kausler, D. and Hakami, M. (1983). Memory for topics of conversation: Adult age differences and intentionality experiments. *Ageing Research*, **9**, 153–157.

Kawabata, S., Higgins, G. and Gordon, J. (1991). Amyloid plaques, neurofibrillary tangles and neuronal loss in brain of transgenic mice overexpressing a C–terminal fragment of human amyloid precursor protein. *Nature*, **354**, 476–478.

Kay, D. and Anglin, J. (1982). Overextension and underextension in the child's expressive and receptive speech. *Journal of Child Language*, **9**, 83–98.

Keane, V. (1972). The incidence of speech and language problems. *Mental Retardation*, **10**, 3–8.

Keenan, E. (1977). Making it last. Uses of repetition in children's discourse. In S. Ervin–Tripp and C. Mitchell-Kernan (Eds.), *Child Discourse* (pp. 125–138). New York: Springer.

Keil, F. (1989). *Concepts, Kinds and Cognitive Development*. Cambridge, MA: MIT Press.

Keilman, P. and Moran, L. (1967). Association structures of mental retardates. *Multivariate Behavioral Research*, **2**, 35–45.

Keiser, H., Montague, J., Wold, D., Mann, S. and Pattison, D. (1981). Hearing loss of Down's syndrome adults. *American Journal of Mental Deficency*, **85**, 467–472.

Kelley, K. (1990, August). *Language Intervention for Children with Williams Syndrome*. Communication presented at the meeting of the National Williams Syndrome Conference, Boston, MA.

Kemper, T. (1988). Neuropathology of Down's syndrome. In L. Nadel (Ed.), *The Psychobiology of Down's Syndrome* (pp. 269–289). Cambridge, MA: MIT Press.

Kempler, D., Curtiss, S. and Jackson, C. (1987). Syntactic preservation in Alzheimer's disease. *Journal of Speech and Hearing Research*, **30**, 343–350.

Kent, R. and Miolo, G. (1995). Phonetic abilities in the first year of life. In P. Fletcher and B. MacWhinney (Eds.), *The Handbook of Child Language* (pp. 303–334). Oxford: Blackwell.

Kernan, K. (1990). Comprehension of syntactically indicated sequence by Down's syndrome and other mentally retarded adults. *Journal of Mental Deficiency Research*, **34**, 169–178.

Kersner, M. (1992). *Test of Voice, Speech and Language*. London: Whurr.

Kertesz, A. (1980). *The Western Aphasia Battery*. London, Ontario: The University of Western Ontario Press.

Kimura, D. (1961). Some effects of temporal lobe damage on auditory perception. *Canadian Journal of Psychology*, **15**, 156–165.

Kimura, D. (1992). Sex differences in the brain. *Scientific American*, September, 119–125.

Kinsbourne, M. and Hicks, R. (1978). Functional cerebral space: A model for overflow, transfer and interference effects in human performance. In J. Requin (Ed.), *Attention and Performance* (Vol. 7, pp. 345–362). New York: Academic.

Kirk, S. and Kirk, W. (1974). *Psycholinguistic Learning Disabilities: Diagnosis and Remediation*. Urbana, IL: University of Illinois Press.

Klee, T. and Fitzgerald, M. (1985). The relation between grammatical development and mean length of utterances in morphemes. *Journal of Child Language*, **12**, 251–269.

Klein, N. and Safford, P. (1977). Application of Piaget's theory to the study of thinking of the mentally retarded: A review of research. *Journal of Special Education*, **11**, 201–216.

Klink, M., Gorstman, L. Raphael, L. Schlanger, B. and Newsome, L. (1986). Phonological process usage by young EMR children and non–retarded preschool children. *American Journal of Mental Deficiency*, **91**, 190–195.

Knox, C. and Kimura, D. (1970). Cerebral processing of non–verbal sounds in boys and girls. *Neuropsychologia*, **8**, 227–237.

Kodman, F. (1958). The incidence of hearing loss in mentally retarded children. *American Journal of Mental Deficiency*, **62**, 675–678.

Koenig, O., Wetzel, C. and Caramazza, A. (1992). Evidence for different types of lexical representations in the cerebral hemispheres. *Cognitive Neuropsychology*, **9**, 33–45.

Kolstoe, O. (1958). Language training of low grade mongoloid children. *American Journal of Mental Deficiency*, **63**, 117–130.

Konopczynski, G. (1986). *Du prélangage au langage: Acquisition de la structure prosodique*. Unpublished doctoral dissertation, University of Strasbourg.

Kosslyn, S. (1980). *Image and Mind*. Cambridge, MA: Harvard University Press.

Kotkin, R., Simpson, A. and Desanto, D. (1978). The effect of sign language on picture naming in two retarded girls possessing normal hearing. *Journal of Mental Deficiency Research*, **22**, 9–25.

Koulischer, L. and Gillerot, Y. (1980). Down's syndrome in Wallonia (South Belgium), 1971–78. Cytogenetics and incidence. *Human Genetics*, **54**, 243–250.

Koulischer, L. and Gillerot, Y. (1984). Epidemiology of Down's syndrome in Wallonia (South Belgium). Recent data (1979–1981). In J. Berg (Ed.), *Perspectives and Progress in Mental Retardation* (Vol. 2, pp. 39–45). Baltimore, MD: University Park Press.

Kounin, J. (1941a). Experimental studies of rigidity: I. The measurement of rigidity in normal and feeble–minded persons. *Character and Personality*, **9**, 251–272.

Kounin, J. (1941b). Experimental studies of rigidity: II. The explanatory power of the concept of rigidity as applied to feeble–mindedness. *Character and Personality*, **9**, 273–282.

Kowall, N., Beal, M., Busciglio, J., Duffy, L. and Yankner, B. (1991). An in vivo model for the neurodegenerative effects of d amyloid and protection by substance P. *Proceedings of the National Academy of Sciences of the United States of America*, **88**, 7247–7251.

Kramer, C. (1974). Women's speech: separate but unequal? *Quarterly Journal of Speech*, **60**, 14–24.

Krashen, S. (1973). Mental abilities underlying linguistic and non–linguistic functions. *Linguistics*, **115**, 39–55.

Krashen, S. (1975). The critical period for language acquisition and its possible basis. In D. Aaronson and R. Rieber (Eds.), *Developmental Psycholinguistics and Communication Disorders. Annals of the New York Academy of Sciences*, **263**, 211–224.

Lackner, J. (1968). A developmental study of language behavior in retarded children. *Neuropsychologia*, **6**, 301–320.

Lai, F. and Williams, R. (1989). A prospective study of Alzheimer disease in Down's syndrome. *Archives of Neurology*, **46**, 849–853.

Lambert, J. L. and Rondal, J. A. (1980). *Le Mongolisme*. Brussels: Mardaga.

Langacker, R. (1987). *Foundations of Cognitive Grammar*. Stanford, CA: Stanford University Press.

Larmat, J. (1979). *La Génétique de l'intelligence*. Paris: Presses Universitaires de France.

Lashley, K. (1930). Basic neural mechanisms in behavior, *Psychological Review*, **37**, 1–24.

Lasnik, H. (1989). On certain substitutes for negative data. In R. Matthews and W. Demopoulos (Eds.), *Learnability and Linguistic Theory* (pp. 89–105). Boston, MA: Kluwer.

La Veck, B. and La Veck, G. (1977). Sex differences in development among young children with Down's syndrome. *The Journal of Pediatrics*, **91**, 767–769.

Layton, T. and Sharifi, H. (1979). Meaning and structure of Down's syndrome and non–retarded children spontaneous speech. *American Journal of Mental Deficiency*, **83**, 139–445.

Leblanc, R. and Page, J. (1989). Autisme infantile précoce. In J. A. Rondal and X. Seron (Eds.), *Troubles du langage. Diagnostic et rééducation* (pp. 299–324). Brussels: Mardaga.

Lebrun, Y. (1992). The language of epilepsy. *Seizure*, **1**, 207–212.

Lebrun, Y. and Van Borsel, J. (1991). Final sound repetitions. *Journal of Fluency Disorders*, **15**, 107–113.

Lee, L. (1975). *Developmental Sentence Analysis*. Boston, MA: Northwestern University Press.

Légé, Y. and Dague, P. (1974). *Test de Vocabulaire en Images*. Paris: Editions du Centre de Psychologie Appliquée.

Lehrke, R. (1974). X–linked mental retardation and verbal ability. *Birth Defects Original Article Series*, **10**, 1–100.

Leifer, J. and Lewis, M. (1983). Acquisition of conversational response skills by young Down's syndrome and non–retarded young children. *American Journal of Mental Deficiency*, **88**, 610–618.

Leiner, H., Leiner, A. and Dow, R. (1986). Does the cerebellum contribute to mental skills? *Behavioral Neuroscience*, **100**, 443–454.

Lejeune, J., Gautier, M. and Turpin, R. (1959). Etudes des chromosomes somatiques de neuf enfants mongoliens. *Comptes rendus de l'Académie des Sciences* de Paris, **248**, 1721–1722.

Lejeune, J., Turpin, R. and Gauthier, M. (1959). Le mongolisme, premier exemple d'aberration autosomique humaine. *L'Année Génétique*, **2**, 41–49.

Lemperle, G. and Radu, D. (1980). Facial plastic surgery in children with Down's syndrome. *Plastic and Reconstruction Surgery*, **66**, 337–342.

Lenneberg, E. (1964). Language disorders in childhood: Mental retardation. *Harvard Educational Review*, **34**, 156–160.

Lenneberg, E. (1966). A biological perspective on language. In E. Lenneberg (Ed.), *New Directions in the Study of Language* (pp. 65–88). Cambridge, MA: MIT Press.

Lenneberg, E. (1967). *Biological Foundations of Language*. New York: Wiley.

Lenneberg E. (1975, February). Personal communication.

Lenneberg, E., Nichols, I. and Rosenberger, E. (1964). Primitive stages of language development in mongolism. In D. McRioch and E. Weinstein (Eds.), *Disorders of Communication. Proceedings of the Association for Research in Nervous and Mental Disease* (Vol. 17, pp. 119–137). Baltimore, MD: Williams and Wilkins.

Lenneberg, E., Rebelski, F. and Nichols, I. (1965). The vocalizations of infants born to deaf and to hearing parents. *Human Development*, **8**, 23–37.

Leonard, L. (1985). Unusual and subtle phonological behavior in the speech of phonologically disordered children. *Journal of Speech and Hearing Disorders*, **50**, 4–13.

Leonard, L. (1992). The use of morphology by children with specific language impairment: Evidence from three languages. In R. Chapman (Ed.), *Processes in Language Acquisition and Disorders*. (pp. 48–65). Chicago: Mosby–Yearbook.

Leonard, L. and Brown, B. (1984). The nature and boundaries of phonological categories: A case study of an unusual phonologic pattern in a language–impaired child. *Journal of Speech and Hearing Disorders*, 49, 419–428.

Leonard, L. Schwartz, R., Swanson, L. and Frome–Loeb, D. (1987). Some conditions that promote unusual phonological behaviour in children. *Clinical Linguistics and Phonetics*, 1, 23–34.

Levelt, W. (1989). *Speaking: From Intention to Articulation*. Cambridge, MA: MIT Press.

Levinson, A., Friedman, A. and Stamps, F. (1955). Variability of mongolism. *Pediatrics*, 16, 43–49.

Levitas, A., McBogg, P. and Hagerman, R. (1983). Behavioral dysfunction in the fragile X syndrome. In R. Hagerman and P. McBogg (Eds.), *The Fragile X Syndrome: Diagnosis, Biochemistry and Intervention* (pp. 153–173). Dillon, CO: Spectra.

Lewis, M. and Freedle, R. (1973). Mother–infant dyad: The cradle of meaning. In P. Pliner, L. Kramer and J. Alloway (Eds.), *Communication and Affect: Language and Thought* (pp. 127–155). New York: Academic Press.

Ley, J. (1929). Un cas d'audi–mutité idiopathique (aphasie congénitale) chez des jumeaux monozygotiques. *Encéphale*, 24, 121–165.

Liberman, A. and Mattingly, I. (1985). The motor theory of speech perception revised. *Cognition*, 21, 1–36.

Liberman, A. and Mattingly, I. (1989). A specialization for speech perception. *Science*, 243, 489–494.

Light, D. and Albertson, S. (1990). Comprehension of pragmatic implications in young and older adults. In D. Burke and L. Light (Eds.), *Language Memory and Ageing* (pp. 174–189). Cambridge: Cambridge University Press.

Light, L. Zelinsky, E. and Moore, M. (1982). Adult age differences in reasoning from new information. *Journal of Experimental Psychology: Learning, Memory and Cognition*, 8, 435–447.

Light, P. Remington, R., Clarke, S. and Watson, J. (1989). Signs of language. In M. Beveridge, G. Conti–Ramsden and Y. Leudar (Eds.), *Language and Communication in Mentally Handicapped People* (pp. 57–59). London: Chapman and Hall.

Light, P., Watson, J. and Remington, R. (1990). Beyond the single sign. II: The significance of sign order in a matrix–based approach to teaching productive sign combinations. *Mental Handicap Research*, 3, 161–178.

Linville, S. (1977). Signed English: A language teaching technique with totally non–verbal, severely mentally retarded adolescents. *Language, Speech and Hearing Services in Schools*, 8, 170–175.

Lipman, R. (1963). Learning: verbal, perceptual–motor and classical conditioning. In N. Ellis (Ed.), *Handbook of Mental Deficiency* (pp. 391–423). New York: McGraw–Hill.

Lipp, J., Myers, G., Graham, E. and Bell, B. (1983). Correlates of intelligence and adaptive behavior in Down's syndrome. *Journal of Mental Deficiency Research*, 27, 205–210.

Lloyd, K., Russel, H. and Garmize, L. (1970). Operant eyelid conditioning in trisomy 18: Replication and extension. *Journal of Abnormal Psychology*, 75, 338–341.

Lloyd, L. (Ed.) (1976). *Communication Assessment and Intervention Strategies*. Baltimore, MD: University Park Press.

Lloyd, L. and Reid, M. (1965). Audiometric studies of mentally retarded subjects: 1951 to present. In L. Lloyd and D. Frisina (Eds.), *The Audiologic Assessment of the Mentally Retarded* (pp. 299–314). Parsons, KS: State Hospital and Training Center.

Locke, J. (1988). The sound shape of early lexical representations. In M. Smith and J. Locke (Eds.), *The Emergent Lexicon* (pp. 3–22). New York: Academic.

Lomonte, V. (1995). *Acquisition de l'ordre des mots chez l'enfant trisomique 21.* Unpublished master's thesis, University of Liège, Belgium.

Lott, I. (1986). The neurology of Down's syndrome. In C. Epstein (Ed.), *The Neurobiology of Down's Syndrome* (pp. 17–27). New York: Raven Press.

Lott, I. (1992). The neurology of Alzheimer's disease in Down's syndrome. *Progress in Clinical Biological Research,* **379,** 1–14.

Lovaas, I. (1987). Behavioral treatment and normal educational and intellectual functioning in young autistic children. *Journal of Consulting and Clinical Psychology,* **55,** 3–9.

Lovelace, E. (Ed.) (1990). *Ageing and Cognition: Mental Processes, Self Awareness and Interventions.* Amsterdam: Elsevier.

Lovelace, E. and Twohig, P. (1990). Healthy older adults' perceptions of their memory functioning and use of mnemonics. *Bulletin of the Psychonomic Society,* **29,** 33–35.

Lovell, K. and Bradbury, B. (1967). The learning of English morphology in educationally subnormal special school children. *American Journal of Mental Deficiency,* **71,** 609–615.

Lovell, K. and Dixon, E.M. (1967). The growth of the control of grammar in imitation, comprehension and production. *Journal of Child Psychology and Psychiatry,* **8,** 31–39.

Lovell, K., Hersee, D. and Preston, B. (1969). A study of some aspects of language development in educationally subnormal pupils. *Journal of Special Education,* **3,** 275–284.

Lozar, B., Wepman, J. and Hass, W. (1972). Lexical use of mentally retarded and non-retarded children. *American Journal of Mental Deficiency,* **76,** 534–539.

Luckasson, R., Coulter, D., Polloway, E., Reiss, S., Schalock, R., Snell, M., Spitalnik D. and Stark, J. (1992). *Mental Retardation: Definition, Classification and Systems of Supports.* Washington, DC: American Association on Mental Retardation

Luria, A.R. (1956). *Problems with the Higher Nervous Activity in Normal and Abnormal Children* (Vol. 1). Moscow: Academy of Pedagogical Sciences Press.

Luria, A. (1959). The directive function of speech, I: Its development in early childhood; II: Its dissolution in pathological states of the brain. *Word,* **15,** 341–352, 453–464.

Luria, A.R. (1961). *The Role of Speech in the Regulation of Normal and Abnormal Behaviour.* London: Pergamon.

Luria, A.R. (1963). *The Mentally Retarded Child.* London: Pergamon.

Luria, A. (1966a). *Higher Cortical Functions in Man.* New York: Consultants Bureau.

Luria, A. (1966b). *Human Brain and Psychological Processes.* New York: Harper and Row.

Luria, A. and Vinogradova, O. (1959). An objective investigation of the dynamics of semantic systems. *British Journal of Psychology,* **50,** 89–105.

Luria, A. and Yudovich, F. (1959). *Speech and the Development of Mental Processes in the Child.* London: Staple Press.

Lutzker, J. and Sherman, J. (1974). Producing generative sentence usage by imitation and reinforcement procedures. *Journal of Applied Behavior Analysis,* **7,** 447–460.

Lyle, J. (1959). The effect of an institutional environment upon the verbal development of institutionalized children. *Journal of Mental Deficiency Research*, 3, 122–128.

Lyle, J. (1960a). The effect of an institutional environment upon the verbal development of institutionalized children, II: Speech and language. *Journal of Mental Deficiency Research*, 4, 1–28.

Lyle, J. (1960b). Some factors affecting the speech development of imbecile children in an institution. *Journal of Child Psychology and Psychiatry*, 2, 121–129.

Lyle, J. (1961a). Comparison of the language of normal and imbecile children. *Journal of Mental Deficiency Research*, 5, 40–50.

Lyle, J. (1961b). A comparison of the verbal intelligence of normal and imbecile children. *Journal of Genetic Psychology*, 99, 237–244.

Lynch, J. and Bricker, W. (1972). Linguistic theory and operant procedures: Toward an integrated approach to language training for the mentally retarded. *Mental Retardation*, 10, 12–17.

Lynch, M., Oller, D., Steffens, M. and Buder, E. (in press). Phrasing in prelinguistic vocalizations. *Developmental Psychology*.

Lynch, M., Oller, D., Steffens, M., Levine, S., Basinger, D. and Umbel, V. (in press). The onset of speech–like vocalizations in infants with Down's syndrome. *American Journal on Mental Retardation*.

Maccoby, E. and Jacklin, C. (1974). *The Psychology of Sex Differences*. Stanford, CA: Stanford University Press.

MacDonald, G. and Roy, D. (1988). Williams syndrome: A neuropsychological profile. *Journal of Clinical and Experimental Neuropsychology*, 10, 125–131.

Macken, M. and Ferguson, C. (1983). Cognitive aspects of phonological development: Model, evidence and issues. In K. Nelson (Ed.), *Children's Language* (Vol. 4, pp. 255–282). Hillsdale, NJ: Erlbaum.

MacKenzie, S. and Hulme, C. (1987). Memory span development in Down's syndrome, severely subnormal and normal subjects. *Cognitive Neuropsychology*, 4, 303–319.

MacMillan, D., Gresham, F. and Siperstein, G. (1993). Conceptual and psychometric concerns about the 1992 AAMR definition of mental retardtion. *American Journal on Mental Retardation*, 98, 325–335.

MacWhinney, B. (1987). The competition model. In B. MacWhinney (Ed.), *Mechanisms of Language Acquisition* (pp. 249–308). Hilldsdale, NJ: Erlbaum.

MacWhinney, B. (1991). *The CHILDES Project: Computational Tools for Analysing Talk*. Hillsdale, NJ: Erlbaum.

Madison, L. George, C. and Moeschler, J. (1986). Cognitive functioning in the fragile–X syndrome: A study of intellectual, memory and communication skills. *Journal of Mental Deficiency Research*, 30, 129–148.

Mahoney, G. (1988). Maternal communication style with mentally retarded children. *American Journal on Mental Retardation*, 92, 352–359.

Mahoney, G., Glover, A. and Finger, I. (1981). Relationship between language and sensorimotor development of Down's syndrome and nonretarded children. *American Journal of Mental Deficiency*, 86, 21–27.

Malec, J., Ivnik, R. and Smith, G. (1993). Neuropsychology and normal ageing: The clinician's perspective. In R. Parks, R. Zec and R. Wilson (Eds.), *Neuropsychology of Alzheimer's Disease and other Dementia* (pp. 81–111). New York: Oxford University Press.

Malone, Q. (1988). Mortality and survival of the Down's syndrome population in Western Australia. *Journal of Mental Deficiency Research*, 32, 59–65.

Malson, L. (1964). *Les Enfants sauvages, mythe et réalité*. Paris: Union Générale d'Editions.

Malzberg, B. (1953). Sex differences in the prevalence of mental deficiency. *America Journal of Mental Deficiency*, **58**, 301–305.

Mann, D. (1988). The pathological association between Down's syndrome and Alzheimer disease. *Mechanisms of Ageing and Development*, **43**, 99–136.

Mann, D. and Esiri, M. (1988). The site of the earliest lesions of Alzheimer's disease. *New England Journal of Medicine*, **318**, 789–790.

Marans, W., Paul, R. and Leckman, J. (1987, May). *Speech and Language Profiles in Males with Fragile X Syndrome*. Paper presented at the Annual Convention of the American Speech and Hearing Association, New Orleans, LA.

Maranto, C., Decuir, A. and Humphrey, T. (1984). A comparison of digit span scores, rhythm span scores and diagnostic factors of mentally retarded persons. *Music Therapy*, **4**, 84–90.

Maratsos, M. (1982). The child's construction of grammatical categories. In E. Wanner and L. Gleitman (Eds.), *Language Acquisition: The State of the Art* (pp. 240–266). New York: Cambridge University Press.

Maratsos, M. and Chalkley, M. (1981). The internal language of children's syntax: The ontogenesis and representation of syntactic categories. In K. Nelson (Ed.), *Children's Language* (Vol. 2, pp. 127–214). New York: Gardner Press.

Maratsos, M., Fox, D., Becker, J. and Chalkley, M. (1985). Semantic restrictions on children's passives. *Cognition*, **19**, 167–191.

Marcell, M. and Armstrong, V. (1982). Auditory and visual sequential memory of Down's syndrome and nonretarded children. *American Journal of Mental Deficiency*, **87**, 86–95.

Marcell, M. and Weeks, S. (1988). Short–term memory difficulties and Down's syndrome. *Journal of Mental Deficiency Research*, **32**, 153–162.

Marcus, G. (1993). Negative evidence in language acquisition. *Cognition*, **46**, 53–85.

Margar–Bacal, M., Witzel, M. and Muaro, L. (1988). Inteligibilidad del habla despues de la glosectomia parcial en niños con sindrome de Down. *Sindrome de Down*, **3**, 1–4 (reproduced from *Plastic and Reconstructive Surgery*, 1987, **79**, 44–47).

Marinosson, G. (1974). Performance profiles of matched normal, educationally subnormal and severely subnormal children on the revised ITPA. *Journal of Child Psychology and Psychiatry*, **15**, 139–148.

Markowitz, J. (1976, June). *The Acquisition of Spatial Adjectives in their Nominal Comparative and Superlative Forms among Moderately Retarded Children*. Paper presented at the 100th Annual Meeting of the American Association on Mental Deficiency, Chicago.

Marshall, J. (1984). Multiple perspectives on modularity. *Cognition*, **17**, 29–242.

Marshall, J. (1990). Foreword to J. Yamada, *Laura. A Case for the Modularity of Language* (pp. VII–XI). Cambridge, MA: MIT Press.

Martin, A. (1987). Representations of semantic and spatial knowledge in Alzheimer's patients: Implications for models of preserved learning and amnesia. *Journal of Clinical and Experimental Neuropsychology*, **9**, 121–124.

Martin, N., Snodgrass B. and Cohen, R. (1984). Ideopathic infantile hypercalcemia – a continuing enigma. *Archives of Disease in Childhood*, **59**, 605–613.

Martinez–Frias, M.–L. (1992). Estudio de la frecuencia del sindrome de Down en España. *Sindrome de Down*, **13**, 1–7.

Matson, J. and Adkins, J. (1980). A self–instructional social skills training program for mentally retarded persons. *Mental Retardation*, **18**, 245–248.

Mattingly, I. and Studdert–Kennedy M. (Eds.) (1991). *Modularity and the Motor Theory of Speech Perception*. Hillsdale, NJ: Erlbaum.

Maurer, H. and Sherrod, K. (1987). Context of directives given to young children with Down's syndrome and non–retarded children. *American Journal of Mental Deficiency*, **91**, 579–590.

Maxim, J. (1982). Language change with increasing age. In M. Edwards (Ed.), *Communication Changes in Elderly People* (pp. 126–148). London: College of Speech Therapists, Monograph N°. 3.

Maxim, J. and Bryan, K. (1994). *Language of the Elderly: A Clinical Perspective*. London: Whurr.

Mayberry, R. (1984, November). *Early and Late Learning of Sign Language: Processing Patterns*. Paper presented at the American Speech-Language-Hearing Association Annual Convention, San Francisco, CA.

Mayberry, R., Fisher, S. and Hatfield, N. (1983). Sentence repetition in American Sign Language. In J. Kyle and B. Woll (Eds.), *Language in Sign: International Perspective on Sign Language* (pp. 206–214). London: Croom Helm.

Mayer, M. (1969). Frogs, Where Are You? New York: Dial Press.

McAlaster, R. (1992). Postnatal cerebral maturation in Down's syndrome children: A developmental EEG coherence study. *International Journal of Neuroscience*, **65**, 221–237.

McCarthy, D. (1930). *Language Development of the Preschool Child*. Institute of Child Welfare Monograph N°. 4. Minneapolis, MN: University of Minnesota Press.

McCarthy, D. (1952a). Le développement du langage. In L. Carmichael (Ed.), *Manuel de psychologie de l'enfant* (pp. 148–196). Paris: Presses Universitaires de France.

McCarthy, D. (1952b). Factors that influence language growth: Home influences. *Elementary English*, **29**, 421–428.

McCarthy, D. (1954). Language development in children. In L. Carmichael (Ed.), *Manual of Child Psychology* (pp. 492–630). New York: Wiley.

McCarthy, J. (1965). *Patterns of Psycholinguistic Development of Mongoloid and Non–mongoloid Severely Retarded Children*. Unpublished doctoral dissertation, University of Illinois, Urbana, IL.

McCarthy, J. and Kirk, S. (1961). *The Illinois Test of Psycholinguistic Abilities*. Urbana, IL: Institute for Research in Exceptional Children.

McCauley, C., Sperber, R. and Roaden, S. (1978). Verification of property statements by retarded and non–retarded adolescents. *American Journal of Mental Deficiency*, **83**, 276–282.

McGuigan, F. (1966). *Thinking: Studies of Covert Language Behavior*. New York: Appleton-Century-Crofts.

McKee, C. (1992). A comparison of pronouns and anaphors in Italian and English acquisition. *Language Acquisition*, **2**, 21–54.

McNamara, P., Obler, L., Au, R., Durso, R. and Albert, M. (1992). Speech monitoring skills in Alzheimer's disease, Parkinson's disease and normal ageing. *Brain and Language*, **42**, 38–51.

McNeil, D. (1966). A study of word association. *Journal of Verbal Learning and Verbal Behavior*, **5**, 548–557.

Mehler, J. (1963). Some effects of grammatical transformations on the recall of English sentences. *Journal of Verbal Learning and Verbal Behavior*, **2**, 346–351.

Mehler, J., Bertoncini, J., Barrière, M. and Jassik–Gerschenfeld, D. (1978). Infant recognition of mother's voice. *Perception*, **7**, 491–497.

Mehler, J. and Dupoux, E. (1990). *Naître humain*. Paris: Jacob.

Mehler, J., Jusczyk, P., Lambertz, G., Halsted, N., Bertoncini, J. and Amiel-Tison, C. (1988). A precursor of language acquisition in young infant. *Cognition*, **29**, 143–178.

Mehler, J., Lambertz, G., Jusczyk, P. and Amiel-Tison, C. (1987). Discrimination de la langue maternelle par le nouveau–né. *Comptes-rendus de l'Académie des Sciences de Paris*, **303**, 637–640.

Mein, R. (1961). A study of the oral vocabularies of severely subnormal patients: II. Grammatical analysis of speech samples. *Journal of Mental Deficiency Research*, **5**, 52–59.

Mein, R. and O'Connor, N. (1960). A study of the oral vocabularies of severely subnormal patients. *Journal of Mental Deficiency Research*, **4**, 130–143.

Melyn, M. and White, D. (1973). Mental and developmental milestones of non–institutionalized Down's syndrome children. *Pediatrics*, **52**, 542–545.

Menn, L. (1978). *Pattern, Control and Contrast in the Development of Word Form and Word Function*. Unpublished manuscript, Indiana University, Bloomington.

Menn, L. (1983). Development of articulatory phonetic and phonological capabilities. In B. Butterworth (Ed.), *Language Production* (Vol. 2, pp. 3–50). New York: Academic.

Menn, L. and C. Stoel-Gammon (1995). Phonological development. In P. Fletcher and B. MacWhinney (Eds.), *The Handbook of Child Language* (pp. 335–359). Oxford: Blackwell.

Menyuk, P. (1969). *Sentences Children Use*. Cambridge, MA: MIT Press.

Menyuk, P. (1977). *Language and Maturation*. Cambridge, MA: MIT Press.

Mervis, C. B. (1984). Early lexical development: The contributions of mother and child. In C. Sophian (Ed.), *Origins of Cognitive Skills* (pp. 339–370). Hillsdale, NJ: Erlbaum.

Mervis, C. B. (1988). Early lexical development. Theory and application. In L. Nadel (Ed.), *The Psychobiology of Down's Syndrome* (pp. 101–143). Cambridge, MA: MIT Press.

Mervis, C. B. (1990). Early conceptual development of children with Down's syndrome. In D. Cicchetti and M. Beeghly (Eds.), *Children with Down's Syndrome: A Developmental Perspective* (pp. 252–301). New York: Cambridge University Press.

Mesulam, M. (1987). Primary progressive aphasia-differentiation from Alzheimer's disease. *Annals of Neurology*, **22**, 533–534.

Meyers, L. (1988). Using computers to teach children with Down's syndrome spoken and written language skills. In L. Nadel (Ed.), *The Psychobiology of Down's Syndrome* (pp. 247–265). Cambridge, MA: MIT Press.

Meyerson, M. and Frank, R. (1987). Language, speech and hearing in Williams syndrome: Intervention approaches and research needs. *Developmental Medicine and Child Neurology*, **29**, 258–270.

Michaelis, C. (1976). The language of a Down's syndrome child. *Dissertation Abstracts International*, **37**, 416.

Michel, J. and Carney, R. (1964). Pitch characteristics of mongoloid boys. *Journal of Speech and Hearing Disorders*, **29**, 121–125.

Michelet, A. and Woodill, G. (1993). *Le Handicap dit mental*. Neuchâtel, Switzerland: Delachaux et Niestlé.

Miezejeski, C., Jenkins, E., Hill, A., Wisniewski, K., French, J. and Brown, W. (1986). Note: A profile of cognitive deficit in females from fragile X families. *Neuropsychologia*, **24**, 405–409.

Milgram, N. (1973). Cognition and language in mental retardation: Distinctions and implications. In D. Routh (Ed.), *The Experimental Psychology of Mental Retardation* (pp. 157–230). Chicago: Aldine.

Miller, G. and McKean, K. (1964). A chronometric study of some relations between sentences. *Quarterly Journal of Experimental Psychology*, **16**, 297–308.

Miller, J. (1981). *Assessing Language Production in Children: Experimental Procedures*. Baltimore, MD: University Park Press.

Miller, J. (1983). Identifying children with language disorders and describing their language performance. In J. Miller, D. Yoder and R. Schiefelbusch (Eds.), *Contemporary Issues in Language Intervention* (pp. 61–74). Rockville, MD: American Speech and Hearing Association.

Miller, J. (1988). The developmental asynchrony of language development in children with Down's syndrome. In L. Nadel (Ed.), *The Psychobiology of Down's Syndrome* (pp. 167–198). Cambridge, MA: MIT Press.

Miller, J. (1992). Lexical development in young children with Down's syndrome. In R. Chapman (Ed.), *Processes in Language Acquisition and Disorders* (pp. 202–216). St Louis, MI: Mosby.

Miller, J. and Chapman, R. (1981). The relation between age and mean length of utterances in morphemes. *Journal of Speech and Hearing Research*, **24**, 154–161.

Miller, J., Chapman, R., Branston, M. and Reichle, J. (1980). Language comprehension in sensorimotor stages V and VI. *Journal of Speech and Hearing Research*, **23**, 284–311.

Miller, J., Chapman, R. and Mackensie, H. (1981). Individual differences in the language acquisition of mentally retarded children. *Proceedings of the Second Wisconsin Symposium on Research in Child Language Disorders*, **2**, 130–147.

Miller, S., Shelton, J. and Flavell, J. (1970). A test of Luria's hypothesis concerning the development of verbal self–regulation. *Child Development*, **41**, 651–665.

Milner, B. (1974). Functional recovery after lesions of the nervous system. 3. Developmental processes in neural plasticity. Sparing of language functions after early unilateral brain damage. *Neuroscience Research Program Bulletin*, **12**, 213–217.

Mittler, P. (1970a). The use of morphological rules by four years old children: An item analysis of the Auditory–Vocal Automatic Test of the ITPA. *British Journal of Disorders of Communication*, **5**, 99–109.

Mittler, P. (1970b, May). *Comprehension of Spoken Language in Normal and Subnormal Children*. Communication to the Medical College Symposium, Royal Society of Medicine, London.

Moerk, E. (1975). Verbal interaction between children and their mothers during the preschool years. *Developmental Psychology*, **11**, 788–794.

Moerk, E. (1976). Processes of language teaching and language learning in the interactions of mother–child dyads. *Child Development*, **47**, 1064–1078.

Moerk, E. (1983). *The Mother of Eve as a First–language Teacher*. New York: Ablex.

Moerk, E. (1992). *First Language Taught and Learned*. Baltimore, MD: Brookes.

Molfese, D., Freeman, R. and Palermo, D. (1975). The ontogeny of brain lateralization for speech and non–speech stimuli. *Brain and Language*, **2**, 356–368.

Montague, J. and Hollien, H. (1973). Perceive voice quality disorders in Down's syndrome. *Training School Bulletin*, **71**, 80–89.

Morais, J., Alegria, J. and Content, A. (1987). The relationship between segmental analysis and alphabetic literacy: An interactive view. *Cahiers de Psychologie Cognitive*, **7**, 415–438.

Morais, J., Cary, L. Alegria, J. and Bertelson, P. (1979). Does awareness of speech as a sequence of phones arise spontaneously? *Cognition*, 7, 323–331.

Moran, M., Money, S. and Leonard, D. (1984). Phonological process analysis in the speech of mentally retarded adults. *American Journal of Mental Deficiency*, 89, 304–306.

Morel, P. (1859). *Traité théorique et pratique des maladies mentales*. Paris: Baillière.

Morris, C., Thomas, I. and Greenberg, F. (in press). Williams syndrome: Autosomal dominant inheritance. *American Journal of Medical Genetics*.

Moscovitch, M. and Umilta, C. (1990). Modularity and neuropsychology: Modules and central processes in attention and memory. In M. Schwartz (Ed.), *Modular Deficits in Alzheimer-type Dementia* (pp. 1–59). Cambridge, MA: MIT Press.

Mueller, M. and Weaver, S. (1964). Psycholinguistic abilities of institutionalized and non-institutionalized trainable mental retardates. *American Journal of Mental Deficiency*, 68, 775–783.

Mulley, J., Kerr, B., Stevenson, R. and Lubs, H. (1992). Nomenclature guidelines for X-linked mental retardation. *American Journal of Medical Genetics*, 43, 383–391.

Mundy, P., Seibert, J. and Hogan, A. (1984). Relationship between sensorimotor and early communication abilities in developmentally delayed children. *Merrill-Palmer Quarterly*, 30, 33–48.

Mundy, P., Sigman, M. and Kasari, C. (1990). A longitudinal study of joint attention and language development in autistic children. *Journal of Autism and Developmental Disorders*, 20, 115–128.

Mundy, P., Sigman, M., Kasari, C. and Yirmiya, N. (1988). Non–verbal communication skills in children with Down's syndrome. *Child Development*, 59, 235–249.

Mussen, P., Conger, J., Kagan, J. and Gewirtz, P. (1978). *Psychological Development: Life-span Approach*. New York: Harper and Row.

Muysken, P. (1988). Are creoles a special type of language? In F. Newmeyer (Ed.), *Linguistics: The Cambridge Survey* (Vol. 2, pp. 285–301). Cambridge: Cambridge University Press.

Nadel, L. (1986). Down syndrome in neurobiological perspective. In C. Epstein (Ed.), *The Neurobiology of Down Syndrome* (pp. 239–251). New York: Raven Press.

Nadel, L. (in press). Learning, memory and neural function in Down syndrome. In J. A. Rondal, J. Perera, L. Nadel and A. Comblain (Eds.), *Down Syndrome: Psychological, Psychobiological and Socio-educational Perspectives*. London: Whurr.

Nelson, K. (1973). Structure and strategy in learning to talk. *Monograph of the Society for Research in Child Development*, 38, 1–2, N°. 149.

Nelson, T., Lott, I., Touchette, P., Satz, P. and D'Elia, L. (1995). Detection of Alzheimer disease in individuals with Down syndrome. *American Journal of Mental Retardation*, 99, 616–622.

Netchine, G. (1969). Idiots, débiles et savants au XIXe siècle. In R. Zazzo (Ed.), *Les Débilités mentales* (pp. 70–107). Paris: Colin.

Neville, H., Mills, D. and Bellugi, U. (1993). Effects of altered auditory sensitivity and age of language acquisition on the development of language–relevant neural systems: Preliminary studies of Williams syndrome. In S. Broman and J. Grafman (Eds.), *Atypical Cognitive Deficits in Developmental Disorders: Implications for Brain Function* (pp. 67–83). Hillsdale, NJ: Erlbaum.

Newell, K., Sanborn, B. and Hagerman, R. (1983). Speech and language dysfunction in the fragile X syndrome. In R. Hagerman and P. McBogg (Eds.), *The Fragile X Syndrome: Diagnosis, Biochemistry and Intervention* (pp. 175–220). Dillon, CO: Spectra.

Newfield, M. and Schlanger, B. (1968). The acquisition of English morphology by normal and educable mentally retarded children. *Journal of Speech and Hearing Research*, 2, 693–708.

Newport, E. (1984). Constraints on learning. Studies in the acquisition of ASL. *Papers and Reports on Child Language Development* (Stanford University), 23, 1–22.

Newport, E. (1990). Maturational constraints on language learning. *Cognitive Science*, 14, 11–28.

Newport, E. (1992). Contrasting conception of the critical period for language. In S. Carey and R. Gelman (Eds.), *The Epigenesis of Mind: Essays on Biology and Cognition* (pp. 111–130). Hillsdale, NJ: Erlbaum.

Newport, E., Gleitman, L. and Gleitman, H. (1977). Mother, I'd rather do it myself: Some effects and non–effects of maternal speech style. In C. Snow and C. Ferguson (Eds.), *Talking to Children* (pp. 109–150). New York: Cambridge University Press.

Nicholson, A. and Alberman, E. (1982). Prediction of the number of Down's syndrome infants to be born in England and Wales up to the year 2000 and their likely survival rates. *Journal of Intellectual Disability Research*, 36, 505–517.

Noizet, G. and Pichevin, L. (1966). Organisation paradigmatique et organisation syntagmatique du discours: Une approche comparative. *L'Année Psychologique*, 61, 91–110.

Nolan Post, K. (1994). Negative evidence in the language learning environment of laterborns in a rural Florida community. In J. Sokolov and C. Snow (Eds.), *Handbook of Research in Language Development Using CHILDES* (pp. 132–153). Hillsdale, NJ: Erlbaum.

Nuccio, J. and Abbeduto, L. (1993). Dynamic contextual variables and the directives of persons with mental retardation. *American Journal of Mental Retardation*, 97, 547–558.

Nurss, J. and Day, D. (1971). Imitation, comprehension and production of grammatical structures. *Journal of Verbal Learning and Verbal Behavior*, 10, 68–74.

Oberlé, I., Rousseau, F., Heitz, D., Kretz, C., Devys, D., Hanauer, A., Boue, J., Bertheas, M. and Mandel, J. (1991). Instability of a 550–base pair DNA segment and abnormal methylation in fragile X syndrome. *Science*, 252, 1097–1110.

Obler, L. and Albert, M. (1981). Language and ageing: A neurobehavioral analysis. In D. Bedsley and G. Davis (Eds.), *Ageing Communication Processes and Disorders* (pp. 26–52). New York: Van Nostrand.

Obler, L. Mildworf, B. and Albert, M. (1977). *Writing Style in the Elderly*. Montreal: Academy of Aphasia Abstracts.

O'Connor, N. (Ed.). (1966). *Present-day Russian Psychology*. London: Pergamon.

O'Connor, N. and Hermelin, B. (1959a). Some effects of word learning in imbeciles. *Language and Speech*, 2, 63–71.

O'Connor, N. and Hermelin, B. (1959b). Discrimination and reversal learning in imbeciles. *Journal of Abnormal and Social Psychology*, 59, 409–413.

O'Connor, N. and Hermelin, B. (1963). *Speech and Thought in Severe Subnormality*. London: Macmillan.

O'Connor, N. and Hermelin, B. (1991). A specific linguistic ability. *American Journal on Mental Retardation*, 95, 673–680.

OECD (Office Européen de Coopération au Développement). (1988). *Ageing Populations: The Social Policy Implications. Demographic Change and Public Policy*. Paris: OECD.

Ogland, V. (1972). Language behavior of the educable mentally retarded children. *Mental Retardation*, 3, 30–32.

Olbrisch, R. (1985). Plastic and aesthetic surgery on children with Down's syndrome. *Aesthetic Plastic Surgery*, 9, 241–248.

Oliver, B. and Buckley, S. (1994). The language development of children with Down's syndrome: First words to two-word phrases. *Down's Syndrome*, 2, 71–75.

Oliver, C. and Holland, A. (1986). Down's syndrome and Alzheimer's disease: A review. *Psychological Medicine*, 16, 307–322.

Oller, K. (1990). The emergence of sounds in speech in infancy. In J. Yeni-Komshian, J. Kavanagh and C. Ferguson (Eds.), *Child Phonology* (Vol. 1, pp. 93–112). New York: Springer.

Oller, K. and Eilers, R. (1988). The role of audition in infant babbling. *Child Development*, 59, 441–449.

Oller, K. and Lynch, M. (1993). Infant vocalizations and innovations in infraphonology: Toward a broader theory of development and disorders. In C. Ferguson, L. Menn and C. Stoel-Gammon (Eds.), *Phonological Development* (pp. 509–536). Parkton, MD: York Press.

Omar, M. (1973). *The Acquisition of Egyptian Arabic as a Native Language*. The Hague: Mouton.

Orlando, R. and Bijou, S. (1960). Single and multiple schedules of reinforcement in developmentally retarded children. *Journal of Experimental Analysis of Behavior*, 3, 339–348.

Osgood, C. (1953). *Method and Theory in Experimental Psychology*. New York: Oxford University Press.

Osgood, C. (1957a). A behavioristic analysis of perception and language as cognitive phenomena. In C. Osgood (Ed.), *Contemporary Approaches to Cognition. The Colorado Symposium* (pp. 75–119). Cambridge, MA: Harvard University Press.

Osgood, C. (1957b). Motivational dynamics of language behavior. In M. Jones (Ed.), *Nebraska Symposium on Motivation* (pp. 348–424). Lincoln, NE: University of Nebraska Press.

Osser, H., Wang, M. and Zaid, F. (1969). The young child's ability to imitate and comprehend speech: A comparison of two subcultural groups. *Child Development*, 40, 1063–1075.

Oster, J. (1953). *Mongolism*. Copenhagen: Danish Science Press Limited.

Owens, J., Harris, F., Walker, S., McAllister, E. and West, L. (1983). The incidence of Down's syndrome over a 19-year period with special reference to maternal age. *Journal of Medical Genetics*, 20, 90–93.

Owens, R. and MacDonald, J. (1982). Communicative uses of the early speech of nondelayed and Down syndrome children. *American Journal of Mental Deficiency*, 86, 503–510.

Owings, N., McManus, M. and Scherer, N. (1981). A deinstitutionalized retarded adult's use of communication functions in a natural setting. *British Journal of Disorders of Communication*, 16, 119–128.

Paine, R. (1963). The future of the 'floppy infant': A follow-up study of 133 patients. *Developmental Medicine and Child Neurology*, 5, 115–124.

Paine, R., Brazelton, T., Donovan, D., Drorbaugh, J., Hubbel, J. and Sears, E. (1964). Evolution of postural reflexes in normal infants and in the presence of chronic brain syndromes. *Neurology*, 14, 1036–1048.

Paivio, A. (1986). *Mental Representations: A Dual-coding Approach*. New York: Oxford University Press.

Papania, N. (1954). A qualitative analysis of the vocabulary responses of institutionalized mentally retarded children. *Journal of Clinical Psychology*, 10, 361–365.

Papile, L,. Burstein, J., Burstein, R. and Koffler, H. (1978). Incidence and evolution of subependymal and intraventricular hemorrhage: A study of infants with birthweights less than 1,500 gm. *The Journal of Pediatrics*, 92, 529–534.

Pareskevopoulos, J. and Kirk, S. (1969). *The Development and Psychometric Characteristics of the Revised Illinois Test of Psycholinguistic Abilities*. Urbana, IL: University of Illinois Press.

Parisi, D. (1971). Development of syntactic comprehension in preschool children as a function of socio–economic level. *Developmental Psychology*, 5, 186–189.

Parsley, K., Powell, M., O'Connor, H. and Deutsch, M. (1963). Are there really sex differences in achievement? *Journal of Educational Research*, 57, 210–212.

Partridge, J., Babcock, D., Steichen, J. and Han, B. (1983). Optimal timing for diagnostic cranial ultrasound in low-birth-weight infants: Detection of intracranial hemorrhage and ventricular dilatation. *The Journal of Pediatrics*, 102, 281–287.

Patterson, D. (1987). The causes of Down syndrome. *Scientific American*, 257, 42–48.

Paul, R., Cohen, D., Breg, R., Watson, M. and Herman, S. (1984). Fragile X syndrome: Its relations to speech and language disorders. *Journal of Speech and Hearing Disorders*, 49, 326–336.

Pavlov, I. (1954). *Oeuvres choisies*. Moscow: Editions en Langues Etrangères.

Pavlov, I. (1962). *Les Reflexes conditionnés*. Paris: Masson.

Pecile, V. and Filippi, G. (1991). Screening for fragile X mutation and Klinefelter syndrome in mental institutions. *Clinical Genetics*, 39, 189–193.

Peins, M. (1962). Mental retardation: A selected bibliography on speech, hearing and language problems. *American Speech and Hearing Association*, 4, 38–40.

Penner, S. (1987). Parental responses to grammatical and ungrammatical child utterances. *Child Development*, 58, 376–384.

Penney, C. (1975). Modality effects in short–term verbal memory. *Psychological Bulletin*, 82, 68–84.

Perera, J. (Ed.). (1995). *Especificidad en el sindrome de Down*. Barcelona: Masson.

Perrett, D., Mistlin, A., Chitty, A., Harries, M., Newcombe, F. and de Haan, E. (1988). Neuronal mechanisms of face perception and their pathology. In C. Kennard and F. Clifford-Rose (Eds.), *Physiological Aspects of Clinical Neuro-ophthalmology* (pp. 137–154). London: Chapman and Hall.

Perron, R. (1969). Attitudes et idées face aux déficiences mentales. In R. Zazzo (Ed.), *Les Débilités mentales* (pp. 41–69). Paris: Colin.

Perron–Borelli, M. and Misès, R. (1974). *Epreuves Différentielles d'Efficience Intellectuelle*. Issy-les-Moulineaux, France: Editions Scientifiques et Psychologiques.

Petersen, G. and Sherrod, K. (1982). Relationship of maternal language to development and language delay of children. *American Journal of Mental Deficiency*, 86, 391–398.

Peterson, R. (1968). Some experiments on the organization of a class of imitative behaviors. *Journal of Applied Behavior Analysis*, 1, 225–235.

Petitto, L. (1987). On the autonomy of language and gesture: Evidence from the acquisition of personal pronouns in American sign language. *Cognition*, 27, 1–50.

Petitto, A. and Marentette, P. (1991). Babbling in the manual mode: Evidence for the ontogeny of language. *Science*, 251, 1493–1496.

Pettigrew, A., Gollin, S., Greenberg, F., Riccardi, V. and Ledbetter, D. (1987). Duplication of proximal 15q as a cause of Prader-Willi syndrome. *American Journal of Medical Genetics*, 28, 791–802.

Phillips, J. (1973). Syntax and vocabulary of mothers' speech to young children: Age and sex comparisons. *Child Development*, 44, 182–185.

Piaget, J. (1936). *La Naissance de l'intelligence chez l'enfant*. Neuchâtel, Switzerland: Delachaux et Niestlé.

Piaget, J. (1937). *La Construction du réel chez l'enfant*. Neuchâtel, Switzerland: Delachaux et Niestlé.

Piaget, J. (1945). *La Formation du symbole chez l'enfant*. Neuchâtel, Switzerland: Delachaux et Niestlé.

Piaget, J. (1968). *Le Structuralisme*. Paris: Presses Universitaires de France.

Piaget, J. (1970). Piaget's theory. In P. Mussen (Ed.), *Manual of Child Psychology* (Vol. 2, pp. 703–792). New York: Wiley.

Piaget, J. (1976). Piaget's theory. In B. Inhelder and H. Chipman (Eds.), *Piaget and his School. A Reader in Developmental Psychology* (pp. 11–23). New York: Springer.

Piaget, J. (1979a). Schèmes d'action et apprentissage du langage. In M. Piattelli-Palmarini (Ed.), *Théorie du langage. Théories de l'apprentissage. Le débat entre Jean Piaget et Noam Chomsky* (pp. 247–251). Paris: Seuil.

Piaget, J. (1979b). La psychogenèse des connaissances et sa signification épistémologique. In M. Piattelli-Palmarini (Ed.), *Théorie du langage. Théories de l'apprentissage. Le débat entre Jean Piaget et Noam Chomsky* (pp. 53–64). Paris: Seuil.

Piattelli-Palmarini, M. (1989). Evolution, selection and cognition. From 'learning' to parameter setting in biology and the study of language. *Cognition*, **31**, 1–44.

Picard, A. (1994). Sequelles intellectuelles et cognitives des leucomalacies périventriculaires chez le prématuré. *Approche Neuropsychologique des Apprentissages chez l'Enfant*, **28**, 132–136.

Pinker, S. (1984). *Language Learnability and Language Development*. Cambridge, MA: MIT Press.

Pinker, S. (1987). The bootstrapping problem in language acquisition. In B. MacWhinney (Ed.), *Mechanisms of Language Acquisition* (pp. 399–441). Hillsdale, NJ: Erlbaum.

Pinker, S. (1989). *Learnability and Cognition. The Acquisition of Argument Structure*. Cambridge, MA: MIT Press.

Pinker, S. (1993). Interview with Jean A. Rondal: Pieces of minds in psycholinguistics. *International Journal of Psychology*, **28**, 459–480.

Pinker, S. and Bloom, P. (1990). Natural language and natural selection. *Behavioral and Brain Sciences*, **13**, 707–727.

Piret, R. (1973). *Psychologie différentielle des sexes*. Paris: Presses Universitaires de France.

Plomin, R. and Defries, J. (1980). Genetics and intelligence: Recent data. *Intelligence*, **4**, 15–24.

Ploog, D. (1984). Comment on J. Leiber's paper. In R. Harre and V. Reynolds (Eds.), *The Meaning of Primate Signals* (p. 88). Cambridge: Cambridge University Press.

Plude, D. and Doussard-Roosevelt, J. (1989). Ageing, selective attention and feature integration. *Psychology and Aging*, **4**, 98–105.

Ponthier, N. (1995). *Différenciation langagière sub–étiologique dans le syndrome de Down: Trisomie standard, translocation, et mosaïcisme*. Unpublished master's thesis, University of Liège, Belgium.

Posner, M. and Raichle, M. (1994). *Images of Mind*. New York: Scientific American Library.

Power, D. and Quigley, S. (1973). Deaf children's acquisition of passive voice. *Journal of Speech and Hearing Research*, **16**, 5–11.

Prasher, V. (1992). Longevity and Down's syndrome. *British Journal of Psychiatry*, **161**, 722.

Précis of the modularity of mind (collective). (1985). *Behavior and Brain Sciences*, **8** (whole issue).

Preus, A. (1972). Stuttering in Down's syndrome. *Scandinavian Journal of Educational Research, 16*, 89–104.

Preus, A. (1984). The Williams syndrome: Objective definition and diagnosis. *Journal of Clinical Genetics*, **25**, 422–428.

Price, P. (1989). Language intervention and mother–child interaction. In M. Beveridge, G. Conti–Rasmden and I. Lendar (Eds.), *Language and Communication in Mentally Handicapped People* (pp. 185–217). London: Chapman and Hall.

Price-Williams, D. and Sabsay, S. (1979). Communicative competence among severely retarded persons. *Semiotica*, **26**, 35–63.

Pryce, M. (1994). The voice of people with Down's syndrome: An EMG biofeedback study. *Down's Syndrome: Research and Practice*, **2**, 106–111.

Psycinfo (1994, November). *Lexical Development and/or Functioning in Mental Retardation*. Base: PI67. Washington, DC: American Psychological Association.

Pueschel, S. (1995). Caracteristicas fisicas de las personas con sindrome de Down. In J. Perera (Ed.), *Especificidad en el sindrome de Down* (pp. 53–63). Barcelona: Masson.

Pueschel, S., Gallagher, P., Zartler, A. and Pezzullo, J. (1987). Cognitive and learning processes in children with Down's syndrome. *Research in Developmental Disabilities*, **8**, 21–37.

Pueschel, S., Padre-Mendoza, T. and Ellenbogen, R. (1980). Partial trisomy 21. *Clinical Genetics*, **18**, 392–395.

Puig–Vergès, N. (1993). *Margaret S. Mahler. Une vie, une oeuvre*. Paris: Desclée de Brouwer.

Purves, D. (1988). *Body and Brain: A Trophic Theory of Neural Connections*. Cambridge, MA: Harvard University Press.

Purves, D. (1994). *Neural Activity and the Growth of Brain*. New York: Cambridge University Press.

Purves, D. and Lichtman, J. (1985). *Principles of Neural Development*. Sunderland, MA: Linauer.

Queixalos, F. (1989). Les conceptions linguistiques des indiens d'Amérique. In S. Auroux (Ed.), *Histoire des idées linguistiques* (Vol. 1, pp. 45–64). Brussels: Mardaga.

Quigley, S., Montanelli, D. and Wilbur, R. (1974). *An Examination of Negation in the Written Language of Deaf Children*. Unpublished manuscript, University of Illinois, Urbana-Champaign.

Quigley, S., Smith, N. and Wilbur, R. (1974). Comprehension of relativized sentences by deaf students. *Journal of Speech and Hearing Research*, **17**, 325–341.

Ramey, C., Bryant, D., Wasik, B., Sparling, J., Fendt, K. and La Vange, L. (1992). Infant health and development program for low birth weight, premature infants: Program elements, family participation and child intelligence. *Pediatrics*, **89**, 454–465.

Rankin, J. and Collins, M. (1985). Adult age differences in memory elaboration. *Journal of Gerontology*, **40**, 451–458.

Rasmussen, D. and Sobsey, D. (1994). Age, adaptive behavior and Alzheimer's disease in Down syndrome: Cross–sectional and longitudinal analyses. *American Journal on Mental Retardation*, **99**, 151–165.

Rast, M. and Meltzoff, A. (1995). Memory and representation in young children with Down syndrome: Exploring deferred imitation and object permanence, *Development and Psychopathology*, **7**, 393–407.

Raven, J. (1981). *Progressive Matrices*. Issy–Les–Moulineaux, France: Editions Scientifiques et Psychologiques.

Raven, J. C. (1965). *Raven's Coloured Progressive Matrices*. London: Lewis.

Reilly, J., Klima, E. and Bellugi, U. (1991). Once more with feeling: Affect and language in atypical populations. *Developmental Psychopathology*, 2, 367–391.

Reiss, S. (1994). Issues in defining mental retardation. *American Journal of Mental Retardation*, 99, 1–7.

Remington, R. and Clarke, S. (in press). Alternative and augmentative systems of communication for children with Down's syndrome. In J.A. Rondal, J. Perera, L. Nadel and A. Comblain (Eds.), *Down's Syndrome: Psychological, Psychobiological and Socio-educational Perspectives*. London: Whurr.

Reuchlin, M. (1979). *Psychologie*. Paris: Presses Universitaires de France.

Reuchlin, M. and Bacher, F. (1989). *Les Différences individuelles dans le développement cognitif de l'enfant*. Paris: Presses Universitaires de France.

Rey, A. (1967). *Les Troubles de la mémoire et leur examen psychométrique*. Brussels: Dessart.

Reynell, J. (1977). *Manual for the Reynell Development Language Scales*. Windsor: NFER.

Rheingold, H. and Bayley, N. (1959). The later effects of an experimental modification of mothering. *Child Development*, 30, 363–372.

Rheingold, H., Gewirtz, J. and Moss, H. (1967). Social conditioning of vocalization in the infant. In S. Bijou and D. Baer (Eds.), *Child Development: Reading in Experimental Analysis* (pp. 128–142). New York: Meredith.

Ribes, E. (1977). Relationship among behavior theory, experimental research and behavior modification techniques. *Psychological Record*, 2, 417–424.

Ribes, E. (1979). El desarollo del lenguaje gramatical en niños: Un analisis teorico y experimental. *Revista Mexicana de Analisis de la Conducta*, 5, 93–112.

Richard, B. (1969). Mosaic mongolism. *Journal of Mental Deficiency Research*, 13, 66–83.

Richards, C. (1967). A test of understanding of the spoken word. *British Journal of Disorders of Communication*, 2, 124–136.

Ricks, J. (1958). Age and vocabulary test performance: A qualitative analysis of the responses of adults. *Dissertation Abstracts*, 19, 182.

Riess, B. (1946). Genetic changes in semantic conditioning. *Journal of Experimental Psychology*, 36, 143–152.

Rigrodsky, S., Prunty, F. and Glovsky, L. (1961). A study of the incidence, types and associated etiologies of hearing loss in an institutionalized mentally retarded population. *Training School Bulletin*, 58, 30–34.

Risley, T. (1966). *The Development and Maintenance of Vocal Verbal Behavior*. Unpublished doctoral dissertation, University of Washington, Seattle.

Risley, T. and Wolf, M. (1967). Establishing functional speech in echolalic children. *Behavior Research and Therapy*, 5, 53–88.

Rittmanic, P. (1958). An oral language program for institutionalized educable mentally retarded children. *American Journal of Mental Deficiency*, 63, 403–407.

Rizzi, L. (1985). Two notes on the linguistic interpretation of Broca's aphasia. In M. Kean (Ed.), *Agrammatism* (pp. 153–164). New York: Academic.

Roberts, G. and Black, K. (1972). The effect of naming and object permanence on toy preferences. *Child Development*, 43, 858–868.

Roberts, T. (1967). An investigation of language abilities and their relation to school achievement in educable mentally retarded children. *Dissertation Abstracts*, 28, 37.

Robinson, H. and Robinson, N. (1965). *The Mentally Retarded Child. A Psychological Approach*. New York: McGraw-Hill.

Roeper, T. (1987). The modularity of meaning in language acquisition. In S. Modgil and C. Modgil (Eds.), *Noam Chomsky, Consensus and Controversy* (pp. 157–172). New York: Falmer.

Rogers, S. (1977). Characteristics of the cognitive development of profoundly retarded children. *Child Development*, 48, 837–843.

Rohr, A. and Burr, D. (1978). Etiological differences in patterns of psycholinguistic development of children of IQ 30 to 60. *American Journal of Mental Deficiency*, 82, 549–553.

Rondal, J. A. (1975). Développement du langage et retard mental: Une revue critique de la littérature en langue anglaise. *L'Année Psychologique*, 75, 513–547.

Rondal, J. A. (1976). Investigation of the regulatory power of the impulsive and meaningful aspects of speech. *Genetic Psychology Monographs*, 94, 3–33.

Rondal, J. A. (1977). Développement du langage et retard mental: Une revue des études ayant utilisé l'Illinois Test of Psycholinguistic Abilities. *Psychologica Belgica*, 17, 24–34.

Rondal, J. A. (1978a). Maternal speech to normal and Down's syndrome children matched for mean length of utterance. In C. Meyers (Ed.), *Quality of Life in the Severely and Profoundly Retarded People: Research Foundations for Improvement* (pp. 193–265). Washington, DC: American Association on Mental Deficiency.

Rondal, J. A. (1978b). Developmental sentence scoring procedure and the delay–difference question in language development of Down's syndrome children. *Mental Retardation*, 16, 169–171.

Rondal, J. A. (1978c). Patterns of correlations for various language measures in mother–child interactions for normal and Down's syndrome children. *Language and Speech*, 21, 242–252.

Rondal, J. A. (1978d). *Langage et éducation*. Brussels: Mardaga.

Rondal, J. A. (1980a). Une note sur la théorie cognitive–motivationnelle d'Edward Zigler en matière de retard mental culturel-familial. *Psychologica Belgica*, 20, 61–82.

Rondal, J. A. (1980b). Fathers' and mothers' speech in early language development. *Journal of Child Language*, 7, 353–369.

Rondal, J. A. (1980c). Language delay and language difference in moderately and severely mentally retarded children. *Special Education in Canada*, 54, 27–32.

Rondal, J. A. (1980d). Verbal imitation by Down's syndrome and non–retarded children. *American Journal of Mental Deficiency*, 85, 318–321.

Rondal, J. A. (1983). Quel rôle peut jouer l'imitation verbale dans l'acquisition du langage pour l'enfant? *Rééducation Orthophonique*, 21, 393–407.

Rondal, J. A. (1984). Linguistic and prelinguistic development in moderate and severe mental retardation. In J. Dobbing, A. Clarke, J. Corbett, J. Hogg and R. Robinson (Eds.), *Scientific Studies in Mental Retardation* (pp. 323–345). London: The Royal Society of Medicine and Macmillan.

Rondal, J. A. (1985a). *Langage et communication chez les handicapés mentaux*. Brussels: Mardaga.

Rondal, J. A. (1985b). *Adult–Child Interaction and the Process of Language Acquisition*. New York: Praeger.

Rondal, J. A. (1985c). *Le Développement du langage chez l'enfant trisomique 21. Manuel pratique d'aide et d'intervention*. Bruxelles: Mardaga.

Rondal, J. A. (1986). Communication et langage. In J.A. Rondal and M. Hurtig (Eds.), *Introduction à la psychologie de l'enfant* (Vol. 1, pp. 455–510). Brussels: Mardaga.

Rondal, J. A. (1987a). *A Longitudinal Study of Maternal Verbal Feedback in First Language Acquisition*. Unpublished manuscript, University of Liège, Belgium.

Rondal, J. A. (1987b). Language development and mental retardation. In W. Yule and M. Rutter (Eds.), Language Development and Disorders (pp. 248–261). Oxford: Blackwell.

Rondal, J. A. (1988a). Indications positives et négatives dans l'acquisition des aspects grammaticaux de la langue maternelle. *European Bulletin of Cognitive Psychology*, **8**, 383–398.

Rondal, J. A. (1988b, 1993). Down's syndrome. In D. Bishop and K. Mogford (Eds.), *Language Development in Exceptional Circumstances* (pp. 165–176). London: Churchill Livingstone. (Republished by Erlbaum, Hillsdale, NJ.)

Rondal, J. A. (1988c). Language development in Down's syndrome: A life-span perspective. *International Journal of Behavioural Development*, **11**, 21–36.

Rondal, J. A. (1994a). Exceptional cases of language development in mental retardation: The relative autonomy of language as a cognitive system. In H. Tager–Flusberg (Ed.), *Constraints on Language Acquisition: Studies of Atypical Children* (pp. 155–174). Hillsdale, NJ: Erlbaum.

Rondal, J. A. (1994b). Exceptional language development in mental retardation: Natural experiments in language modularity. *Current Psychology of Cognition (Cahiers de Psychologie Cognitive)*, *13*, 427–467.

Rondal, J. A. (1995a). *Exceptional Language Development in Down Syndrome. Implications for the Cognition–Language Relationship*. New York: Cambridge University Press.

Rondal, J. A. (1995b). Especificidad sistemica del lenguaje en el sindrome de Down. In J. Perera (Ed.), *Especifidad en el sindrome de Down* (pp. 91–107). Barcelona: Masson.

Rondal, J. A. (1995c). *Educar y hacer hablar al niño Down. Un guia al servico de padres y profesores*. Mexico, D.F.: Trillas.

Rondal, J. A. (1995d, August 1996). *Language Development and use in Down Syndrome Persons*. Invited address to the Third European Down Syndrome Conference, Dublin, Ireland. (Reproduced in *Leben mit Down–syndrom*,22, 10–16).

Rondal, J. A. (in press–a). *Faire parler l'enfant retardé mental. Un programme d'intervention psycholinguistique*. Brussels: Labor; Lyon, France: Chronique Sociale; Lausanne, Switzerland: LEP.

Rondal, J. A. (in press–b). Interactions verbales adulte–enfant et construction du langage. Le problème de l'informaiton en retour. In A. Trognon, J. Bernicot and J. Caron–Pargue (Eds.), *Conversation, interaction, et fonctionnement cognitif*. Nancy, France: Presses Universitaires de Nancy.

Rondal, J. A., Adrao, M. and Neves, S. (1980, 1981). Classe sociale, langage, et instruction: La compréhension du langage de l'enseignant par l'enfant au niveau de l'école maternelle et élémentaire inférieure. *Les Sciences de l'Education pour l'Ere Nouvelle*, **17**, 245–264 (republished in G. Gagné and M. Pagé (Eds), *Etudes sur la langue des jeunes québécois, 1967–1979*, Montréal, Presses de l'Université de Montréal, pp. 40–64.)

Rondal, J. A., Bachelet, J. F. and Perée, F. (1986). Analyse du langage et des interactions verbales adulte–enfant. *Bulletin d'audiophonologie*, *5–6*, 507–535.

Rondal, J. A., Bragard–Ledent, A., Bastyns, A., Montulet, I., Fonsny, H., Goffard, F., Devel, F. and Krins, A. (1988). *Aide et intervention précoce à domicile. La méthode psycho-educative de l'APEM*. Heusy-Verviers, Belgium: APEM.

Rondal, J. A., Cession, A. and Vincent, E. (1988). *Compréhension des phrases déclaratives selon la voix et l'actionalité du verbe chez un groupe d'adultes trisomique 21.* Unpublished manuscript, University of Liège, Belgium.

Rondal, J. A., Coquiart, P., Crommen, T., Marissiaux, P., Neuville, P., Rolin, K. and Thonon, C. (1981). *Aspects du langage de sujets handicapés mentaux adolescents.* Unpublished manuscript, University of Liège, Belgium.

Rondal, J. A., Ghiotto, M., Brédart, S. and Bachelet, J. F. (1987). Age-relation, reliability and grammatical validity of measures of utterance length. *Journal of Child Language*, **14**, 433–446.

Rondal, J. A., Ghiotto, M., Brédart, S. and Bachelet, J.F. (1988). Mean length of utterance of children with Down's syndrome. *American Journal on Mental Retardation*, **93**, 64–66.

Rondal, J. A. and Hoffmeister, R. (1976). Sign language as an alternative language system for the mentally retarded. *Philippine Journal of Mental Health*, **7**, 52–62.

Rondal, J. A. and Lambert, J. L. (1982). *Questions et réponses sur le mongolisme.* Québec: Les Editions La Liberté; Paris: Maloine.

Rondal, J. A. and Lambert, J. L. (1983). The speech of mentally retarded adults in a dyadic communication situation: Some formal and informative aspects. *Psychologica Belgica*, **23**, 49–56.

Rondal, J. A., Lambert, J. L. and Sohier, C. (1980a). Analyses des troubles articulatoires chez des enfants arriérés mentaux mongoliens et non-mongoliens. *Bulletin d'Audiophonologie*, **10**, 13–20.

Rondal, J. A., Lambert, J. L. and Sohier, C. (1980b). L'imitation verbale et non-verbale chez l'enfant retardé mental mongolien et non-mongolien. *Enfance*, **3**, 107–122.

Rondal, J. A., Lambert, J. L. and Sohier, C. (1981). Elicited verbal and non–verbal imitation in Down's syndrome and other mentally retarded children: A replication and an extension of Berry. *Language and Speech*, **24**, 245–254.

Rondal, J. A. and Perera, J. (1995). *Como hacer hablar al nino con sindrome de Down y mejorar su language.* Madrid: Cepe.

Rondal, J. A. and Rondal, R. (1975). Bibliography on speech and language in mental retardation 1900–1975 (Part 1: Descriptive studies). *Philippine Journal of Mental Health*, **6**, 39–62.

Rondal, J. A. and Rondal, R. (1976). Bibliography on speech and language in mental retardation 1900–1975 (Part 2: Intervention studies). *Philippine Journal of Mental Health*, **7**, 51–64.

Rondal, J. A., Thibaut, J. P. and Cession, A. (1990). Transitivity effects on children's sentence comprehension. *European Bulletin of Cognitive Psychology*, **10**, 385–400.

Rondal, J. A., Thibaut, J. P., Fayasse, M., Comblain, A., Javaux, D. and Ferrara, A. (1995). *Computer–Enhanced Language Intervention Program for Mentally Retarded Children* (CELIP/MRC). Unpublished manuscript, University of Liège, Belgium.

Rönne–Jeppesen, E. (1971). Psychological and pedagogical studies of low birth weight children. *Skolepsyckologie*, **3**, 145.

Rosch, E. (1977). Principles of categorization. In E. Rosch and B. Lloyd (Eds.), *Cognition and Categorization* (pp. 27–48). Hillsdale, NJ: Erlbaum.

Rosch, E. (1978). Human categorization. In N. Warren (Ed.), *Advances in Cross–cultural Psychology* (Vol. 1, pp. 122–148). New York: Academic.

Rosecrans, C. (1971). A longitudinal study of exceptional cognitive development in a partial translocation Down's syndrome child. *American Journal of Mental Deficiency*, **76**, 291–294.

Rosenbaum, B. and Sonne, H. (1986). *The Language of Psychosis*. New York: New York University Press.

Rosenberg, S. (1982). The language of the mentally retarded: Development, processes, intervention. In S. Rosenberg (Ed.), *Handbook of Applied Psycholinguistics: Major Thrusts of Research and Theory* (pp. 329–392). Hillsdale, NJ: Erlbaum.

Rosenberg, S. and Abbeduto, L. (1993). *Language and Communication in Mental Retardation. Development, Processes and Intervention*. Hillsdale, NJ: Erlbaum.

Rosenberg, S., Spradlin, J. and Mabel, S. (1961). Interaction among retarded children as a function of their relative language skills. *Journal of Abnormal and Social Psychology*, **63**, 402–410.

Rosin, M., Swift, E. and Bless, D. (1987, May). *Communication Profiles of People with Down's Syndrome*. Communication presented at the Annual Convention of the American Speech and Hearing Association, New Orleans.

Rosin, M., Swift, E., Bless, D. and Vetter, D. (1988). Communication profiles of adolescents with Down's syndrome. *Journal of Childhood Communication Disorders*, **12**, 49–64.

Ross, M., Galaburda, A. and Kemper, T. (1984). Down's syndrome: Is there a decreased population of neurons? *Neurology*, **34**, 909–916.

Roth, M. (1993). Foreword. In J. Berg H., Karlinsky and A. Holland (Eds.), *Alzheimer's Disease, Down's Syndrome and their Relationship* (pp. V–XI). Oxford: Oxford University Press.

Routh, D. (Ed.). (1973). *The Experimental Psychology of Mental Retardation*. Chicago: Aldine.

Rozner, L. (1983). Facial plastic surgery for Down's syndrome. *Lancet*, **11**, 1320–1323.

Rusch, J. and Karlan, G. (1983). Language training. In J. Matson and J. Mulick (Eds.), *Handbook of Mental Retardation* (pp. 397–409). New York: Pergamon.

Rushton, D., Preston, P. and Durbin, G. (1985). Structure and evolution of echodense lesions in the neonatal brain. *Archives of Diseases in Children*, **60**, 798–808.

Rutter, T. and Buckley, S. (1994). The acquisition of grammatical morphemes in children with Down's syndrome. *Down's Syndrome*, **2**, 76–82.

Ryan, J. (1975, 1977). Mental subnormality and language development. In E. Lenneberg (Ed.), *Foundations of Language Development: A Multidisciplinary Approach* (Vol. 2, pp. 269–277). New York: Academic.

Rynders, J. (1994, July). *Supporting the Educational Development and Progress of Individuals with Down's Syndrome*. Communication to the Third Ross Roundtable on Critical Issues in Family Medicine, Washington, DC.

Sailor, W. (1971). Reinforcement and generalization of productive plural allomorphs in two retarded children. *Journal of Applied Behavior Analysis*, **4**, 305–310.

Sailor, W., Guess, D. and Baer, D. (1973). Instructional language for verbally deficient children: An experimental program. *Mental Retardation*, **11**, 27–35.

Salkie, R. (1987). Core grammar and periphery. In S. Modgil and C. Modgil (Eds.), *Noam Chomsky, Consensus and Controversy* (pp. 109–117). New York: Falmer.

Salthouse, T. and Babcock, R. (1991). Decomposing adult age differences in working memory. *Developmental Psychology*, **26**, 763–776.

Sampson, G. (1985). *Writing Systems*. Stanford, CA: Stanford University Press.

Sander, E. (1972). When are speech sounds learned? *Journal of Speech and Hearing Disorders*, **37**, 55–63.

Savic, S. (1975). Aspects of adult–child communication: The problem of question acquisition. *Journal of Child Language*, **2**, 251–260.

Savin, H. and Bever, T. (1970). The non–perceptual reality of the phoneme. *Journal of Verbal Learning and Verbal Behavior*, **9**, 295–302.

Scarborough, H. (1985, May). *Measuring Syntactic Development: The Index of Productive Syntax*. Paper presented at the Biennial Meeting of the Society for Research in Child Development, Toronto.

Scarborough, H., Rescorla, L. Tager–Flusberg, H., Fowler, A. & Sudhalter, V. (1991). The relation of utterance length to grammatical complexity in normal and language–disordered groups. *Applied Psycholinguistics*, **12**, 23–45.

Schaeffer, M. and Shearer, W. (1968). A survey of mentally retarded stutterers. *Mental Retardation*, **6**, 44–45.

Schaffer, H. and Emerson, P. (1964). The development of social attachment in infancy. *Monographs of the Society for Research in Child Development*, **29**, N°. 3.

Schapiro, M., Haxby, J. and Grady, C. (1992). Nature of mental retardation and dementia in Down syndrome: Study with PET, CT and neuropsychology. *Neurobiology of Aging*, **13**, 723–734.

Scheibel, A. (1984). A dendritic correlate of human speech. In N. Geschwind and A. Galaburda (Eds.), *Cerebral dominance: The Biological Foundations* (pp. 43–52). Cambridge, MA: Harvard University Press.

Scherer, N. and Owings, N. (1984). Learning to be contingent: Retarded children's responses to their mothers', requests. *Language and Speech*, **27**, 255–267.

Schiefelbusch, R. (1965). A discussion of language treatment methods for mentally retarded children. *Mental Retardation*, **3**, 4–7.

Schiefelbusch, R. (1974). Language. In J. Wortis (Ed.), *Mental Retardation and Developmental Disabilities: An Annual Review* (Vol. 5, pp. 142–175). New York: Brunner/Mazel.

Schiefelbusch, R. and Lloyd, L. (Eds.). (1974). *Language Perspectives: Acquisition, Retardation and Intervention*. Baltimore, MD: University Park Press.

Schlanger, B. (1953). Speech examination of a group of institutionalized mentally handicapped children. *Journal of Speech and Hearing Disorders*, **18**, 339–349.

Schlanger, B. (1958). Speech therapy with mentally retarded children. *Journal of Speech and Hearing Disorders*, **23**, 298–301.

Schlanger, B. and Gottsleben, R. (1957). Analysis of speech defects among the institutionalized mentally retarded. *Journal of Speech and Hearing Disorders*, **22**, 98–103.

Schoenberg, B. (1986). Epidemiology of Alzheimer's disease and other dementing illnesses. *Journal of Chronic Diseases*, **39**, 1095–1104.

Scholes, R. (1978). Syntactic and lexical components of sentence comprehension. In A. Caramazza and E. Zurif (Eds.), *Language Acquisition and Language Breakdown* (pp. 78–94). Baltimore, MD: Johns Hopkins University Press.

Schulman, M. and Havighurst, R. (1947). Relations between ability and social status in a midwestern community. Size of vocabulary. *Journal of Educational Psychology*, **38**, 437–442.

Schumaker, J. and Sherman, J. (1970). Training generative verb usage by imitation and reinforcement procedures. *Journal of Applied Behavior Analysis*, **3**, 273–287.

Schwartz, M. (Ed.). (1990). *Modular Deficits in Alzheimer-type Dementia*. Cambridge, MA: MIT Press.

Schwartz, M. and Chawluk, J. (1990). Deterioration of language in progressive aphasia: A case study. In M. Schwartz (Ed.), *Modular Deficits in Alzheimer-type Dementia* (pp. 207–244). Cambridge, MA: MIT Press.

Schwartz, M., Marin, D. and Saffran, E. (1979). Dissociations of language function in dementia: A case study. *Brain and Language*, **7**, 277–306.

Schwartz, R. and Terrell, B. (1983). The role of input frequency in lexical acquisition. *Journal of Child Language*, **10**, 57–64.

Seagoe, M. (1965). Verbal development in a mongoloid. *Exceptional Children*, 6, 229–275.

Searle, J. (1969). *Speech Acts*. Cambridge: Cambridge University Press.

Seckel, H. (1960). *Bird–head Dwarfs: Studies in Developmental Anthropology Including Human Proportions*. Springfield, IL: Thomas.

Seguin, E. (1846). *Idiocy: Its Treatment by the Physiological Method*. New York: Wood.

Seitz, S., Goulding, P. and Conrad, R. (1969). The effects of maturation on word associations of the mentally retarded. *Multivariante Behavioral Research*, 4, 79–88.

Seitz, S. and Stewart, C. (1975). Imitations and expansions: Some developmental aspects of mother–child communications. *Developmental Psychology*, **11**, 763–768.

Seltzer, M. and Krauss, M. (1987). *Ageing and Mental Retardation. Extending the Continuum*. Washington, DC: American Association on Mental Retardation.

Semmel, E. and Wiig, E. (1980). *Clinical Evaluation of Language Functions* (CELF). Columbus, OH: Merrill.

Semmel, E., Wiig, E. and Secord, W. (1980). *CELF–R: Clinical Evaluation of Language Fundamentals – Revised*. San Antonio, TX: The Psychological Corporation.

Semmel, M., Barritt, L. and Bennet, S. (1970). Performance of educable mentally retarded children and non–retarded children on a modified cloze–task. *American Journal of Mental Deficiency*, **74**, 681–688.

Semmel, M., Barrit, L. Bennet, S. and Perfetti, C. (1968). A grammatical analysis of word associations of educable mentally retarded and normal children. *American Journal of Mental Deficiency*, **72**, 567–576.

Semmel, M. and Bennet, S. (1970). Effects of linguistic structure and delay of presentation on memory recall of educable mentally retarded children. *American Journal of Mental Deficiency*, **74**, 674–680.

Semmel, M. and Dooley, D. (1971). Comprehension and imitation of sentences by Down's syndrome children as a function of transformational complexity. *American Journal of Mental Deficiency*, **75**, 739–745.

Sersen, E., Astrup, E., Floistad, I. and Wortis, J. (1970). Motor conditioned reflexed and word association in retarded children. *American Journal of Mental Deficiency*, **74**, 495–501.

Shallice, T. (1988). *From Neuropsychology to Mental Structure*. New York: Cambridge University Press.

Shapiro, B. (1970). Prenatal dental abnormalities in mongolism. *Annals of the New York Academy of Sciences*, **171**, 562–564.

Shapiro, T., Roberts, A. and Fish, B. (1970). Imitation and echoing. *Journal of the American Academy of Child Psychiatry*, **9**, 421–439.

Share, J. (1975). Developmental progress in Down's syndrome. In R. Koch and F. de la Cruz (Eds.), *Down's Syndrome (Mongolism): Research, Prevention and Management* (pp. 78–86). New York: Brunner and Mazel.

Share, J., Koch, R., Webb, A. and Graliker, B. (1963). The longitudinal development of infants and young children with Down's syndrome (mongolism). *American Journal of Mental Deficiency*, **68**, 685–692.

Shatz, M. and Gelman, R. (1973). The development of communication skills: Modification in the speech of young children as a function of listener. *Monographs of the Society for Research in Child Development*, **38**, N°. 152.

Sherman, J. (1971). Imitation and language development. In H. Reese (Ed.), *Advances in Child Development* (Vol. 6, pp. 239–272). New York: Academic.

Sherman, S. (1992, June). *Epidemiology and Screening*. Paper presented at the Third International Fragile X Conference, Snowmass Resort, CO.

Shotwell, A. and Shipe, D. (1964). Effect of out-of-home care on mongoloid children. *American Journal of Mental Deficiency*, 68, 693–699.

Shriberg, L. and Widder, C. (1990). Speech and prosody characteristics of adults with mental retardation. *Journal of Speech and Hearing Research*, 33, 627–653.

Shubert, O., Vanden Heuvel, C. and Fulton, R. (1966). Effects of speech improvement on articulatory skills in institutionalized retardates. *American Journal of Mental Deficiency*, 71, 274–278.

Shvarts, L. (1954). Conditioned responses to verbal stimuli. *Soviet Psychology and Psychiatry*, 2, 3–14.

Siegel, G. (1967). Interpersonal approaches to the study of communication disorders. *Journal of Speech and Hearing Disorders*, 32, 112–120.

Siegel, P. and Foshee, J. (1960). Molar variability in the mentally defective. *Journal of Abnormal and Social Psychology*, 61, 141–143.

Sievers, D. and Essa, S. (1961). Language development in institutionalized children. *American Journal of Mental Deficiency*, 66, 413–420.

Silverman, H., McNaughton, S. and Kates, B. (1978). *Handbook of Blissymbolics*. Toronto: Blissymbolics Communication Institute.

Silverstein, A., Legutki, G., Friedman, S. and Takayama, D. (1982). Performance of Down's syndrome individuals on the Stanford–Binet Intelligence Scale. *American Journal of Mental Deficiency*, 86, 548–551.

Sinclair, H. (1970). The transition from sensori-motor behaviour to symbolic activity. *Interchange*, 1, 119–126.

Sinclair, H. (1971). Sensorimotor action patterns as a condition for the acquisition of syntax. In R. Huxley and E. Ingram (Eds.), *Language Acquisition: Models and Methods* (pp. 121–135). New York: Academic.

Sinclair, H. (1973). Language acquisition and cognitive development. In T. Moore (Ed.), *Cognitive Development and the Acquisition of Language* (pp. 9–25). New York: Academic.

Sinclair, H. and Ferreiro, E. (1970). Etude génétique de la compréhension, production et répétition des phrases au mode passif. *Archives de Psychologie*, 40, 1–42.

Sinclair, H., Sinclair, A. and de Marcellus, O. (1971). Young children's comprehension and production of passive sentences. *Archives de Psychologie*, 39, 1–22.

Singer, N. and Goodman, J. (1992, June). *Developmental Trajectories of Language and Cognitive Function in Two Syndromes: Opposite Patterns of Decoupling*. Paper presented at the Symposium 'Two genetic syndromes of contrasting cognitive profiles: A neuropsychological and neurobiological dissection' of the American Psychological Society, San Diego, CA.

Singh, K. (1990). Trisomy 13 (Patau's syndrome): A rare case of survival into adulthood. *Journal of Mental Deficiency Research*, 34, 91–93.

Singleton, D. (1989). *Language Acquisition: The Age Factor*. Cleveland, OH: Multilingual Matters.

Sinha, S., D'souza, S., Rivlin, E. and Chiswick, M. (1990). Ischaemic brain lesions diagnosed at birth in preterm infants: Clinical events and developmental outcome. *Archives of Disease in Childhood*, 65, 1017–1020.

Skinner, B.F. (1938). *The Behavior of Organisms*. New York: Appleton-Century-Crofts.

Skinner, B.F. (1953). *Science and Human Behavior*. New York: MacMillan.

Skinner, B.F. (1957). *Verbal Behavior*. Englewood Cliffs, NJ: Prentice-Hall.

Skuse, D. (1993). Extreme deprivation in early childhood. In D. Bishop and K. Mogford (Eds.), *Language Development in Exceptional Circumstances* (pp. 29–46). Hove: Erlbaum.

Slater, E. and Cowie, V. (1971). *The Genetics of Mental Disorders*. New York: Oxford University Press.

Sloane, H., Johnston, M. and Harris, F. (1968). Remedial procedures for teaching verbal behavior to speech deficient or defective young children. In H. Sloane and B. MacAulay (Eds.), *Operant Procedures in Remedial Speech and Language Training* (pp. 77–101). Boston, MA: Houghton Mifflin, 1968.

Slobin, D. (1968). Imitation and grammatical development in children. In N. Endler, L. Bowler and H. Osser (Eds.), *Contemporary Issues in Developmental Psychology* (pp. 437–443). New York: Academic.

Slobin, D. (Ed.). (1971). *The Ontogenesis of Language. A Theoretical Symposium*. New York: Academic.

Slobin, D. (1973). Cognitive prerequisites for the development of grammar. In C. Ferguson and D. Slobin (Eds.), *Studies of Child Language Development* (pp. 607–619). New York: Holt, Rinehart and Winston.

Slobin, D. (1981). L'apprentissage de la langue maternelle. *La Recherche*, **12**, 572–578.

Slobin, D. and Welsch, C. (1973). Elicited imitation as a research tool in developmental psycholinguistics. In C. Ferguson and D. Slobin (Eds.), *Studies of Child Language Development* (pp. 485–497). New York: Holt, Rinehart and Winston.

Smith, A., Volato, F. and Trent, R. (1988). Correlation of cytogenetic and DNA findings in Prater–Willi syndrome. In W. Fraser (Ed.), *Key Issues in Mental Retardation Research* (pp. 57–63). London: Routledge.

Smith, B. (1977, August). *Phonological Development in Down's Syndrome Children*. Communication presented at the 85th Annual convention of the American Psychological Association, San Francisco, CA.

Smith, B. and Oller, K. (1981). A comparative study of pre-meaningful vocalizations produced by normally developing and Down's syndrome infants. *Journal of Speech and Hearing Disorders*, **46**, 46–51.

Smith, B. and Stoel-Gammon, C. (1983). A longitudinal study of the development of stop consonant production in normal and Down's syndrome children. *Journal of Speech and Hearing Disorders*, **48**, 114–118.

Smith, F. and Miller, G. (Eds.). (1966). *The Genesis of Language*. Cambridge, MA: MIT Press.

Smith, J. (1962). Group language development for educable mental retardates. *Exceptional Children*, **29**, 95–101.

Smith, L. and Von Tetzchner, S. (1986). Communicative, sensori-motor and language skills of young children with Down's syndrome. *American Journal of Mental Deficiency*, **91**, 57–66.

Smith, L. Von Tetzchner, S. and Michalsen, B. (1988). The emergence of language skills in young children with Down's syndrome. In L. Nadel (Ed.), *The Psychobiology of Down's Syndrome* (pp. 145–165). Cambridge, MA: MIT Press.

Smith, N. and Tsimpli, I. M. (1995). *The Mind of a Savant. Language Learning and Modularity*. Oxford: Blackwell.

Snow, C. (1977). Mothers' speech research: From input to interaction. In C. Snow and C. Ferguson (Eds.), *Talking to Children* (pp. 31–51). New York: Cambridge University Press.

Snow, C. (1990). The development of definitional skill. *Journal of Child Language*, **17**, 68–697–710.

Snow, C., Arlman–Rupp, A., Hassing, J., Jobse, J., Joosten, J. and Vorster, J. (1976). Mothers' speech in three social classes. *Journal of Psycholinguistic Research*, **5**, 1–20.

Snyder–McLean, L. and McLean, J. (1987). Effectiveness of early intervention for children with language and communication disorders. In M. Guralnick and F. Bennett (Eds.), *The Effectiveness of Early Intervention for At-risk and Handicapped Children* (pp. 213–274). New York: Academic.

Sokolov, A. (1972). *Inner Speech and Thought*. New York: Plenum.

Sokolov, J. (1992). Linguistic imitation in children with Down's syndrome. *American Journal on Mental Retardation*, **97**, 209–221.

Sollier, P. (1891). *Psychologie de l'idiot et de l'imbecile*. Paris: Alcan.

Sommers, R. (1962). Factors in the effectiveness of mothers trained to aid in speech correction. *Journal of Speech and Hearing Disorders*, **27**, 178–187.

Sommers, R. and Shilling, S. (1959). Training parents of children with functional misarticulation. *Journal of Speech and Hearing Research*, **2**, 258–265.

Sorg, A. (1979). Acquisition and use of Blissymbols by severely mentally retarded adolescents. *Mental Retardation*, **17**, 253–255.

Sparrow, S., Balla, D. and Cicchetti, D. (1984). *Vineland Adaptive Behavior Scales*. Circle Pines, MN: American Guidance Corporation.

Spearman, C. (1904). General intelligence objectively determined and measured. *American Journal of Psychology*, **15**, 201–292.

Spearman, C. (1927). *The Abilities of Man*. New York: Macmillan.

Speidel, G. and Nelson, K. (1989). *The Many Faces of Imitation in Language Learning*. New York: Springer.

Sperber, R., Ragain, R. and McCauley, C. (1976). Reassessment of category knowledge in retarded individuals. *American Journal of Mental Deficiency*, **81**, 227–234.

Spitz, H. (1973). The channel capacity of educable mental retardates. In D. Routh (Ed.), *The Experimental Psychology of Mental Retardation* (pp. 133–156). Chicago: Aldine.

Spitz, R. (1958). *La Première année de vie de l'enfant*. Paris: Presses Universitaires de France.

Spitzer, R., Rabinowitch, J. and Wybar, K. (1961). A study of the abnormalities of the skull, teeth and lenses in mongolism. *Canadian Medical Association Journal*, **84**, 567–572.

Spradlin, J. (1963). Language and communication of mental defectives. In N. Ellis (Ed.), *Handbook of Mental Deficiency: Psychological Theory and Research* (pp. 512–555). New York: McGraw-Hill.

Spradlin, J. (1968). Environmental factors and the language development of retarded children. In S. Rosenberg and J. Koplin (Eds.), *Development in Applied Psycholinguistics Research* (pp. 178–215). New York: Macmillan.

Spradlin, J., Girardeau, F. and Corte, E. (1967). Social and communication behavior of retarded adolescents in a two person situation. *American Journal of Mental Deficiency*, **73**, 473–481.

Spradlin, J. and Rosenberg, S. (1964). Complexity of adult verbal behavior in a dyadic situation with retarded children. *Journal of Abnormal and Social Psychology*, **68**, 694–698.

Spreen, D. (1965). Language functions in mental retardation: A review. I. Language development, types of retardation and intelligence level. *American Journal of Mental Deficiency*, **69**, 482–494.

Staats, A. (1971). Linguistic–mentalistic theory versus explanatory S–R learning theory of language development. In D. Slobin (Ed.), *The Ontogenesis of Grammar: A Theoretical Symposium* (pp. 103–150). New York: Academic.

Staats, A. (1975). *Social Behaviorism*. Chicago: Dorsey.

Staats, A. (1976). Social behaviorism and neo–psycholinguistics. *Die Neueren Sprachen, April*, 127–141.

Stampe, D. (1972). *A Dissertation on Natural Phonology*. Unpublished doctoral dissertation, University of Chicago.

Stansfield, J. (1990). Prevalence of stuttering and cluttering in adults with mental handicaps. *Journal of Mental Deficiency Research*, **34**, 287–307.

Stedman's Medical Dictionary (1990). Baltimore, MD: Williams and Wilkins.

Steele, J. and Stratford, B. (1995). The United Kingdom population with Down syndrome: Present and future projections. *American Journal on Mental Retardation*, **99**, 664–682.

Steffelaar, J. and Evenhuis, H. (1989). Life expectancy, Down syndrome and dementia. *Lancet*, 492–493.

Steffens, M., Oller, D., Lynch, M. and Urbano, R. (1992). Vocal development in infants with Down syndrome and infants who are developing normally. *American Journal on Mental Retardation*, **97**, 235–246.

Sternberg, R. (1988a). Intelligence. In R. Sternberg and E. Smith (Eds.), *The Psychology of Human Thought* (pp. 267–308). New York: Cambridge University Press.

Sternberg, R. (1988b). *The Triarchic Mind: A New Theory of Human Intelligence*. New York: Viking.

Stickland, C. (1954). Two mongols of unusually high mental status. *British Journal of Medical Psychology*, **27**, 80–83.

Stoel-Gammon, C. (1980). Phonological analysis of four Down's syndrome children. *Applied Psycholingustics*, **1**, 31–48.

Stoel-Gammon, C. (1981). Speech development of infants and children with Down's syndrome. In J. Darby (Ed.), *Speech Evaluation in Medicine* (pp. 341–360). New York: Grune and Stratton.

Stokes, T. and Baer, D. (1977). An implicit technology of generalization. *Journal of Applied Behavior Analysis*, **10**, 349–367.

Stowe, L. Wijers, A., Willemsen, A., Reuland, E., Paans, A. and Vaalburg, W. (1994). PET studies of language: An assessment of the reliability of the technique. *Journal of Psycholinguistic Research*, **23**, 499–527.

Strazzulla, M. (1953). Speech problems of the mongoloid child. *Quarterly Review of Pediatrics*, **8**, 268–273.

Stremel, K. (1972). Language training: A program for retarded children. *Mental Retardation*, **10**, 47–49.

Sudhalter, V. and Braine, M. (1985). How does passive develop? A comparison of actional and experiential verbs. *Journal of Child Language*, **12**, 455–470.

Sudhalter, V., Cohen, I., Silverman, W. and Wolf–Schein, E. (1990). Conversational analyses of males with Fragile X, Down syndrome and autism: Comparison of the emergence of deviant language. *American Journal on Mental Retardation*, **94**, 431–441.

Sudhalter, V., Scarborough, H. and Cohen, I. (1991). Syntactic delay and pragmatic deviance in the language of males with fragile X syndrome. *American Journal of Medical Genetics*, **43**, 65–71.

Sunderland, A., Watts, K., Baddeley, A. and Harris, J. (1986). Subjective memory assessment and test performance in elderly adults. *Journal of Gerontology*, **41**, 376–384.

Swann, W. and Mittler, P. (1976). Language abilities of ESN(s) pupils. *Special Education Forward Trend*, **13**, 24–27.

Swetlik, B. and Brown, L. (1977). Teaching severely handicapped students to express selected first, second and third person singular pronoun responses in answer to 'who doing' questions. In N. Haring and L. Brown (Eds.), *Teaching the Severely Handicapped* (Vol. 2, pp. 15–62). New York: Grune and Stratton.

Sylvester, P. (1983). The hippocampus in Down's syndrome. *Journal of Mental Deficiency Research*, **27**, 227–236.

Tager-Flusberg, H. (1981). On the nature of linguistic functioning in early infantile autism. *Journal of Autism and Developmental Disorders*, **11**, 45–56.

Tager-Flusberg, H. (1985a). Psycholinguistic approaches to language and communication in autism. In E. Shopler and G. Mesibov (Eds.), *Communication Problems in Autism* (pp. 69–87). New York: Plenum.

Tager-Flusberg, H. (1985b). The conceptual basis for referential word meaning in children with autism. *Child Development*, **56**, 1167–1178.

Tager-Flusberg, H. (1986). Constraints on the representation of word meaning: Evidence from autistic and mentally retarded children. In S. Kuczaj and M. Barrett (Eds.), *The Development of Word Meaning* (pp. 69–81). New York: Springer.

Tager-Flusberg, H. (1994). Dissociations in form and function in the acquisition of language by autistic children. In H. Tager-Flusberg (Ed.), *Constraints on Language Acquisition. Studies of Atypical Children* (pp. 175–194). Hillsdale, NJ: Erlbaum.

Tager-Flusberg, H. and Calkins, S. (1990). Does imitation facilitate the acquisition of grammar? Evidence from a study of autistic, Down's syndrome and normal children. *Journal of Child Language*, **17**, 591–606.

Takuma, S., Narita, S., Nakamura, H., Matsumoto, H. and Munekata, T. (1992). Analysis of computer software development for the learning of handicapped children. NISE (National Institute of Special Education) *Bulletin*, **4**, 1–5.

Tannock, R. (1988). Mother directiveness in their interactions with their children with and without Down's syndrome. *American Journal on Mental Retardation*, **93**, 154–165.

Tannock, R., Kershner, J. and Oliver, J. (1984). Do individuals with Down's syndrome possess right hemisphere language dominance? *Cortex*, **20**, 221–231.

Tauber, M. (1979). Sex differences in parent-child interaction styles during a free play session. *Child Development*, **50**, 981–988.

Taylor, D. (1969). Differential rates of cerebral maturation between sexes and between hemispheres. *Lancet*, **2**, 140–142.

Taylor, D. (1974). The influence of sexual differentiation on growth, development and disease. In J. Davis and J. Dobbing (Eds.), *Scientific Foundations of Paediatrics* (pp. 29–44). Philadelphia: Saunders.

Templin, M. (1957). *Certain Language Skills in Children: Their Development and Interrelationship*. Minneapolis, MN: University of Minnesota Press.

Terman, L. (1952). Différences psychologiques dues au sexe. In L. Carmichael (Ed.), *Manuel de psychologie de l'enfant* (Vol. 3, pp. 1510–1596). Paris: Presses Universitaires de France.

Terman, L. and Merrill, M. (1960). *Stanford-Binet Intelligence Scale. Manual for the Third Revision*. Boston, MA: Houghton-Mifflin.

Tew, B. (1979). The 'cocktail party syndrome' in children with hydrocephalus and spina bifida. *British Journal of Disorders of Communication*, **14**, 89–101.

Tezner, D., Tzaveras, S., Gruner, J. and Hecaen, H. (1972). L'asymétrie droite-gauche du planum temporale, à propos de l'étude anatomique de cent cerveaux. *Revue Neurologique*, **126**, 444–449.

Thal, D., Bates, E. and Bellugi, U. (1989). Language and cognition in two children with Williams syndrome. *Journal of Speech and Hearing Research*, 32, 489–500.

Thase, M. (1988). The relationship between Down syndrome and Alzheimer's disease. In L. Nadel (Ed.), *The Psychobiology of Down Syndrome* (pp. 345–368). Cambridge, MA: MIT Press.

Thesaurus of Psychological Index Terms (1994). Washington, DC: American Psychological Association.

Thibaut, J. P. and Rondal, J. A. (in press). Differences in the processing of action versus non–action verbs: Formal or procedural explanations? *Psychologica Belgica*.

Thibaut, J. P., Rondal, J. A. and Kaens, A. M. (1995). Actionality and mental imagery in children's comprehension of declaratives. *Journal of Child Language*, 22, 189–209.

Thompson, M. (1963). Psychological characteristics relevant to the education of the pre-school mongoloid child. *Mental Retardation*, 1, 148–151.

Thorndike, R. and Gallup, G. (1944). Verbal intelligence of the American adult. *Journal of General Psychology*, 30, 75–78.

Thurstone, L. (1938). *Primary Mental Abilities*. Chicago: University of Chicago Press.

Tissot, R., Mounin, G. and Lhermitte, F. (1973). *L'Agrammatisme*. Brussels: Mardaga.

Tizard, B. and Hughes, M. (1984). *Young Children Learning*. London: Fontana.

Tomblin, B. (1989). Familial concentration of developmental language impairment. *Journal of Speech and Hearing Disorders*, 54, 287–285.

Tourrette, C. (1991). *D'un bébé à l'autre. Les différences individuelles au début du développement*. Paris: Presses Universitaires de France.

Trahan, D. and Quintana, J. (1990). Analysis of gender effects upon verbal and visual memory performance in adults. *Archives of Clinical Neuropsychology*, 5, 325–334.

Tufts, L. and Holliday, A. (1959). Effectiveness of trained parents as speech therapists. *Journal of Speech and Hearing Disorders*, 24, 395–401.

Tulkin, S. and Kagan, J. (1972). Mother–child interaction in the first year of life. *Child Development*, 43, 31–41.

Tulving, E. (1983). *Elements of Episodic Memory*. New York: Oxford University Press.

Tulving, E. (1987). Multiple memory systems and consciousness. *Human Neurobiology*, 6, 67–80.

Turk, J., Hagerman, R., Barnicoat, A. and McEvoy, J. (1994). The fragile X syndrome. In N. Bonras (Ed.), *Mental Health in Mental Retardation: Recent Advances and Practices* (pp. 135–153). Cambridge, UK: Cambridge University Press.

Udwin, O. and Yule, W. (undated) *Infantile Hypercalcaemia and Williams Syndrome. Guidelines for Parents*. Old Harlow, UK: The Infantile Hypercalcaemia Foundation.

Uecker, A., Maugan, P., Obrzut, J. and Nadel, L. (1993). Down's syndrome in neurobiological perspective: An emphasis on spatial cognition. *Journal of Clinical Child Psychology*, 22, 266–276.

U.S. National Center for Health Statistics (1980). *Basic Data on Hearing Levels of Adults 25–74 Years*. U.S. 1971–75 series U, N°. 215. Washington, DC: Department of Health, Education and Welfare.

Uzgiris, I. and Hunt, J. (1975). *Assessment in Infancy: Ordinal Scales of Psychological Development*. Urbana, IL: University of Illinois Press.

Valleur-Masson, D. and Vaivre-Douret, L. (1994). Periventricular leukomalacia in the preterm. The state of the art. *Approche Neuropsychologique des Apprentissages chez l'Enfant*, 28, 137–145.

Van Borsel, J. (1988). An analysis of the speech of five Down's syndrome adolescents. *Journal of Communication Disorders*, 21, 409–422.

Van Borsel, J. (1991, August). Personal communication.

Van Borsel, J. (1993). *De articulatie bij adolescenten en volwassenen met het syndroom van Down.* Unpublished doctoral dissertation, Vrije Universiteit Brussels.

Vanderheiden, G. and Harris-Vanderheiden, D. (1976). Communication techniques and aids for the non–vocal severely handicapped. In L. Lloyd (Ed.), *Communication Assessment and Intervention Strategies* (pp.607–652). Baltimore, MD: University Park Press.

Vanderheiden, G. and Lloyd, L. (1986). Overview. In S. Blackstone (Ed.), *Augmentation Communication : An Introduction* (pp. 201–234). Rockville, MD: American Association on Speech, Language and Hearing.

Van der Linden, M. (1994a). Mémoire de travail et vieillissement. In M. Van der Linden and M. Hupet (Eds.), *Le Vieillissement Cognitif* (pp. 37–85). Paris: Presses Universitaires de France.

Van der Linden, M. (1994b). Mémoire à long terme et vieillissement. In M. Van der Linden and M. Hupet (Eds.), *Le Vieillissement Cognitif* (pp. 87–140). Paris: Presses Universitaires de France.

Van Dyke, D., Lang. J., Heide, F., Van Duyne, S. and Soucek, M. (1990). *Clinical Perspectives in the Management of Down's Syndrome.* New York: Springer.

Van Hout, A. and Seron, X. (1983). *L'Aphasie de l'enfant et les bases biologiques du langage.* Brussels: Mardaga.

Venita, J., Chan, F. and Becker, L. (1990). Dendritic arborization in the human fetus and infant with the trisomy 18 syndrome. *Developmental Brain Research*, **54**, 291–294.

Verloes, A., Schoos, R., Herens, C., Vintens, A. and Koulischer, L. (1995). A prenatal trisomy 21 screening program using alpha-fetoprotein, human chorionic gonadotropin and free estril on maternal dried blood. *American Journal of Obstetrical Gynecology*, **172**, 167–174.

Vernant, P., Corone, P., Rossignol, A. and Bielman, C. (1980). Etude de 120 observations de syndrome de Williams et Beuren. *Archives des Maladies du Coeur*, **73**, 661–666.

Vernon, P. (1971). *The Structure of Human Abilities.* London: Methuen.

Vernon, P. (1979). *Intelligence: Heredity and environment.* San Francisco, CA: Freeman.

Vial, M. (1990). *Les Enfants anormaux à l'école. Aux origines de l'éducation spécialisée* 1882–1909. Paris: Colin.

Vilkman, E., Niemi, J. and Ikonen, U. (1988). Fragile X speech phonology in Finnish. *Brain and Language*, **34**, 203–221.

Villiers, J. de and Villiers, P. de (1973). A cross-sectional study of the acquisition of grammatical morphemes in child speech. *Journal of Psycholinguistic Research*, **2**, 267–278.

Vygotsky, L. (1962). *Thought and Language.* Cambridge, MA: MIT Press (first published in Russian, 1929).

Wada, J., Clark, R. and Hamm, A. (1975). Cerebral hemispheric asymmetry in humans. *Archives of Neurology*, **32**, 239–246.

Walker, M. (1978). The Makaton vocabulary. In T. Tebbs (Ed.), *Ways and Means* (pp. 172–183). Basingstoke, UK: Globe Education.

Wang, P. (1992, June). *Relationship of Neuropsychological and Neurobiological Profiles in Williams and Down's Syndromes.* Paper presented at the Symposium 'Two genetic syndromes of contrasting cognitive profiles: A neuropsychological and neurobiological dissection' of the American Psychological Society, San Diego, CA.

Wang, P. and Bellugi, U. (1993). Williams syndrome, Down's syndrome and cognitive neuroscience. *American Journal of Diseases of Children*, **147**, 1246–1251.

Wang, P. and Bellugi, U. (in press). Evidence from two genetic syndromes for a dissociation between verbal and visual-spatial short-term memory. *Journal of Clinical and Experimental Neuropsychology*.

Wang, P., Doherty, S., Hesselink, J. and Bellugi, U. (1992). Callosal morphology concurs with neuropathological findings in two neurodevelopmental disorders. *Archives of Neurology*, **49**, 407–411.

Wang, P., Hesselink, J., Jernigan, T., Doherty, S. and Bellugi, U. (1992). Specific neurobehavioral profile of Williams syndrome is associated with neocerebellar hemispheric preservation. *Neurology*, **42**, 1999–2002.

Warren, S. (1992, June). *Discovery of the FMR-1 Gene*. Paper presented at the Third International Fragile X Conference, Snowmass Resort, CO.

Warren, S. and Kaiser, A. (1988). Research in early language intervention. In S. Docom and M. Karnes (Ed.), *Research in Early Childhood Special Education* (pp. 89–108). Baltimore, MD: Brookes.

Waters, G., Caplan, D. and Rochon, E. (1995). Processing capacity and sentence comprehension in patients with Alzheimer's disease. *Cognitive Neuropsychology*, **12**, 1–30.

Waters, T. (1956). Qualitative vocabulary responses in three etiologies of mental defectives. *Training School Bulletin*, **53**, 151–156.

Watson, M., Breg, W., Pauls, D., Brown, W., Carroll, A., Howard-Peebles, P., Meryash, D. and Shapiro, L. (1988). Aneuploidy and the fragile X syndrome. *American Journal of Medical Genetics*, **30**, 115–121.

Waugh, R. (1973). Comparison of revised and experimental editions of the Illinois Test of Psycholinguistic Abilities. *Journal of Learning Disabilities*, **6**, 39–41.

Webb, C. and Kinde, S. (1967). Speech, language and hearing of the mentally retarded. In A. Baumeister (Ed.), *Mental Retardation* (pp. 86–119). Chicago: Aldine.

Webb, T., Bundey, S., Thake, A. and Todd, J. (1986). Population incidence and segregation ratios in Martin-Bell syndrome. *American Journal of Medical Genetics*, **23**, 573–580.

Wechsler, D. (1958). *The Measurement and Appraisal of Adult Intelligence*. New York: Baillière, Tindall and Cox.

Weener, P., Barritt, L. and Semmel, M. (1967). A critical evaluation of the ITPA. *Exceptional Children*, **33**, 382–384.

Weinberg, B. and Zlatin, M. (1970). Speaking fundamental frequency characteristics of five- and six-year-old children with mongolism. *Journal of Speech and Hearing Research*, **13**, 418–425.

Weir, C. (1990). *Communicative Language Testing*. Englewood Cliffs, NJ: Prentice-Hall.

Weiss, A. (1925). Linguistics and psychology. *Language*, **1**, 52–57.

Weiss, D. (1964). *Cluttering*. Englewood Cliffs, NJ: Prentice-Hall.

Weiss, H. and Born, B. (1967). Speech training or language acquisition? A distinction when speech training is taught by operant conditioning procedures. *American Journal of Orthopsychiatry*, **37**, 49–55.

Weisz, J. and Zigler, E. (1979). Cognitive development in retarded and non-retarded persons: Piagetian tests of the similar sequence hypothesis. *Psychological Bulletin*, **86**, 831–851.

Werker, J., Gilbert, J., Humphreys, G. and Tees, R. (1981). Developmental aspects of cross-language speech perception. *Child Development*, **52**, 349–355.

Werker, J. and Tees, R. (1984). Cross-language speech perception: Evidence for perceptual reorganization during the first year of life. *Infant Behavior and Development*, 7, 49–63.

Werner, H. (1948). *Comparative Psychology of Mental Development*. New York: International Universities Press.

West, R. (1947). Speech defects of the feeble-minded. In R. West, L. Kennedy and A. Carr (Eds.), *The Rehabilitation of Speech* (pp. 209–215). New York: Harper.

Wexler, K. (1994). Interview with Jean A. Rondal. *International Journal of Psychology*, 29, 147–164.

Wexler, K. and Culicover, P. (1980). *Formal Principles of Language Acquisition*. Cambridge, MA: MIT Press.

Wexler, M., Peled, I., Rand, Y., Mintzker, Y. and Feuerstein, R. (1986). Rehabilitation of the face in patients with Down's syndrome. *Plastic and Reconstruction Surgery*, 77, 383–391.

Whalen, D., Levitt, A. and Wang, Q. (1991). Intonational differences between the reduplicative babbling of French- and English-learning infants. *Journal of Child Language*, 18, 501–516.

Wheeler, A. (1972). Using attendants to build a verbal repertoire in a profoundly retarded adolescent. *Journal of Applied Behavior Analysis*, 5, 140–144.

Wheeler, A. and Sulzer, B. (1970). Operant training and generalization of a verbal response form in a speech-deficient child. *Journal of Applied Behavior Analysis*, 3, 139–147.

Wheldall, K. (1976). Receptive language in the mentally handicapped. In P. Berry (Ed.), *Language and Communication in the Mentally Handicapped* (pp. 36–55). Baltimore, MD: University Park Press.

Whitaker, H. (1976). A case of the isolation of the language function. In H. Whitaker and H. A. Whitaker (Eds.), *Studies in Neurolinguistics* (Vol. 2, pp. 1–58). New York: Academic.

Wiegel–Crump, C. (1981). The development of grammar in Down's syndrome children between the mental ages of 2–0 and 6–11 years. *Education and Training of the Mentally Retarded*, 16, 24–30.

Wilkins, L., Brown, J., Nance, W. and Wolf, B. (1982). Clinical heterogeneity in 86 home-reared children with the Cri-du-chat syndrome. *Journal of Pediatrics*, 102, 528–533.

Wilkins, L., Brown, J. and Wolf, B. (1981). Psychomotor development in 65 home–reared children with Cri-du chat syndrome. *Journal of Pediatrics*, 97, 401–405.

Williams, J., Barrett–Boyes, B. and Lowe, J. (1961). Supravalvular aortic stenosis. *Circulation*, 24, 1311–1318.

Willott, J. (1991). *Ageing and the Auditory System: Anatomy, Physiology and Psychophysics*. London: Whurr.

Winters, J. and Brzoska, M. (1976). Development of formation of categories by normal and retarded persons. *Developmental Psychology*, 12, 125–131.

Winters, J. and Hoats, D. (1986). Comparison of mentally retarded and non–retarded persons' organization of semantic memory. *American Journal of Mental Deficiency*, 91, 102–104.

Wishart, J. (1988). Early learning in infants and young children with Down syndrome. In L. Nadel (Ed.), *The Psychobiology of Down Syndrome* (pp. 7–50). Cambridge, MA: MIT Press.

Wishart, J. (1993). The development of learning difficulties in children with Down's syndrome. *Journal of Intellectual Disability Research*, 37, 389–403.

Wishart, J. (1994). Reactions of young children with Down's syndrome to an impossible task. *British Journal of Developmental Psychology*, 12, 485–489.

Wishart, J. (in press). Cognitive abilities in children with Down syndrome: Developmental instability and motivational deficits. In C. Epstein (Ed.) *Proceedings of the 1994 Conference of the National Down Syndrome Society* (provisional title). New York: Wiley.

Wisniewski, H., Dalton, A., Crapper-McLachlan, D., Wen, G. and Wisniewski, K. (1985). Alzheimer's disease in Down's syndrome: Clinicopathological studies. *Neurology*, 35, 957–961.

Wisniewski, H. and Silverman, W. (in press). Alzheimer's disease, neuropathology and dementia in Down's syndrome. In J. A. Rondal, J. Perera, L. Nadel and A. Comblain (Eds.), *Down's Syndrome: Psychobiological, Psychological and Socio-educational Perspectives*. London: Whurr.

Wisniewski, K. (1990). Down syndrome children often have brain with maturation delay, retardation of growth and cortical dysgenesis. *American Journal of Medical Genetics Supplement*, 7, 274–281.

Wisniewski, K., French, J., Fernando, S., Brown, W., Jenkins, E. Friedman, E., Hill, A. and Miezejeski, C. (1985). The fragile X syndrome: Associated neurological abnormalities and developmental disabilities. *Annals of Neurology*, 18, 665–669.

Wisniewski, K. and Kida, E. (1994). Abnormal neurogenesis and synaptogenesis in Down syndrome brain. *Development Brain Dysfunction*, 17, 1–12.

Wisniewski, K., Kida, E. and Brown, W. (in press). Consequences of genetic abnormalities in Down syndrome on brain structure and function. In J. A. Rondal, J. Perera, L. Nadel and A. Comblain (Eds.), *Down Syndrome: Psychological, Psychobiological and Socio-educational Perspectives*. London: Whurr.

Wisniewski, K., Laure-Kamionowska, M., Connell, F. and Wen, G. (1986). Neuronal density and synaptogenesis in the postnatal stage of brain maturation in Down syndrome. In C. Epstein (Ed.), *The Neurobiology of Down Syndrome* (pp. 29–44). New York: Raven.

Wisniewski, K., Miezejeski, C. and Hill, A. (1988). Neurological and psychological status of individuals with Down syndrome. In L. Nadel (Ed.), *The Psychobiology of Down Syndrome* (pp. 315–343). Cambridge, MA: MIT Press.

Witelson, S. and Pallie, W. (1973). Left hemisphere specialization for language in the newborn: Neuroanatomical evidence of asymmetry. *Brain*, 96, 641–646.

Wode, H. (1980). Grammatical intonation in child language. In L. Waugh and C. Van Schooneveld (Eds.), *The Melody of Language: Intonation and Prosody* (pp. 331–345). New York: Academic.

Wolfensberger, W., Mein, R. and O'Connor, N. (1963). A study of the oral vocabularies of severely subnormal patients. III. Core vocabulary, verbosity and repetitiousness. *Journal of Mental Deficiency Research*, 7, 38–45.

Wolf-Schein, E., Sudhalter, V., Cohen, I., Fish, G., Hanson, D., Pfadt, A., Hagerman, R., Jenkins, E. and Brown, W. (1987). Speech-language and the fragile X syndrome: Initial findings. *Journal of the American Speech and Hearing Association*, 29, 35–38.

Woodward, A., Markman, E. and Fitzsimmons, C. (1994). Rapid word learning in 13- and 18-month-olds. *Developmental Psychology*, 30, 553–566.

Woodward, M. (1959). The behaviour of idiots interpreted by Piaget's theory of sensori-motor development. *British Journal of Educational Psychology*, 29, 60–71.

Woodward, M. (1963). The application of Piaget's theory to research in mental deficiency. In N. Ellis (Ed.), *Handbook of Mental Deficiency* (pp. 297–325). New York: McGraw-Hill.

Woodward, M. and Stern, D. (1963). Developmental patterns of severely subnormal children. *British Journal of Educational Psychology*, **33**, 10–21.

Wooster, A. (1970). Social and ethnic differences in understanding the spoken word. *British Journal of Disorders of Communication*, **5**, 118–125.

Wozniak, R. (1972). Verbal regulation of motor behavior. Soviet research and non-Soviet replication. A review and an explication. *Human Development*, **15**, 13–57.

Yairi, E. and Clifton, N. (1972). Disfluent speech behaviour of preschool children, high school seniors and geriatric persons. *Journal of Speech and Hearing Research*, **15**, 714–719.

Yamada, J. (1981). Evidence for the independence of language and cognition: A case study of a 'hyperlinguistic' adolescent. *UCLA Working Papers in Cognitive Linguistics*, **3**, 121–160.

Yamada, J. (1983). *The Independence of Language: A Case Study*. Unpublished doctoral dissertation. University of California, Los Angeles..

Yamada, J. (1990). *Laura. A Case for the Modularity of Language*. Cambridge, MA: MIT Press.

Yarrow, L. (1972). Attachment and dependency. In J. Gewirtz (Ed.), *Attachment and Dependency* (pp. 81–95). New York: Winston.

Yoder, D. and Miller, J. (1972). What we may know and what we can do: Input towards a system. In J. McLean, D. Yoder and R. Schiefelbusch (Eds.), *Language Intervention with the Retarded: Developing Strategies* (pp. 89–107). Baltimore, MD: University Park Press.

Young, E. and Kramer, B. (1991). Characteristics of age-related language decline in adults with Down syndrome. *Mental Retardation*, **29**, 75–79.

Young, F. (1941). An analysis of certain variables in a developmental study of language. *Genetic Psychology Monographs*, **23**, 3–141.

Youssef, V. (1988). The language bioprogram hypothesis revisited. *Journal of Child Language*, **15**, 451–458.

Yu, S., Pritchard, M., Kremer, E., Lynch, M., Nancarrow, J., Baker, E. and Holman, E. (1991). Fragile X genotype characterized by an unstable region of DNA. *Science*, **252**, 1179–1181.

Yule, W. and Berger, M. (1972). Behaviour modification principles and speech delay. In W. Yule and Rutter (Eds.), *The Child with Delayed Speech* (pp. 204–219). London: Heinemann.

Zappella, M. (1964). Postural reactions in 100 children with cerebral palsy and mental handicap. *Developmental Medicine and Child Neurology*, **6**, 475–484.

Zappella, M., Foley, J. and Cookson, M. (1964). The placing and supporting reactions in children with mental retardation. *Journal of Mental Deficiency Research*, **8**, 1–16.

Zazzo, R. (Ed.) (1969). *Les Débilités mentales*. Paris: Colin.

Zeaman, D. (1959). Discrimination learning in retardates. *Training School Bulletin*, **56**, 62–67.

Zellweger, H. (1990). Foreword to Van Dyke et al. *Clinical Perspectives in the Management of Down Syndrome* (pp. VI–IX). New York: Springer.

Zetlin, A. and Sabsay, S. (1980, March). *Characteristics of Verbal Interaction among Moderately Retarded Peers*. Paper presented at the Gatlinburg Conference on Research in Mental Retardation, Gatlinburg, TN.

Zigler, E. (1966). Mental retardation: Current issues and approaches. In M. Hoffman and L. Hoffman (Eds.), *Review of Child Development Research* (Vol. 2, pp. 107–168). New York: Russel Sage Foundation.

Zigler, E. (1967). Familial mental retardation: A continuing dilemma. *Science*, **155**, 292–298.

Zigler, E. (1969). Developmental versus difference theories of mental retardation and the problem of motivation. *American Journal of Mental Deficiency*, 73, 536–556.

Zigler, E. (1973). The retarded child as a whole person. In D. Routh (Ed.), *The Experimental Psychology of Mental Retardation* (pp. 231–322). Chicago: Aldine.

Zigler, E. and Hodapp, R. (1986). *Understanding Mental Retardation*. New York: Cambridge University Press.

Zisk, P. and Bialer, I. (1967). Speech and language problems in mongolism: A review of the literature. *Journal of Speech and Hearing Disorders*, 32, 228–241.

Name Index

Dielkens, A., 253
Ding, X., 252
Diniz, F., 82, 163, 164, 229, 232
Dixon, E., 24, 260
Dobbs, J., 61, 239
Dobkin, C., 252
Dodd, B., 99, 135, 148, 158, 242
Doherty, S., 230, 286
Dolk, H., 38, 242
Donahue, M., 47, 250
Donovan, D., 143, 268
Dooley, D., 101, 102, 177, 278
Dooley, J., 100, 170, 173, 175, 242
Dooling, E., 125, 237
Dore, J., 160, 242
Doussard-Roosevelt, J., 205, 270
Dow, R., 63, 258
Dowing, J., 54, 242
Down, L., 40, 41, 242
Drorbaugh, J., 143, 268
Dubbler, C., 241
Duchan, J., 100, 174, 242
Duckett, D., 239
Duffen, L., 219, 243
Duffy, L., 210, 257
Duncan, C., 254
Dunn, L., 234
Dupoux, E., 126, 145, 263
Durand, C., 147, 233, 148, 251
Durbin, G., 75, 276
Durso, R., 208, 263
Dykens, E., 57, 68, 79, 80, 214, 243, 253
Dykstra, R., 46, 243

Edwards, D., 108, 189,243
Edwards, J., 77, 238
Edwards, S., 159, 160, 243
Eels, K., 53, 243
Eilers, R., 145, 146, 147, 149, 243, 268
Eimas, P., 144, 243
Einfeld, S., 69, 243
Eisele, J., 126, 243
Elitzur, A., 238
Ellenbogen, R., 77, 271
Elliott, C., 183, 185, 186, 243
Elliott, D., 183, 184, 185, 186, 243
Ellis, N., 29, 105, 243
Emerson, P., 142, 277
Engler, M., 13, 244
Ensminger, E., 32, 250
Entus, A., 126, 244

Entwistle, D., 171, 244
Epstein, C., 114, 244
Erickson, J., 100, 174, 242
Erwin, S., 171, 172, 244
Esiri, M., 6, 262
Esperet, E., 46, 53, 55, 244
Esposito, A., 119, 232
Esquirol, J., 40, 41, 244
Essa, S., 20, 279
Evans, D., 11, 48, 49, 50, 51, 52, 82, 83, 206, 210, 244
Evans, J., 245
Evenhuis, H., 6, 153, 209, 244, 282

Facon, B., 166, 244
Fagan, J., 2, 244
Fantz, R., 2, 244
Farber, B., 52, 244
Farmer, A., 196, 197, 244
Farrel, M., 10, 255
Fay, W., 119, 244
Fayasse, M., 137, 177, 225, 238, 239, 275
Feifel, H., 128, 207, 245
Fein, D., 234
Feldman, H., 75, 125, 245
Fendt, K., 217, 171
Fenson, L., 182, 245
Ferguson, C., 157, 261
Fernando, S., 210, 288
Ferrara, A., 225, 275
Ferreiro, E., 108, 109, 245
Ferri, R., 10, 153, 245, 248
Ferrier, L., 72, 245
Feuerstein, R., 147, 287
Filippi, G., 69, 269
Fillmore, C., 173, 245
Finer, D., 111, 130, 245, 249
Finger, I., 82, 261
Finley, S., 77, 245
Finley, W., 245
Firman, D., 39, 230
Fisch, G., 69, 245
Fish, B., 119, 278
Fish, G., 234, 288
Fisher, H., 245
Fisher, M., 131, 245
Fisher, S., 127, 263
Fishler, K., 13, 77, 78, 178, 245
Fishman, M., 121, 212, 228
Fitzgerald, M., 134, 238
Fitzsimmons, C., 165, 288

Subject Index

deficits in motor coordination, 154
delay-difference question, 105–107
dementia, 121
developmental-organizational
approach, 2–4
dichotic listening, 183–186
discursive capacities, 179–181
dissociation tendencies in the language
of mentally retarded subjects,
98–105, 119–120
Down's syndrome (trisomy 21)
cognitive functions, 77
etiology, 77
hearing problems, 10
language, 77–78, 81–85
life expectancy, 5–6
mean length of utterance, 84–85
mosaicism subtype, 77
neurology and brain, 81–82, 114–116
occurrence, 38–39
short term memory, 83–84
standard trisomy, 77
translocation subtype, 77
voice, 11
dual-task studies, 184–186
dyslexia, 125

early language studies, 12–14
early speech studies
hearing problems, 10
speech sounds, 9–10
stuttering, 10
voice problems, 11
Edwards syndrome (trisomy 18), 76
exceptional language in mentally retarded individuals (case studies)
Anderson and Spain's, 89, 96
Bellugi et al.'s, 87–88
Cromer, 89, 96–97
Curtiss, Yamada, and associates, 88,
99–92
Hadenius et al.'s, 89, 96
O'Connor and Hermelin's, 89, 97
Rondal's, 88, 92–96, 98
Seagoe's, 89, 96
Smith and Tsimpli's, 97–98
Tew's, 89, 96
explaining individual differences in the
language of mentally retarded
individuals, 183–187

feedback problem in language development, 189–192, 194–195
Fodorian modules, 116–117, 122
Fragile-X syndrome
autistic-like behaviours, 72
cognitive functions, 69–70
etiology, 67–68
hyperactivity, 72
language, 70–73, 81
occurrence, 68
physical appearence, 69
psychological profile, 68

grammatical morphology, 26–27
grammatical predispositions, 114–116
hearing problems, 153
Huntington's disease, 206
hypotonia, 154
Illinois Test of Psycholinguistic
Abilities, 20–21, 83
individual differences in morphosyntactic development, 181–183
informational encapsulation,
117–118
inner speech, 18
Intraventricular haemorrhage, 76

Klinefelter's syndrome, 69

language learnability, 189
language pragmatics, 139–141, 193,
201–204
lexical definition, 167–168
lexical development and problems,
162–173
lexical diversity, 50, 100, 166, 198–199,
202–203
life-span developmental perspective, 5
literacy training, 215, 219–221

maternal hyperphenylalaninaemia, 73
mean length of utterances, 84–85,
132–134, 137–138, 175, 194–195,
199, 202–203
memory
episodic, 206
long-term, 205–206
procedural, 206
proper nouns, 208
short-term, 83, 205–206
working, 206

memory and language, 221–224
mild and other forms of mental retarda-
    tion, 39–41
minimal cerebral dysfunction, 119
modularity of intelligence, 38
modularity of language, 1,86, 116–122,
    213, 227
morphosyntactic development, 174–181

naming explosion, 165
negative evidence problem, 189–191
non-Fodorian modules, 117, 122
non-segmental phonological develop-
    ment, 158–162

operant conditioning of verbal
    responses, 29–35

paradigmatic associations, 171–172
Parkinson's disease, 206
passive sentences, 178–179
Patau syndrome (trisomy 13), 76
periventricular leukomalacia, 75–76
phenylketonuria, 73
phonological awareness, 220–221
phonological development, 155–158
phonological problems in mentally
    retarded children, 158
Piaget's theory, 19–20, 108–111,
    142–143, 157
Pick's disease, 121
Positron Emission Tomography, 116
Prader-Willi syndrome, 73
prelinguistic development, 142–152
prelinguistic phrasing, 149–150
prevalence of mental retardation, 38
primary degenerative diseases, 120–122
process-oriented approach, 5

remediation of language problems
    computer-enhanced intervention
    dimensions and contents, 213, 227
    early intervention, 214
    efficiency issue, 216–217, 227
    improving working memory, 223–224
    individual differences, 213–214
    life-span perspective, 213–215
    older studies, 28–35
    syndromic differences, 213–214

role of intelligence in language
    acquisition, 23

schizophrenia, 119
Seckel syndrome, 73
semantic conditioning, 14–16
semantic lexical categories, 168–171
semantic structural development,
    173–174
sensorimotor development, 143
sensorimotor intelligence, 142–143
sex differences in language functioning
    of mentally retarded individuals,
    48–53
sex differences in language functioning
    of non-retarded individuals, 45–48
social class differences in language func-
    tioning of mentally retarded indi-
    viduals, 55–56
social class differences in language func-
    tioning of non-retarded individu-
    als, 53–55
sound discrimination, 143–146
specific language impairment, 117–118
speech acts, 139–141
speech perception, 148
stuttering, 10, 118–119
syndromic specificity, 79–81
syndromic specificity of language prob-
    lems, 56–57, 81–85, 226
syntagmatic associations, 171–172

verbal regulation of behaviour, 16–18
voice problems, 154

Williams syndrome
    etiology, 58–59
    interindividual variability, 64–65
    language, 59–62, 81
    neurology and brain, 62–64, 66–67,
    81–82
    occurrence, 58
    physical appearance, 58
    psychological profile, 59
    short-term memory, 84
word learning, 162–171

Zigler's two-group approach of mental
    retardation, 41–44